Local and Systemic Management

of Primary Breast Cancers

Local and Systemic Management
of Primary Breast Cancers

edited by

Masakazu Toi

and

Eric P. Winer

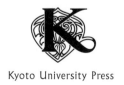

Kyoto University Press

First published in 2010 jointly by:

Kyoto University Press
Kyodai Kaikan
15-9 Yoshida Kawara-cho
Sakyo-ku, Kyoto 606-8305, Japan
Telephone: +81-75-761-6182
Fax: +81-75-761-6190
Email: sales@kyoto-up.or.jp
Web: http://www.kyoto-up.or.jp

Trans Pacific Press
PO Box 164, Balwyn North, Melbourne
Victoria 3104, Australia
Telephone: +61 3 9859 1112
Fax: +61 3 9859 4110
Email: tpp.mail@gmail.com
Web: http://www.transpacificpress.com

Distributors

Australia and New Zealand
DA Information Services/Central Book Services
648 Whitehorse Road
Mitcham, Victoria 3132
Australia
Telephone: +61(0)3-9210-7777
Fax: + 61(0)3-9210-7788
Email: books@dadirect.com
Web: www.dadirect.com

USA and Canada
International Specialized Book Services (ISBS)
920 NE 58th Avenue, Suite 300
Portland, Oregon 97213-3786
USA
Telephone: (800) 944-6190
Fax: (503) 280-8832
Email: orders@isbs.com
Web: http://www.isbs.com

Taiwan and Southeast Asia
Kinokuniya Company Ltd.

Head office:
38-1 Sakuragaoka 5-chome
Setagaya-ku, Tokyo 156-8691
Japan
Telephone: +81(0)3-3439-0161
Fax: +81(0)3-3439-0839
Email: bkimp@kinokuniya.co.jp
Web: www.kinokuniya.co.jp

Asia-Pacific office:
Kinokuniya Book Stores of Singapore Pte., Ltd.
391B Orchard Road #13-06/07/08
Ngee Ann City Tower B
Singapore 238874
Telephone: +65 6276 5558
Fax: +65 6276 5570
Email: SSO@kinokuniya.co.jp

ISBN   978–1–920901–22–6

Contents

Shortened Forms

ABCSG	Austrian Breast and Colorectal Cancer Study Group
AGO	Arbeitsgemeinschaft Gynäkologische Onkologie (Breast Study Group)
AI	aromatase inhibitor
AJCC	American Joint Committee on Cancer
ALND	axillary lymph node dissection
APBI	accelerated partial breast irradiation
ASCO	American Society of Clinical Oncology
ASTRO	American Society for Radiation Oncology
ATAC	Arimidex, Tamoxifen, Alone or in Combination [trial]
Ax	axillary lymph node dissection
BCS	breast-conserving surgery
BCT	breast-conserving therapy
BIG	Breast International Group
BRCA1/2	breast cancer 1 and 2
CAP	College of American Pathologists
cCR	clinical complete response
CHF	chronic heart failure
CI	confidence interval
CMF	cyclophosphamide + methotrexate + 5-fluorouracil
CNB	core needle biopsy
CPM	contralateral prophylactic mastectomy
cRR	clinical response rate
CT (scan)	computed tomography
CT	chemotherapy
DBCG	Danish Breast Cancer Cooperative Group
DCIS	ductal carcinoma in situ
DDFS	distant disease-free survival
DFS	disease-free survival
EBCTCG	Early Breast Cancer Trialists' Collaborative Group
ECOG	East Cooperative Oncology Group
EFC	fluorouracil/epirubicin/cyclophosphamide
EIA	enzyme immunoassay

EORTC	European Organisation for Research and Treatment of Cancer
ER	estrogen receptor
ER +	estrogen receptor positive
FAC	fluorouracil + adriamycin + cyclophosphamide
FEC	fluorouracil + epirubicin + cyclophosphamide
FISH	fluorescence in situ hybridization
FNA	fine needle aspiration
FNAC	fine needle aspiration cytology
FNR	false-negative rate
GBG	German Breast Group
GWAS	genome-wide association study
H&E	hematoxylin and eosin
HER	epidermal growth factor receptor
HERA	Herceptin Adjuvant [trial]
HR	hazard ratio (in chapter 7)
HR	hormone receptor
HRT	hormone replacement therapy
IBC	ipsilateral breast cancer
IBCSG	International Breast Cancer Study Group
IBTR	Ipsilateral breast tumor recurrence
ICG	indocyanine green
IDC	invasive ductal cancer
IHC	immunohistochemical (chemistry)
ILC	invasive lobular cancer
IMC	internal mammary chain
IMN	internal mammary node
IORT	Intraoperative radiotherapy (radiation therapy)
IR	identification rate
JBCRG	Japan Breast Cancer Research Group
JBCS	Japanese Breast Cancer Society
JCOG	Japan Clinical Oncology Group
KBCCC	Kyoto Breast Cancer Consensus Conference
KROG	Korean Society for Therapeutic Radiology and Oncology
LABC	locally advanced breast cancer
LATER	Later Adjuvant Aromatase Inhibitor Therapy for Postmenopausal Women with Endocrine Responsive Tumor [trial]
LCIS	lobular carcinoma in situ
LR	local recurrence
LRR	local recurrence rates

LVI	lymphovascular invasion
MDACC	MD Anderson Cancer Center
MMG	mammography
MRC	Medical Research Council
MRI	magnetic resonance imaging
MSBR	modified Scarff-Bloom-Richardson
N −	negative axillary nodes
N +	positive axillary nodes
NAC	neoadjuvant chemotherapy
NACT	neoadjuvant chemotherapy
NCCN	National Comprehensive Cancer Network
NCI	National Cancer Institute
NEAT	National Epirubicin Adjuvant Trial
NICE	National Institute for Health and Clinical Excellence
NIH	National Institutes of Health
NSABP	National Surgical Adjuvant Breast and Bowel Project
OR	odds ratio
OS	overall survival
PBC	primary breast cancer
PBI	partial-breast irradiation
PBM	prophylactic bilateral mastectomy
PBSO	prophylactic bilateral salpingo-oophorectomy
pCR	pathologic complete response (remission)
PCR	polymerase chain reaction
PET	positron emission tomography
PMRT	postmastectomy radiotherapy
PPV	positive predictive value
PR	progesterone receptor
PST	preoperative systemic therapy
RCB	residual cancer burden
RCT	randomized clinical trial
RFS	recurrence-free survival
RI	radioisotope
RM	radical mastectomy
RR	relative risk (also risk ratio)
RT	radiotherapy
RTOG	Radiation Oncology Therapy Group
SCTBG	Scottish Cancer Trials Breast Group
SEER	Surveillance, Epidemiology, and End Results [program]
SLNB	sentinel lymph node biopsy

SNPs	single-nucleotide polymorphisms
START	Trial Standardisation of Breast Radiotherapy Trial
SUPREMO	Selective Use of Postoperative Radiotherapy after Mastectomy [trial]
SUV	standardized uptake volume
SWOG	South Western Oncology Group
TARGIT	Targeted Intraoperative Radiotherapy Trial
Tc-99m	technetium-99m
TNBC	triple negative breast cancer
TNM	tumor-nodes-metastasis [stage]
TROG	Trans Tasman Radiation Oncology Group
UICC	Union Internationale Contre le Cancer
US	ultrasound, or ultrasonography
US-FNAC	ultrasound-guided fine-needle aspiration cytology
VEGF	vascular endothelial growth factor
WB	whole breast
WBRT	whole breast radiotherapy
WLE	wide local excision

List of Figures

List of Tables

Foreword

It is our great pleasure to issue this textbook on Local and Systemic Management of Primary Breast Cancers. Its authors were notable presenters at the Kyoto Breast Cancer Consensus Conference (KBCCC) 2009, where we discussed the algorithm forms of breast cancer treatment, especially pathologic analysis, axillary surgery, breast surgery, radiation therapy, and preoperative systemic therapy (PST).

At the KBCCC 2009, we found that the management of such cancers was often controversial and lacked evidence. For example, in axillary management, we found no clear evidence about tracers, site of injection, lymphatic mapping, adequate number of sentinel lymph nodes, availability of ultrasound-guided fine needle aspiration biopsy, definition of positive node, sparing of axillary lymph node dissection for sentinel lymph node-positive cases, significance of sentinel lymph node biopsy in ductal carcinoma in situ, and timing of sentinel lymph node biopsy in preoperative systemic therapy.

We also had questions on PST, including who needs PST, how to detect a pathologic complete response after PST, how to manage patients who do not respond to initial PST, how to manage patients with residual disease in the breast after maximum PST, and how to use biologicals — trastuzumab, lapatinib, or bevacizumab — for PST. Furthermore, we concluded that there was neither exact indication of increasing hypofractionated whole breast radiation therapy and accelerated partial breast irradiation after breast-conserving surgery, nor sufficient information about the management of hereditary breast cancer.

This textbook therefore provides up-to-date answers to such questions, given the emergence at the conference of new evidence or consensus in cases of no evidence.

Promising techniques and drugs for local and systemic management of primary breast cancer have been developed recently, but many issues remain without evidence. The KBCCC held in Japan showed us that optimal local management of early breast cancer is indeed possible. This textbook, written by specialists who participated in the KBCCC, therefore contains neo-standard information for the local and systemic management of early breast cancer. We believe that this textbook will assist practitioners and specialists in their decision making on the local and systemic management of early breast cancer.

Hiroshi Sonoo
Kawasaki Medical University, Kurashiki, Japan
April 2010

Preface

This handbook deals with local and systematic management of primary breast cancers. It provides information on current topics in surgery, radiation therapy, pathology, and multidisciplinary approaches, and gives preoperative therapy guidance to clinicians for the management of the disease in patients.

The handbook is divided into seven key sections: Overview and Future Perspectives of Primary Breast Cancer, Axillary Diagnosis and Treatment, Optimal Breast Surgery, Pathology, Genetics — Personal Genomics Data, Radiation Therapy, and Preoperative Therapy.

The handbook's structure and content are based on medical papers presented at the *Kyoto Breast Cancer Consensus Conference (KBCCC) International Convention 2009.*

The conference convention through its high-quality presentations and discussions sought to establish a consensus, or agreement, among participant members sharing the same fundamentals about the best practical ways of treating breast cancer. The central principle of the consensus approach at the conference was the strong desire to improve the quality of life of patients, as well as the effectiveness of the breast cancer treatments.

The twenty-one articles in this handbook reflect and capture that consensus as an ongoing global development. Together, the articles represent a medical record of current diagnostic and treatment approaches to the disease, and point to future possibilities in standard of care.

Our intention with this handbook is to share the latest fundamentals discussed and collated as a group to be put into practice by medical professionals. The collaboration and sequencing of different types of disciplines, such as surgery, chemotherapy, radiotherapy, and pathological diagnosis during individual clinical practice, indicates the ongoing importance of creating understanding of, and unification between, methodologies.

We hope that this handbook will help medical professionals and students better appreciate, identify, and understand the various research approaches, medical issues and perspectives, and treatment options available for the effective management of breast cancer in patients.

Importantly, through the pursuit and practice of ongoing knowledge, shared globally through and across our many disciplines that constitute breast cancer prediction, diagnosis, treatment, and care, we will continue to make purposeful inroads into the control of this difficult disease.

Eric P. Winer
Harvard Medical School, Harvard University, Boston, USA
Masakazu Toi
Postgraduate School of Medicine, Kyoto University, Kyoto, Japan
April 2010

Acknowledgments

Acting as Executive Advisors to this handbook project were Professor Masahiro Hiraoka of Kyoto University, and Professor Fabrizio Michelassi, Chairman of the Department of Surgery, NewYork-Presbyterian Hospital/Weill Cornell Medical Center. Professor Michelassi also kindly guided development of the consensus questionnaire, which formed an integral part of the project.

The authors contributing to this handbook comprised the invited specialists and other colleagues of the *Kyoto Breast Cancer Consensus Conference (KBCCC) International Convention 2009*. To them, we give our heart-warm thanks for their insightful contributions.

The conference itself was part of the Raising Proficient Oncologists program run by the Japanese Ministry of Education, Culture, Sports, Science and Technology. Kyoto University's Graduate School of Medicine was invited by the Ministry to join the program, and contributed time and resources to this important conference project.

We would like to thank the Kyoto University Foundation, without whose generous donation of funds the conference would not have been possible. Also, we thank the Japan Breast Cancer Society for their constant and kind support.

Many thanks to the invited KBCCC faculty members, including speakers, chairpersons, and panelists, who contributed their valuable time to participate in the conference; the key participating doctors at the conference, who voted on the consensus questions; the doctors, specialists, and experts who completed the consensus questionnaire before the conference; and the major supporters of the conference. Their names can be found at: http://www.kyoto-breast-cancer.org/international/info.php.

A special thank you must go to the conference's Scientific Committee member, Dr. Hiroshi Ishiguro, whose tireless efforts contributed greatly to the success of the conference. Also, ours thanks go to Professor Akira Yamauchi for his most valuable help and wealth of scientific and technical advice.

We also wish to extend our great appreciation to the administrative support members of the KBCCC Conference Secretariat staff, namely, Aya Morotomi, David Graham, Mihoko Yamamoto, Nastajia Burke, Chisa Takano, and Nobuko Yagi for making the whole conference run smoothly and trouble free.

Finally we are grateful to Dr. Naoko Abe, whose tireless assistance in editing this handbook has proven invaluable. We are indebted to the professionalism of Kyoto University Press staff members involved in this handbook project, especially, Tetsuya Suzuki in his capacity as chief compiler of this handbook, Itaru Saito who acted as the book's main organizer, and Sayoko Yamawaki for her help with promotion activities. Our thanks also go to Trans Pacific Press for their editorial work on this project.

Contributors

(in alphabetical order by surname)

Ahmadiyeh, Nasim
  Brigham and Women's Hospital and Dana-Farber Cancer Institute, Boston, USA

Arriagada, Rodrigo
  Institut Gustave Roussy, Villejuif, France; Karolinska Institutet, Stockholm, Sweden

Benson, John R.
  Cambridge Breast Unit, Addenbrooke's Hospital; University of Cambridge, Cambridge, United Kingdom

Chen, Jiayi
  Department of Radiation Oncology, Fudan University, Shanghai, China

Forbes, John F.
  The University of Newcastle, Newcastle, Australia; Department of Surgical Oncology, Calvary Mater Newcastle Hospital; and Australian New Zealand Breast Cancer Trials Group

Golshan, Mehra
  Brigham and Women's Hospital and Dana-Farber Cancer Institute, Boston, USA

Ha, Sung Whan
  Department of Radiation Oncology, Seoul National University College of Medicine, Seoul, Korea

Huang, Chiun-Sheng
  National Taiwan University, Taiwan

Inamoto, Takashi
  Department of Breast Surgery, Tazuke Kohukai Medical Research Institute, Kitano Hospital, Osaka, Japan

Jakesz, Raimund
  Department of Surgery, Vienna Medical School, University of Vienna, Vienna, Austria

Kitai, Toshiyuki
  Department of Surgery, Nara Social Insurance Hospital, Nara, Japan

Kunkler, Ian

Edinburgh Cancer Research Unit, Western General Hospital, The University of Edinburgh, Edinburgh, United Kingdom

Lee, Eun Sook

Department of Breast and Endocrine Surgery, College of Medicine, Korea University, Seoul, Korea

Linder, Mattea

German Breast Group, Neu-Isenburg, Germany

Mitsumori, Michihide

Department of Radiation Oncology and Image Applied Therapy, Kyoto University, Kyoto, Japan

Mikami, Yoshiki

Department of Diagnostic Pathology, Kyoto University, Kyoto, Japan

Nakamura, Seigo

Department of Breast Surgical Oncology, St. Luke's International Hospital, Tokyo, Japan

Roukos, Dimitrios H.

Personalized Cancer Medicine, Biobank, Department of Surgery, Ioannina University, School of Medicine, Ioannina, Greece

Sakita, Nobuko

Department of Breast Surgery, Kyoto University, Kyoto, Japan

Sasano, Hironobu

Department of Pathology, School of Medicine, Tohoku University, Sendai, Japan

Shafir, Michail

Clinical Professor of Surgery and Oncological Sciences, Mount Sinai School of Medicine; Attending Surgeon, The Mount Sinai Hospital, New York, USA

Sonoo, Hiroshi

Chairman of the Board of Directors, Japanese Society of Breast Cancer; Kawasaki Medical University, Kurashiki, Japan

Strom, Eric A.

Department of Radiation Oncology, The University of Texas MD Anderson Cancer Center, Houston, USA

Sugie, Tomoharu

Department of Breast Surgery, Kyoto University, Kyoto, Japan

Takada, Masahiro

Department of Breast Surgery, Kyoto University, Kyoto, Japan

Thomanek, Karl

Department of Surgery, Vienna Medical School, University of Vienna, Vienna, Austria

Toi, Masakazu

Department of Breast Surgery, Kyoto University, Kyoto, Japan

Ueno, Takayuki
Department of Breast Surgery, Kyoto University Kyoto, Japan

von Minckwitz, Gunter
Centre of Gynaecology and Obstetrics, University of Frankfurt; German Breast Group, Neu-Isenburg, Germany

Winer, Eric P.
Director, Breast Oncology Center at Dana-Farber Cancer Institute, Harvard Medical School, Boston, USA

Yamashiro, Hiroyasu
Department of Breast Surgery, Kyoto University, Kyoto, Japan

Ziogas, Dimosthenis
Personalized Cancer Medicine, Biobank, Department of Surgery, Ioannina University, School of Medicine, Ioannina, Greece

Chapter 1

Overview

Overview and Future Perspectives of Primary Breast Cancer

John F. Forbes

Summary

Medical advances result from insights, new technologies, and rigorous research, including clinical trials. Guidelines translate advances from trials into new community standards and better community outcomes. We need effective targeted treatments for better outcomes, and avoidance of costs and morbidity from ineffective treatments. Reliable biomarkers of sensitivity and resistance are also required. Potential strategies, particularly for the management of hormone-sensitive (estrogen receptor positive, or ER+) breast cancer (BC), are discussed. The importance of prospective randomized clinical trials (RCTs) is stressed.

Strategies for diagnosis and treatments that may improve outcomes for women include:

1. Presurgical diagnosis by biopsy and molecular characterization of tumors facilitates early evaluation of sensitivity and resistance for targeted systemic treatments. Gene expression signatures need careful evaluation before routine adoption.

2. Tailoring of surgery and radiotherapy (RT) for breast and nodes depends on the likelihood of tumor presence in sentinel nodes and the ipsilateral and contralateral breast and sensitivity of BC to RT.

3. Emerging technologies, including dynamic positron emission tomography (PET) scanning, may improve assessment of sentinel nodes and presurgical systemic treatments. Intraoperative RT (IORT) uses systems, such as IntraBeam®, Mobetron or Novac 7; and clinical trials, for example, the Targeted Intraoperative Radiotherapy Trial (TARGIT), are in progress to evaluate IORT and aim to improve RT delivery by reducing costs and morbidity without loss of efficacy.

4. Preoperative molecular diagnoses, multidiscipline review, and presurgical

systemic treatment should be standard of care. Currently, many women do not know that their chemotherapy was ineffective until BC recurs. We must do better.

5. Early diagnosis will be improved by the use of biomarkers for riskdapted screening, and for targeted prevention strategies for women at high risk. Both are important for the improved management of primary BC.

6. The most important long-term survivorship issue is the very high, long-term risk of recurrence, particularly for women who had an ER+ primary tumor. We have models for endocrine control of BC, which provide a scientific basis for testing new control strategies for long-term survivors. The clinical trial, Later Adjuvant Aromatase Inhibitor Therapy for Postmenopausal Women with Endocrine Responsive Tumor (LATER), addresses these issues.

Evolution of Current Treatment Paradigms

Local management of BC has evolved over a long period of time. Surgery became more precise when the disease's anatomy was documented, and painless after the introduction of anesthesia. Japanese surgeon, Seishu Hanaoka, was the first to succeed in the excision of BC from a 60-year old woman named Kan Aiya under general anesthesia using an oral preparation 'Tsusensan (or Mafutsu-To)' on Oct. 13, 1804 (Figures 1–1 and 1–2).[1] Anesthesia was first described in the United States in 1846, after William Morton, a dentist, administered ether inhalation to a patient operated on by John Collins Warren for the removal of a small neck lump (Figures 1–3).[2,3]

However, it was still potentially contaminated surgery until Ignaz Phillip Semmelweis (Figure 1–4) showed by a classical 'before and after' clinical trial that handwashing using a solution of chlorinated lime reduced the incidence of neonatal infection — 'puerperal fever' — and perinatal mortality for pregnant women.[4] The scientific basis for clean surgery was established when Louis Pasteur, Joseph Lister, and others developed the germ theory of disease, and clean surgery became the standard. Hence, by the beginning of the 20th century, William Halsted and others were able to use clean, painless, anatomically based surgery to apply radical mastectomy as the major treatment of BC. Marie Curie's discovery of radium led to the first use of RT in treatments.

Throughout much of the 20th century, local treatments alone continued as the paradigm for treatment of BC. If treatment failed, it was believed that the surgery should have been more extensive, so extended radical mastectomy was used. High BC mortality rates continued, as the problem was not control of

Special Contribution

Medical History: Seishu Hanaoka and His Success in Breast Cancer
Surgery Under General Anesthesia Two Hundred Years Ago

Masaru Izuo

Former President of The Japanese Breast Cancer Sociely Professor Emeritus, Gunma University (Breast and Endocrine Surgery, Shorakudo Hospital, Japan)

In 1804, Seishu Hanaoka performed the first successful surgical treatment of breast cancer under general anesthesia in the world. It preceeded by 38 years CW Long's trial of ether anesthesia in 1842, In this paper, Hanaoka's biography and his contributions to surgery and anesthesiology in those days, and alsohis advanced ideas about medicine and sanitation are presented.

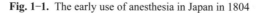

Fig. 1–1. The early use of anesthesia in Japan in 1804

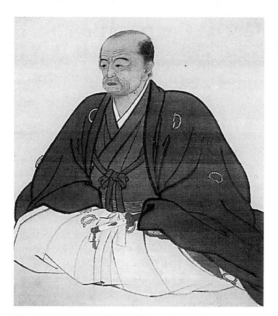

Fig. 1–2. Portrait of Seishu Hanaoka
The portrait was drawn apparently in commemoration of his
70th birthday.

disease in the breast alone.

The Cambridge mathematician, Ronald A. Fisher (Figure 1–5), introduced the concept of randomization in 1925.[5] This was a landmark step, as together with the availability of systemic treatments — in particular, tamoxifen and combination cytotoxic chemotherapy regimens such as 'CMF' (cyclophosphamide, methotrexate, and fluorouracil) — large prospective RCTs could be undertaken to test the concept that systemic treatments would

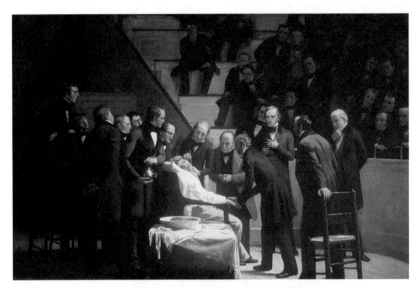

Fig. 1–3. A depiction of the first ether anesthetic in Boston in 1842

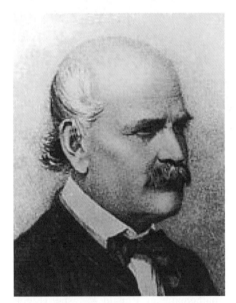

Fig. 1–4. Ignaz Phillip Semmelweis introduced
a treatment for 'puerperal fever' in
1847

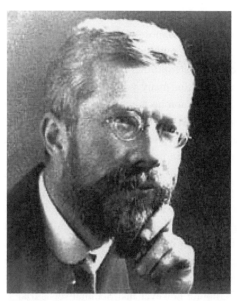

Fig. 1–5. Ronald A. Fisher introduced randomization and the concept of controlled experiments in 1925

improve outcomes beyond surgery and RT alone. These RCTs, which were not undertaken until effective systemic agents became available close to fifty years later, were successful, leading to the modern era where local treatments and systemic therapy are standard of care for women diagnosed with early BC.

The Oxford-based Early Breast Cancer Trialists' Collaborative Group (EBCTCG), in overviewing the documented outcomes for both adjuvant tamoxifen and adjuvant chemotherapy, showed that both approaches would lead to significant reductions in the risk of recurrent disease and deaths from BC beyond local treatment alone.[6] Surgery for early BC has evolved further, and breast preservation — partial mastectomy with removal of all evident tumor — and sentinel node biopsy as an alternative to full axillary dissection have become standards of care for many women. The introduction of mammography screening to detect primary BC earlier has led to more women having breast preservation treatment.

The Current Paradigm of Management of Early Breast Cancer

The current management paradigm in breast centers throughout the world involves early detection by mammography for many women and clinical detection for others. After diagnosis is confirmed, surgery usually follows soon afterwards, and subsequent multidisciplinary discussions consider the potential benefit of the role of systemic therapy and RT. Although primary systemic treatment has been used for many years for large or inflammatory BCs, such tumors are now less common because of screening and early detection. Hence, the most common sequence is detection and diagnosis, followed by surgery, and then systemic treatment. This paradigm of care needs critical review to facilitate further improvement in outcomes for many women.

Some problems with current management

We must constantly address new research questions to ensure that progress continues. New questions usually follow recognition of current problems. Close attention to rigorous research methodology is essential to address these problems. Researchers must aim to obtain reliable, interpretable, and relevant data, and design their research to meet this goal. This will usually involve prospective RCTs, noting however that Semmelweis's trial was a beforendfter controlled trial. Randomized trials are still the best approach when one is questioning the prevailing paradigm. There are times, however, when such trials cannot be done, and in these settings other designs can be substituted, but with an understanding that the conclusions may be less robust. Preoperative systemic therapy (PST) can be used in such a model for both the discovery of a new biology and for the assessment of an early response to systemic treatment (Figure 1–6).

It follows that a search for biomarkers of risk of BC — risk for both development of primary BC and for later recurrence of BC — and for biomarkers of response to treatment can only be evaluated reliably in the context of RCTs. Retrospective studies, subgroup analyses, and nonrandomized controls may identify a possible biomarker, but the value of the biomarker must then be evaluated in a prospectively controlled setting if reliable conclusions are to be obtained. Only after such prospective controlled evaluation can the biomarker be used in clinical practice as a standard of care.

Below are four key management problems associated with breast cancer treatment regimes:

1. *We currently screen 1,000 normal women to diagnose three BCs.* In developed countries with large mammography screening programs, close to 1,000 postmenopausal women need to be screened to detect three BCs. Some of these screen-detected cancers may have continued without causing a clinical problem for many years. The ratio of cancers detected to women screened is even smaller in premenopausal women. This is clearly

unacceptable and highlights the high priority of research to identify reliable biomarkers of risk. It would be a great advance if the clinically important BCs could be found in 100 or even 500 women, let alone 10 or 20, with very substantial savings in morbidity and costs. Hence, tissue specimens, including serial blood samples, should be collected where possible within randomized controlled prevention trials for women at increased risk. This will provide reliable information concerning the relationship between risk biomarkers and detection of BC. If technology is not yet ready for routine use, for example, in proteomics or circulating tumor cells, specimens can be stored for testing in the future when reliable technology becomes available (see below, International Breast Intervention Studies (IBIS) I and II. Collecting tissue — for example, serial blood samples — and mammograms for evaluation of breast density in a normal screening population also may be valuable, but this is less efficient and less reliable than testing samples in the prevention RCT model, due to the many uncontrolled variables in a large population of screened women.

2. *BC recurrences continue at a very high rate over the very long term.* Many women have a high risk of new BC events in the very long term, many years after their treatment for early BC is completed. This risk is about 2% annually over more than fifteen years post diagnosis for women who have had an ER+ primary BC and is similar for node positive (N+) and node negative (N–) BCs (Figure 1–7).[6–8] This long-term annual risk of 2% is comparable to the annual risk of BC for a woman with a breast cancer (BRCA) gene mutation; however, women with a BRCA mutation receive substantially better surveillance than women on long-term follow-up. It is clear that the risk management for women on long-term follow-up has been inadequate, and this must be changed. Close surveillance of such women in a prospective RCT would create a unique opportunity for identification of risk biomarkers, and would set new standards of care for these women. The LATER trial addresses these issues (see below).

3. *Late diagnosis of failed systemic therapy.* A frustrating and distressing current problem is that many women do not know for several years that their adjuvant systemic treatment did not work. It would be better to know early that a systemic treatment was ineffective, and introduce new treatment accordingly. Identification of reliable biomarkers to predict response and resistance would be valuable, and this is particularly important for women diagnosed with triple negative BC where the tumor does not express the estrogen receptor (ER), the progesterone receptor (PR) or the HER-2 receptor, and there is uncertainty as to which chemotherapy treatment will be effective. If systemic treatment is not planned until after surgery

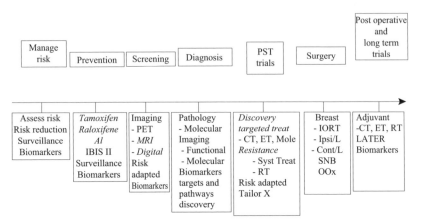

Fig. 1–6. Management of early breast cancer: A continuum of strategies

Strategies involve risk management and early detection before diagnosis, PST at diagnosis, and long-term risk management after diagnosis.

is completed, a valuable opportunity to assess tumor response is lost.[9-11] If, however, the sequence of care is diagnosis, PST, followed by surgery, the response to chemotherapy can be assessed in situ while treatment is being given, and also subsequently by testing the surgery specimen. This sequence may involve dynamic imaging and molecular pathology of the resected specimen. The sequence also enables discovery research, as molecular analysis of the tumor tissue before and after exposure to treatment will allow the biology of tumor response to be studied. This model is an example of a controlled clinical trial using a beforendfter treatment, or PST, design. This management sequence is challenging for many surgeons and requires that the multidisciplinary meeting is held after diagnosis but before surgery. Some of the research opportunities created by this model are summarized below in Figure 1–6.

4. *Cost and morbidity of adjuvant RT after breast conserving surgery.* For many years, the strategy of RT for BC has been to deliver the maximum tolerated RT dose. Today, we need a new approach to deliver the minimum effective dose. Several current trials are investigating IORT strategies designed to deliver a lower total RT dose in a shorter time. The potential gains, if IORT is shown to be effective, would include substantial savings in cost and reduction of morbidity. One example is the TARGIT trial, in which good-prognosis patients having breast preservation are randomized to IORT alone or to conventional whole breast radiation.[12,13] Completion of the accrual is anticipated in 2010.

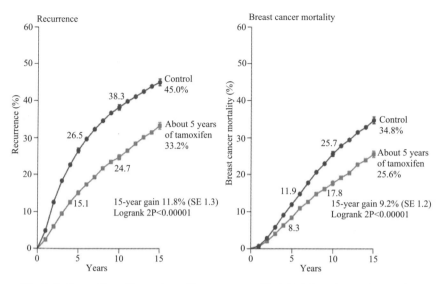

Fig. 1−7. Tamoxifen efficacy, tamoxifen carryover effect, high long-term relapse rates, and deaths[7]

Management of Endocrine Sensitive Breast Cancer

The tamoxifen overview

The EBCTCG has conducted overviews of RCTs testing adjuvant tamoxifen, in addition to local treatments, for early BC, establishing tamoxifen as a standard of care for pre- and postmenopausal women with early ER+ BC. There are important biological aspects of these trials that impact on current and future management of hormone-sensitive early BC (Figure 1−7).[7,8]

Adjuvant tamoxifen is effective treatment

Adjuvant tamoxifen given for five years reduces the risk of relapse from 26.5%, after local treatment alone, to 15.2% (difference of 11.4%) and from 38.3% to 24.7% after ten years follow-up (difference 13.6%). The risk of dying from BC is reduced from 11.9% to 8.3% at five years (difference 2.6%) and from 25.7% to 17.8% at ten years (difference 7.9%). After fifteen years follow-up, the absolute reduction for BC deaths has increased to 9.2%. Tamoxifen is effective both for women aged fifty years and over and for those women aged under fifty years.[7] As tamoxifen blocks the ER at the tumor cell, it is effective in both postmenopausal women and premenopausal women with functioning ovaries. Not all ER+ tumors respond to tamoxifen, and there is no reliable biomarker to predict responsiveness to tamoxifen among the population of women with ER+

BCs.

High long-term relapse rates

Despite this beneficial effect of adjuvant tamoxifen, new BC events and deaths after BC continue long term. At fifteen years follow-up, the BC relapse rate was 33.2% — an average annual rate of just over 2%. This high rate continues long term without evidence that rates will be lower after fifteen years. The BC mortality curve has a similar shape, with annual death rates after BC recurrence close to 1.6%.[7] Management of this high long-term risk has been neglected, but it is now being addressed by a new approach to BC control in the LATER protocol, described below.

The carryover effect and tamoxifen

The effect of adjuvant tamoxifen continues long term, with the absolute benefit for recurrence and mortality reduction being greater at ten years than at the completion of treatment, mostly about five years after diagnosis. The hazard rate (HR) of BC events after adjuvant tamoxifen remains lower than the HR after local treatment alone. Hence, the HR in the two populations is less than 1.0, and the curves continue to diverge (if the HR was 1.0, the curves would be parallel).

The biological basis of this phenomenon is not known. It is plausible that tamoxifen destroys or slows the rate of growth of the residual tumor that remains present after local treatments, and that if tamoxifen was not given, this residual tumor would have continued to grow and been detected some years after diagnosis. It is also plausible that the biology of a premalignant lesion has been changed by exposure to tamoxifen, possibly resulting in the primary prevention of a new BC. There is evidence consistent with this possible prevention role, as tamoxifen also reduces the risk of new contralateral BCs.

Reduction of contralateral breast cancer by tamoxifen

The overview data showed that women treated with adjuvant tamoxifen had a lower risk of subsequent contralateral BC. This risk reduction was greater after longer duration of adjuvant tamoxifen and was close to a 50% reduction of contralateral BC risk after five years of tamoxifen and longer term follow-up. These observations led to the investigation of tamoxifen as a primary prevention drug.[7]

Prevention of endocrine sensitive breast cancer

International Breast Intervention Study (IBIS) I and the overview of selective estrogen receptor modulators (SERMs) prevention. Several prospective

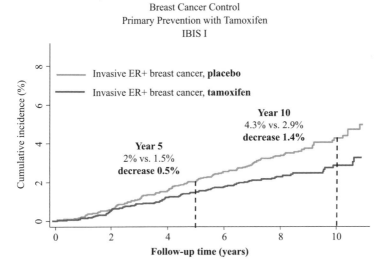

Breast Cancer Control
Primary Prevention with Tamoxifen
IBIS I

Cuzick, Forbes, Howell et al; JNCI 2007

Fig. 1–8. IBIS I tamoxifen prevention outcome
Tamoxifen is effective and has a substantial carryover effect.[14]

RCTs and an overview have established that about five years of adjuvant tamoxifen reduces the risk of primary ER+ BC by up to 50% in women at increased risk. Long-term follow-up data from the IBIS I trial showed that the tamoxifen prevention effect had a marked carryover for at least several years after treatment ended (absolute differences in BC event rates for placebo and tamoxifen were 0.5% at five years and 1.4% at ten years) (Figure 1–8).[14,15]

This tamoxifen primary prevention carryover effect was very similar to the large carryover effect seen with adjuvant tamoxifen. Although the biology is different, as the women on IBIS I had not had any prior BC, it is plausible that the women in the primary prevention trials may have a similar precancerous biology to that of the contralateral breast of woman treated with adjuvant tamoxifen for an ER+ primary cancer. Hence, the tamoxifen prevention carryover effect might result from modification of a precursor lesion.

Approaches to endocrine control 1: The IBIS II Primary Prevention Trial. This IBIS II trial is based, first, on the biology of tamoxifen as a treatment and preventative agent, and second, the observation that the aromatase inhibitor (AI), anastrozole (Arimidex®), is more effective than tamoxifen as adjuvant treatment of postmenopausal women with ER+ primary BC, in both reducing BC recurrence and, importantly, in preventing contralateral BC. Anastrozole not only has a significantly greater effect than tamoxifen in preventing contralateral BC, it also has a much greater carryover effect.[16] Further, an overview of trials

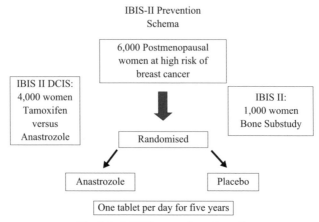

IBIS-II Prevention
Schema

6,000 Postmenopausal
women at high risk of
breast cancer

IBIS II DCIS:
4,000 women
Tamoxifen
versus
Anastrozole

IBIS II:
1,000 women
Bone Substudy

Randomised

Anastrozole   Placebo

One tablet per day for five years

Fig. 1–9. IBIS II prevention schema[18]

evaluating AIs against tamoxifen as adjuvant therapy demonstrated that AIs as a class of drug were about twice as good as tamoxifen in reducing contralateral BC rates.[17] Hence, it is plausible that AIs may have a greater effect as a primary prevention agent than tamoxifen.

The IBIS II trial is an international prospective double-blind primary prevention trial, testing the efficacy of anastrozole. The target population is postmenopausal women with increased risk, based predominantly on family history and breast density, with risk at least double that of an aged matched population. Women take placebo or anastrozole for a planned period of five years (Figure 1–9).[18]

IBIS II has an optional separate bone substudy for women taking part in the main prevention trial, where serial dual-energy X-ray absorptiometry (DXA) scans are completed for all women. Women with osteoporosis are provided with a bisphosphonate, and women with osteopenia have a separate and additional randomization to a bisphosphonate or placebo. Women with normal bone density have serial DXA scans (years one, three, and five). IBIS II also has a separate trial for women with ductal carcinoma in situ (DCIS), where anastrozole is being compared with tamoxifen in a double-blind prospective RCT.

Given the efficacy of tamoxifen for primary prevention and the superiority of anastrozole over tamoxifen in Arimidex, Tamoxifen, Alone or in Combination (ATAC) for prevention of contralateral BC, anastrozole theoretically could prevent several hundred thousand of the ER+ primary BCs diagnosed globally each year in postmenopausal women. The insurmountable problem, however, is that this would require the treatment of several hundred million women at risk, a clearly implausible proposition, which highlights the importance of finding

ANZ 0501 / LATER
Schema

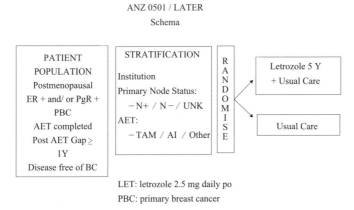

LET: letrozole 2.5 mg daily po
PBC: primary breast cancer

Fig. 1–10. Schema for the LATER trial[19]

biomarkers of risk. In IBIS II, mammograms, serial blood samples, and newly diagnosed BC tissue are being collected, and will be evaluated in the ideal context of a controlled prospective trial. IBIS II has accrued more than 5,000 women.

Approaches to endocrine control 2: The LATER protocol for prevention of late recurrence of breast cancer. Women previously diagnosed with ER+ BC have a high rate of new BC events long term, close to 2% per year for fifteen years or more post diagnosis and for at least ten years after adjuvant tamoxifen is completed. There are a large number of women in this category, and many do not receive regular surveillance, with or without a mammogram. Most women who were treated with tamoxifen did not have access to an AI at the time of diagnosis. Hence, it is plausible that late treatment with an AI may substantially reduce the risk of new BC events for these women on long-term follow-up. Surveys regularly show that the greatest survivorship concern of these women is fear of recurrence of BC.

A new prospective RCT, called LATER, recently has commenced for these women. LATER is testing whether later treatment with the AI, letrozole (Femara ®), can reduce the very high risk of later recurrence. The eligible population are postmenopausal women previously diagnosed with an ER+ primary BC at least six years previous, who received adjuvant tamoxifen for up to five years and who have completed their adjuvant endocrine treatment at least one year previous (Figure 1–10). To date, most women entering the trial already had completed their adjuvant endocrine treatment several years previous.[19]

LATER is an important proof-of-principle trial. A positive result would lead to a new paradigm of care and testing of new strategies to reduce the high risk of recurrence for other women, including those who have had an estrogen receptor negative (ER-) primary BC.

Future Directions

This paper has identified some current problems with the management of BC treatments, and has considered some relevant aspects of control of ER+ BC. Strategies to address problems of BC control have been outlined, including the important clinical trials IBIS II and LATER. It is likely that BC mortality will continue to fall, as new and recently introduced effective treatments have not yet been widely applied in the community outside of clinical trials. Community benefits will come from the wider availability of trastuzumab for treatment of HER-2 positive BC and to a lesser extent from tamoxifen for prevention. New agents such as poly (ADP-ribose) polymerase, or PARP, inhibitors may also impact on outcomes in the community, but first they must be subjected to rigorous evaluation in Phase III trials as a targeted treatment for selected women with early BC.[20,21] Potentially, screening could save more lives, and identification of women at risk using biomarkers must remain a very high priority (Table 1-1).

It is instructive to consider factors that have contributed to the long-term downward linear trend for cardiac mortality over more than fifty years. This trend projects to zero mortality by 2027 (in practice, a long exponential tail-off would be likely, but for the present, the fall is clearly linear) (Figure 1-11). The key components include a substantial risk factor (smoking) that can be managed; excellent biomarkers of risk, including blood pressure and cholesterol; sophisticated diagnostic tools; a wide array of effective treatments, including treatment of the biomarkers; many additional strategies, such as organ replacement; effective lifestyle intervention; and very long-term care that is also delivered within the community.

As breast oncologists, we have many opportunities to improve outcomes, and we have much to learn. The future is now, and the strategies to improve management of BC are clear.

Table 1–1. Current and future goals in breast cancer research, treatments, and management

1. Scientific rigor and optimal use of statistics as a standard for clinical research.
2. Discovery of reliable biomarkers of risk and response to treatment and development of reliable, universal, risk assessment tools.
3. Use of breast density and other risk biomarkers for riskdapted screening.
4. Understanding of breast stem cell biology and the implications for progression to cancer and metastases.
5. Tissue collection and molecular analyses for all new patients diagnosed with breast cancer (BC) as a standard of care.
6. Clinical trials, including new designs, such as adaptive preoperative systemic therapy (PST) trials, as a standard of care for discovery and treatment.
7. Simplified ethics and administrative approval for research, and increased involvement of patients in research planning and conduct.
8. Optimal use of targeted therapies with effective targeting of critical pathways, in addition to single molecular targets.
9. Effective local treatment with minimal cost and morbidity for all women.
10. Optimization of gene expression and pathway analysis for a greater understanding of efficacy, resistance, and tumor biology.
11. Optimal use of aromatase inhibitors (AIs), and new endocrine strategies, for prevention and treatment of estrogen receptor positive (ER+) early and late BC.
12. Discovery of effective strategies to prevent estrogen receptor negative (ER −) and other BC types.

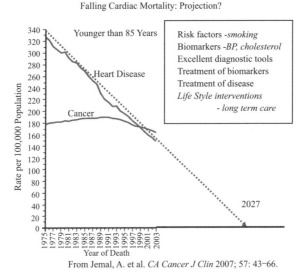

From Jemal, A. et al. *CA Cancer J Clin* 2007; 57: 43−66.

Fig. 1–11. Falling heart disease mortality and projection of 50-year trend[22]

Chapter 2

Axillary Diagnosis and Treatment

Ultrasound for Axillary Staging

Chiun-Sheng Huang

Summary

A large cancer of the breast is not a contra-indication of sentinel lymph node biopsy (SLNB). However, due to the high prevalence of positive nodes in large breast cancers, ultrasound and ultrasound-guided fine-needle aspiration cytology (US-FNAC) should be done to detect metastatic nodes, so that SLNB can be avoided. For patients receiving neoadjuvant chemotherapy, axillary staging by ultrasound can also be helpful in saving patients from SLNB before chemotherapy. If there is no metastatic node detected before chemotherapy, SLNB can be tried after chemotherapy. For patients with positive nodes and T3 operable breast cancer before chemotherapy, SLNB may be tried if ultrasound axillary staging after chemotherapy is negative.

Introduction: Current Status of Sentinel Lymph Node Biopsy (SLNB) in Axillary Staging

Even though most early breast cancers appear to be localized to the breast when diagnosed, one-quarter of node-negative women and more than one-half of node-positive women will develop metastatic disease within ten years of surgery without adjuvant systemic chemotherapy.[1,2] These estimates are over several decades of trials but are probably overly pessimistic given today's availability of adjuvant antibody and hormonal treatments with or without surgery. Nevertheless, postoperative systemic therapy still can be considered a mandatory part of the management of primary early breast cancer in the majority of women patients.[3] Several prognostic factors are used to decide whether a woman needs systemic adjuvant therapy. These include age, tumor size, histologic grade, hormone receptor expression, and axillary lymph node status. Among these prognostic factors, the status of axillary lymph node involvement is the most important one.

SLNB was proposed for axillary staging in the management of breast cancer in the mid-1990s by A. E. Giuliano and co-workers.[4] The sentinel lymph node (SLN) is supposed to be the first lymph node that drains the primary breast cancer. As lymphatic spread is supposed to be stepwise, if there is no metastasis detected in the SLN the rest of the axillary lymph nodes should be free of metastasis. Hence, axillary lymph node dissection (ALND) can be spared, and the patient would be saved from complications.

The incidence of axillary recurrence after a negative SLNB is comparable to the incidence of axillary recurrence following ALND. In a recent report of a randomized trial of 749 patients with tumors not larger than 3 cm, although more loco-regional recurrences were observed in patients receiving only SLNB compared with patients receiving SLNB and ALND, the false-negative rate of SLNB in SLN-negative patients was high at 16.7%[5], in contrast to false-negative rates of about 10% recorded in earlier trials[6-11]. In another randomized trial of 516 patients with tumors not larger than 2 cm, the recurrent events and overall 5-year survival were not significantly different between patients receiving ALND and patients receiving only SLNB, when SLN was negative after a median follow-up of seventy-nine months. Only one axillary recurrence was observed in the patients receiving SLNB only, although eight were expected.[12] Another randomized trial revealed no axillary recurrence in patients receiving SLNB only, at a median follow-up of 5.5 years.[13] Two nonrandomized studies, each including more than 2,200 patients with negative SLN and without ALND, demonstrated that only 0.6% of patients developed axillary recurrence without relapse in other sites after a median follow-up of more than two-and-half years.[14,15]

Although the long-term survival results of large randomized trials are not available yet, SLNB is widely accepted by physicians and patients as an option of axillary staging due to its low incidence of morbidity, compared with ALND. SLNB is safe without significant radiation risk associated with radioisotope and has a low incidence of allergic reaction to the blue dye (with severe anaphylaxis less than 1%)[11] In its SLNB guidelines, the American Society of Clinical Oncology concludes that SLNB is an appropriate alternative to axillary staging for patients with early breast cancers not larger than 5 cm and clinically negative axillary lymph nodes, and that ALND can be spared if the SLN is negative, but the guidelines also advise that a surgeon should not hesitate to convert to ALND if he or she thinks it necessary.[16]

SLNB for Large Breast Cancer

The incidence of lymph node metastasis demonstrated by ALND in breast cancer patients for different tumor sizes as report by Melvin J. Silverstein and co-workers was 5%, 16%, 28%, 47%, 68%, and 86% in T1a, T1b, T1c, T2, T3, and T4 tumors, respectively.[17] Since the chance of lymph node involvement is low in small tumors, which makes the complications associated with ALND more undesirable, SLNB was first applied in small tumors to replace ALND.[5,11,12] Currently, in daily practice, SLNB generally has been applied to small invasive breast cancer, tumors not larger than 2 cm or 3 cm, without clinical evidence of lymph node involvement.[12,15,18] Tumor size is limited to 3 cm or smaller for several reasons: first, nearly half of the T2 tumor may develop lymph node metastasis, which would necessitate a second procedure of ALND after SLNB; second, the cost of SLNB is high; and third, the incorrect perception that the high false-negative rate of SLNB in a large tumor results from the complete occupancy of cancer in the lymph node preventing the radiotracer's entrance into the lymph node.

Several studies have focused on the accuracy of SLNB in large breast cancers. The identification rates of SLN (93%~100%) and false-negative rates of SLNB (3%~6.8%) were not worse in T2 and T3 tumors than those of T1 tumors (Table 2−A−1).[19-22] In a prospective multi-institutional study of 2,085 breast cancer patients with tumor sizes available, the identification rates of SLN and the false-negative rates were not significantly different among patients with T1, T2, and T3 tumors.[22] All patients received SLNB using the combined guidance method of radioactive colloid and blue dye, followed by ALND. The identification rates of SLN were 93.2% and 97.8% for T2 and T3 tumors, respectively, compared with that of 92.1% for T1 tumors, and the false-negative rates were 6.8% and 3.0% for T2 and T3 tumors, respectively compared with 9.2% for T1 tumors. When tumor size was categorized into a 1-cm difference, the SLN identification rate tended to be higher and the false-negative rate lower in patients with larger tumors. In one study of 218 patients with T2 and T3 tumors and in the other study of forty-eight patients with tumor larger than 3 cm, both with negative SLN and not receiving ALND, none of the patients developed isolated axillary recurrence at a median follow-up of thirty-one months and forty-three months, respectively.[14,23] Based on the findings in these studies, it seems that SLNB is as accurate an axillary staging procedure in T2 and T3 breast cancers as it is for T1 cancers.

Table 2–A–1. Summary of SLN identification rate and false-negative rate of SLNB in different reports on large invasive breast cancer

Author	Wong et al[22]	Bedrosian et al[19]	Bedrosian et al[19]	Lelievre et al[21]	Chung et al[20]	Wong et al[22]
Tumor Size	≦2cm	>2,≦5cm	≧2,<5cm	≧3,<5cm	≧3cm (median4.2cm)	≧5cm	>5cm
Total no. patients (cancers)	1496	545	104	56	152	41	44
Overall rate of LN involvement	25%	52%	59%	63%	69%	73%	77%
SLN identification rate (%)	92%	93%	99%	98%	97%	100%	98%
False-negative rate (%)	9%	7%	3%	3%	4%[+]	3%	3%

The Use of Ultrasound in Axillary Staging

Although SLNB is feasible in invasive breast cancers of all sizes and without clinical nodal involvement, a certain percentage of patients, especially those with large tumor, still needs to undergo ALND, once SLNB reveals metastatic SLN. Recently, several studies have reported that ultrasound evaluation of axillae can help to identify metastatic lymph nodes preoperatively, so that SLNB can be spared in those patients with positive lymph nodes proved by core needle biopsy (CNB) (Table 2–A–2).[24-35] Among different studies of different incidences of lymph node involvement in axillae, metastases were detected preoperatively by ultrasound-guided biopsy, and 1.4%–45% of SLNB could be avoided. In one large series of 726 patients (consisting of 732 axillae) with 67% of T1 tumor, 30% of T2 tumors, and 2.7% of T3 or T4 tumors reported by Maartje C. van Rijk and co-workers, about one-quarter of axillae were found by ultrasound to have suspicious lymph node involvement, and of these, about one-third were proved by US-FNAC to have metastatic lymph node involvement by SLNB.[31] Those patients with normal ultrasound did not receive FNAC. The sensitivity and specificity was 35% and 82%, respectively, for ultrasound, and 21% and 99.8%, respectively, for US-FNAC. In this series, 58 of 732 (8%) of axillae were diagnosed preoperatively to have lymph node metastasis. Therefore, 8% of patients can be saved from SLNB and receive ALND directly.

Among the studies shown in Table 2–A–2, the percentage of metastatic lymph nodes diagnosed preoperatively by ultrasound-guided biopsy ranged from 5.7% to 80%, and the percentage of SLNB avoided ranged from 1.4% to 45%.[24-35] The explanation for the wide variation of rates among these studies could be due to differences in the following factors: whether only the suspicious nodes or all of the visualized nodes are biopsied; the biopsy method (CNB or FNAC); the percentage of lymph nodes visualized; the criteria for suspicious nodes detected by ultrasound; and the incidences of metastatic lymph nodes.

Table 2-A-2. Studies of preoperative axilla staging by ultrasound-guided biopsy

Studies	Case number	Biopsy tool	Incidence of involved LN	% of LN Visualized by US	Biopsy criteria	% of involved LN diagnosed by US guided biopsy	% of SLNB avoided
Damera et al[24]	166	CNB/FNAC (FNAC if CNB not feasible)	39%	62%	one, most suspicious	42%	16%
Abe et al[25]	144	CNB	56%	only cases with node visualized and suspicious enrolled	one, suspicious (only US-suspicious cases enrolled)	80%	44%
Bonnema et al[26]	150	FNAC	41%	62%	all visible nodes	63%	26%
de Kanter et al[27]	185	FNAC	47%	37%	one, most suspicious	36%	17%
Swinson et al[35]	369	FNAC	31%	33%	one, most suspicious	55%	11%
Keunen-Boomeester et al[28]	180	FNAC	46%	NR	all visible nodes	44%	20%
Bedrosian et al[29]	208	FNAC	25%	retrospective study	suspicious node	5.70%	1.40%
Deurloo et al[30]	268	FNAC	45%	35%	one, most suspicious	31%	14%
van Rijk et al[31]	732	FNAC	37%	100%	all suspicious nodes	21%	8%
Hinson et al[32]	112	FNAC	52%	NR	suspicious node	59%	30%
Koelliker et al[33]	75	FNAC	68%	retrospective study	most suspicious or largest node	67%	45%
Gilisson et al[34]	195	FNAC	48%	100%	suspicious nodes	56%	27%

Ideally, the sensitivity of US-FNAC in the detection of metastatic nodes needs to be as high as possible, which probably necessitates increasing the use of US-FNAC procedures. The tradeoff could be a decrease in the positive predictive value (PPV) of US-FNAC. Some institutes implement US-FNAC on every lymph node visualized, whether the ultrasound pattern of the lymph node is suspicious or not. When the PPV becomes too low, each institute needs to evaluate if its efforts to diagnose lymph node involvement preoperatively by ultrasound-guided biopsy are still worthwhile.

False-negative rates of US-FNAC were observed in these studies, and the sensitivity of ultrasound is higher than that of US-FNAC generally, which implies that the false-negative rates of US-FNAC may be due to FNAC but not to ultrasound. Two studies reported on the use of CNB in the biopsy of the lymph node.[24,25] Complications associated with the CNB procedure seem acceptable. Just like in the diagnosis of primary tumor, the false-negative rate is expected to be lower with CNB than with FNAC.

Frequent Locations of Sentinel Lymph Nodes

To increase the percentage of metastatic lymph nodes diagnosed preoperatively, one needs to know how to visualize a lymph node. In the early reports, the percentage of lymph node visualized in axillae was only 35%–37%,[27,30] while in more recent reports, it was 100%.[31] A normal lymph node has a central fatty hilum and thin cortex, which sometimes is hard to detect from the surrounding fatty tissue of the axilla (Figure 2–A–1). To find a lymph node, or even an SLN, in the axilla, one also needs to be aware of the frequent location of an SLN. According to a study by C. E. Cox and co-workers, 94% of SLNs were detected in the cross of the axillary hair line and the mid-axillary line, with a 5-cm diameter area.[36] In our unpublished data of 291 SLNB procedures, about 97% of SLNs are located 1 cm–2 cm below the hair line and between the mid-axillary line and the pectoralis muscle (Figure 2–A–2).

Ultrasound Criteria for Metastatic Lymph Nodes

The diagnostic criteria for a metastatic lymph node by ultrasound vary between reports (Table 2–A–3).[24–26,29–31,33,34,39] The following characteristics suggest that a lymph node could be metastasized: absence of or a narrow fatty hilum; eccentrically or concentrically increased thickness of cortex (2 mm); atypical cortex appearance (echo poor, nonhomogeneous); smallest diameter of lymph node larger than or equal to 5 mm; and the ratio of longitudinal to transverse axis less than two (Figure 2–A–1). In addition, if ultrasound examination is done after excisional biopsy, a benign axillary lymph node may look suspicious (with an increased thickening of cortex).[29]

In one study using ultrasound alone without biopsy to evaluate axillary status, Kazuhiko Sato and co-workers chose absence of hilum as the criteria for lymph node involvement.[37] In fifty-four patients with abnormal ultrasound, fifty had lymph node metastasis, and in 208 patients with normal ultrasound, only sixty-two had lymph node involvement. The PPV, sensitivity, and specificity calculated from these data was 93%, 45%, and 97%, respectively. Maximum cortex thickness was the most significant feature in a study by Eline E. Deurloo and co-workers to predict lymph node metastasis.[30] To obtain a high sensitivity at 95%, and a low specificity at 44%, a maximum cortex thickness of 2.3 mm

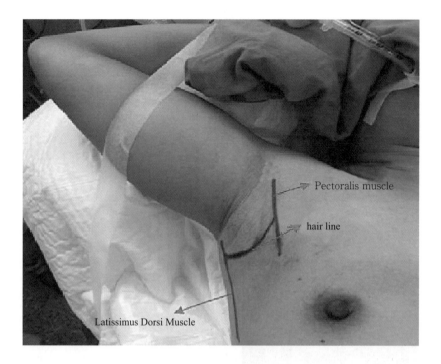

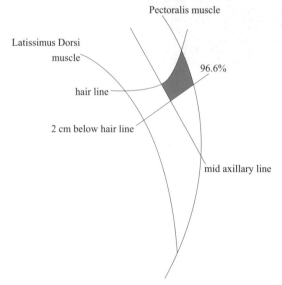

Fig. 2−A−1. Frequent locations of axillary sentinel lymph node

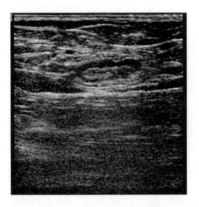 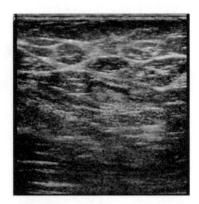

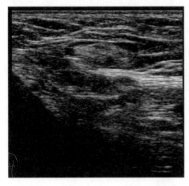

(a) Normal lymph node with preserved fatty hilum and thin cortex. (Hilum is where the efferent lymphatic vessel leaves the lymph node. Each lymph node receives many afferent lymphatic vessels entering the cortex. When there is cancer cell metastasis, it will deposit at the cortex.)

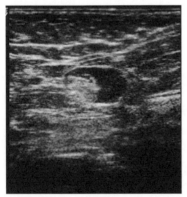

(b) Lymph node with eccentrically thickened cortex proved to be benign

Fig. 2–A–2. Ultrasound images and photos of normal and abnormal axillary lymph nodes (continued)

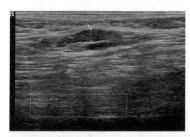

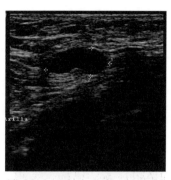

(c) Lymph node with increased thickening of cortex but not hypoechoic in patient post-excision, proved to be benign

(d) Metastatic lymph node with thickened and hypoechoic (lower echogenecity than surrounding fat tissue) cortex

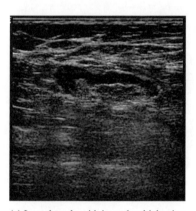

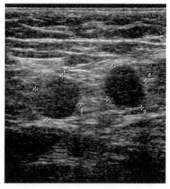

(e) Lymph node with irregular thickening or lobulation of cortex, proved to be metastatic

(f) Metastatic node with round shape and loss of fatty hilum

Fig. 2–A–2. Ultrasound images and photos of normal and abnormal axillary lymph nodes (continued)

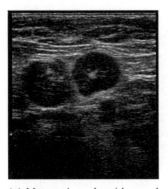

(g) Metastatic node with round
shape and compressed hilum

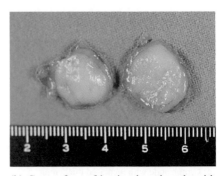

(h) Cut surface of benign lymph node with
thin cortex and predominant fatty hilum

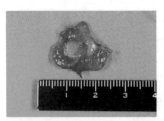

(i) Cut surface of lymph node
with thickened cortex

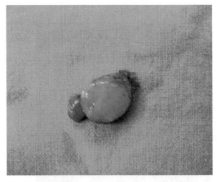

(j) Cut surface of metastatic lymph node
occupied by cancer and loss of fatty hilum

Fig. 2–A–2. Ultrasound images and photos of normal and abnormal axillary lymph nodes
（continued）

was shown to be the most important criteria for biopsy. In a recent study by
Susan L. Koelliker and co-workers, the PPV for absence of hilum, eccentric
hilum, hypoechoic cortex, and thick or lobular cortex was 100%, 94%, 97%,
and 73%, respectively.[33]

In a study using ultrasound-guided CNB, increased cortical thickness and
overall size of lymph node are considered two significant factors to differentiate
metastatic from nonmetastatic nodes.[25] However, the range, mean, and median
of cortical thickness was 2.7 mm–27.3 mm, 10.3 mm, and 8.1 mm, respectively,
for metastatic nodes, and 2.8 mm–12.7 mm, 5.3 mm, and 4.5 mm, respectively,
for nonmetastatic nodes. The range, mean, and median of overall size was
6.9 mm–39.4 mm, 16.5 mm, and 12.9 mm, respectively, for metastatic nodes,

Table 2–A–3. Ultrasound criteria for suspicious lymph nodes, and sensitivity and specificity of ultrasound for axilla staging among different studies

Studies	Ultrasound criteria of suspicious LN	Specificity	Sensitivity
Damera et al[24]	Cortex concentrically or eccentrically thickened ≧2mm longitudinal / transverse axis <2	82%	55%
Abe et al[25]	Cortical thickening[1] (10.3 mm, 8.1 mm), size[2] (mean 16.5 mm, median 12.9 mm), absence of hilum[3], NHBF[4]	64%[1], 97%[3], 81%[1+4]	79%[1], 33%[3], 65%[1+4]
Bonnema et al[26]	Echo poor, inhomogeneous pattern[4], or smallest node>5 mm[5]	95%[4], 56%[5]	36%[4], 87%[5]
Bedrosian et al[29]	Eccentric cortical enlargement, hilum displaced, hypoechoic round nodes	91%	26%
Deurloo et al[30]	Max.cortex smallest diameter≧5 mm, thickness≧2.3 mm atypical cortex appearance	44%	95%
van Rijk et al[31]	Max.cortex smallest diameter≧5 mm, thickness≧2.3 mm atypical cortex appearance	82%	35%
Koelliker et al[33]	Eccentric or replaced hilum, markedly hypoechoic cortex, thick or lobulated cortex	73%	71%
Gilisson et al[34]	LN shortest diameter>5 mm, cortex >2.3 mm, eccentric	NR	NR
Krishnamurthy et al[39]	Disappearance of fatty hilum, eccentric lobulation or increased thickening of cortex	35–67%	96–100%

and 6.2 mm–22.6 mm, 15.0 mm, and 12.0 mm, respectively, for nonmetastatic nodes. Since the ranges for metastatic and nonmetastatic nodes overlap, deciding when to biopsy based on these two factors is difficult. The sensitivity of ultrasound to diagnose metastatic lymph node based on cortical thickening, absence of fatty hilum, and nonhilum blood flow was 79%, 33%, and 65%, respectively, and the PPV was 73%, 93%, and 78%, respectively. The higher the sensitivity, the more metastatic lymph nodes are detected, and the fewer metastatic nodes are missed. The higher the PPV, unnecessary biopsies are fewer, and the higher the percentage of metastatic nodes proved by ultrasound. Since SLNB is the standard for axillary staging in cases with negative ultrasound, a criteria with high PPV and low sensitivity is better than a criteria of low PPV and moderate sensitivity, so that a negative ultrasound-guided biopsy can be saved.

Ultrasound Sensitivity in Detecting Lymph Node Metastasis Increases As Tumor Size Increases

Since a larger tumor is associated with a higher incidence of axillary lymph node metastasis, studies with higher incidences of lymph node metastasis indicate the inclusion of more large tumors. The sensitivity of ultrasound in detecting lymph node metastasis has been shown to increase as the tumor size increases. Koelliker and co-workers reported that the sensitivity of ultrasound for T1, T2, T3, and T4 tumor was 56%, 64%~73%, 82%, and 100%, respectively, while Ponnandai Somasundar and co-workers reported 35% and 67% for T1 and T2 tumors, respectively.[33,38] The sensitivities can be explained by a larger metastasis depositing in lymph nodes of a larger cancer, making it easier to be detected by ultrasound.[32,35] Therefore, if more small breast cancers are evaluated by ultrasound for axillary lymph node metastasis, a lower percentages of lymph node involvement will be diagnosed preoperatively, and fewer SLNBs will be avoided.

Ultrasound Evaluation Decreases False-Negative Rate of SLNB

Importantly, pre-SLNB evaluation of axillary lymph node by ultrasound will help to decrease the false-negative rate of SLNB. As demonstrated in the study by Sato and co-workers, the SLN identification rate for 262 total patients and for 208 patients with negative ultrasound was 88.2% and 98.6%, respectively, while for twenty-three patients with T3 tumors and for six patients with T3 tumors but negative ultrasound, the identification rate was 65.2% and 100%, respectively.[37] The false-negative rate of SLNB for all 262 patients and for 208 patients with negative ultrasound was 10.8% and 1.7%, respectively, while for twenty-three patients with T3 tumors and for six patients with T3 tumors but negative ultrasound, the false-negative rate was 35.7% and 0%, respectively.

Negative Ultrasound Indicates Fewer Nodal Metastases

Reports also suggest that when ultrasound or US-FNAC reveals that axillary lymph nodes is negative, the chance of having more than three positive lymph nodes or tumor deposits in lymph node greater than 5 mm is low. The study by van Rijk and co-workers demonstrated that patients, whose axillary lymph node involvement was diagnosed by preoperative US-FNAC, had more positive nodes than patients whose axillary lymph node involvement could not be detected by US-FNAC (4.3 vs. 2.2, median 3 vs.1.5; p<0.001).[31] The study by Jorien Bonnema and co-workers also demonstrated that the chance to detect metastatic lymph nodes by US-FNAC was higher when there were four or more positive nodes compared with when there was only one positive node.[26] In a study by J. L. Hinson and co-workers., patients without a palpable axillary lymph node and with grade-3 tumors (size not smaller than 1 cm), and patients without a palpable axillary node and with grade-2 tumors (size not smaller than 1.5 cm), were considered as high risk in having axillary lymph node involvement and receiving ultrasound evaluation.[32] US-FNAC detected all patients with more than three positive nodes. Among patients with negative ultrasound but metastatic nodes diagnosed by SLNB, the tumor deposits in lymph node were less than or equal to 5 mm. Separate studies by A. Damera, Savitri Krishnamurthy, and co-workers also showed that all patients with more than three positive nodes were detected by ultrasound-guided biopsy; in Krishnamurthy's study, 93% of the fifty-three patients with cancer deposits larger than 5 mm were detected by US-FNAC.[24,39] In one study series by C. Swinson and co-workers, none of fourteen cases with micrometastasis (0.2 mm−2 mm) of the lymph node was detected by US-FNAC, but thirty-eight of 102 (37%) cases with lymph node metastasis larger than or equal to 2 mm was detected by US-FNAC.[35] Fifty percent of cases with more than three positive nodes were detected preoperatively by US-FNAC, while only 15% of cases with one positive node were diagnosed by US-FNAC. In this study series, 278 of 369 (75%) breast cancers were detected by screening.

Ultrasound for Axillary Staging Before Neoadjuvant Chemotherapy

Whether SLNB is done before or after neoadjuvant chemotherapy remains a controversial issue. Concerns are raised about the lack of data on SLNB alone after neoadjuvant chemotherapy in patients with prechemotherapy diagnosis of positive lymph node, the relatively high false-negative rate of SLNB, and the high frequency of positive nodes after neoadjuvant chemotherapy, especially for locally advanced breast cancer.

No axillary staging was required before chemotherapy in the National Surgical Adjuvant Breast and Bowel Project (NSABP) B-27. No information about the correlation between the SLNB successful rate and nodal status before neoadjuvant chemotherapy was available in the meta-analysis.

Ultrasound is also helpful for axillary staging before neoadjuvant chemotherapy. If SLNB is done before chemotherapy, repeating SLNB after chemotherapy may not be successful, and ALND will be required. When a metastatic lymph node is diagnosed before chemotherapy by ultrasound-guided biopsy, SLNB can be spared. Neoadjuvant chemotherapy may convert one-third of node-positive cancers to a node-negative disease, so that when SLNB is done after neoadjuvant chemotherapy, a certain percentage of patients can be saved from ALND. Different identification rates of SLN and false-negative rates of SLNB reported in the literatures are probably related to the different extent of nodal involvement of cancers in different series. When ultrasound does not detect a suspicious node and US-FNAC does not diagnose a metastatic lymph node, the chance of having more than three positive nodes is low, and conversion from node-positive status, if positive nodes do exist, to node-negative disease should be high. Ultrasound also can be done after chemotherapy to evaluate axillary status, so that false-negative SLNB can be prevented. Therefore, axillary staging by ultrasound before neoadjuvant chemotherapy may save more patients from ALND than initial axillary staging by SLNB.

The following studies show an example of axillary staging by ultrasound before neoadjuvant chemotherapy. Amina Khan and co-workers reported a series of ninety-one patients receiving neoadjuvant chemotherapy.[45] There were 42% (38/91) of patients diagnosed to have lymph node metastasis before chemotherapy either by SLNB (twenty patients) or by US-FNAC (eighteen patients). SLNB followed by ALND was done after chemotherapy on thirty-three prechemotherapy diagnosed node-positive patients (13 US-FNAC, 20 SLNB) and revealed a 97% identification rate (SLN not identified in one case with prechemotherapy diagnosis by US-FNAC) and a 4.5% false-negative rate (in one case, prechemotherapy diagnosis by SLNB). One-third of these thirty-three patients (5/13 in US-FNAC and 6/20 in SLNB) became node-negative after chemotherapy. Another series of sixty-one patients receiving neoadjuvant chemotherapy was reported by Somasundar.[38] US-FNAC was done for axillary staging and identified that 77% of patients were node-positive and 23% were node-negative. After chemotherapy, 28% were node-negative proved by SLNB or ALND. Erika A. Newman and co-workers reported fifty-three node-positive breast cancers treated by neoadjuvant chemotherapy.[46] Thirteen patients were diagnosed to be node-positive by SLNB before chemotherapy, and forty patients by US-FNAC. SLNB was done after chemotherapy and 32% of patients (17/53) became node-negative. The false-negative rate of SLNB among patients diagnosed to be node-positive by US-FNAC before chemotherapy was 11% (3/28) and 0% in patients by SLNB. In 219 patients with an initially palpable

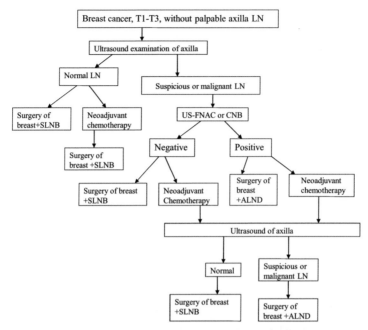

Fig. 2–A–3. Flowchart of proposed algorithm using ultrasound, US-FNAC and SLNB for axilla staging among patients receiving primary surgery or neoadjuvant chemotherapy

or positive node, proved by US-FNAC, or with a highly suspicious node on ultrasound, Seeyoun Lee and co-workers reported that 78.5% of patients remained node-positive after neoadjuvant chemotherapy.[47] The identification rate of SLN after neoadjuvant chemotherapy was 77.6% only, but the false-negative rate was 5.6%. Jeannie Shen and co-workers reported a high false-negative rate (25%) of SLNB after neoadjuvant chemotherapy in sixty-nine patients with initially node-positive cancers proved by US-FNAC.[48] Jyh-Chern Yu and co-workers reported an identification rate of SLN of 91% and a false-negative rate of SLNB at 9.6% in 127 T3 locally advanced breast cancers after neoadjuvant chemotherapy. Intraoperative ultrasound identified five cases with a non-SLN that were missed in SLN mapping, which decreased the false-negative rate of SLNB from 9.6% to 1.4%.[49]

Concluding Remark

An algorithm of ultrasound, US-FNAC, and SLNB is proposed for axillary staging among breast cancer patients with T1–T3 tumors (Figure 2–A–3).

Bio-optical Aspects in Indocyanine Green Fluorescence for Sentinel Node Biopsy in Breast Cancer

Toshiyuki Kitai

Summary

The indocyanine green (ICG) fluorescence method is more reliable, and less training is required, than the conventional dye-guided method, for detecting, assessing, and biopsy-ing sentinel nodes. The ICG technique is useful in making sentinel node biopsy (SNB) more popular, especially in small-volume hospitals where radioisotope facilities are unavailable. This paper describes the principles and clinical presentation of the ICG fluorescence method, and introduces bio-optical devices that overcome difficulties with the ICG fluorescence method.

Introduction: The Emerging Technology of Fluorescence

SNB is an established procedure to assess the lymph node status of patients with early breast cancer, so as to avoid unnecessary axillary dissection.[1-4] There are two methods of SNB: radioisotope-guided method[5] and dye-guided method.[6] The radioisotope method is the worldwide standard, because little training is required and satisfactory results can be obtained. The dye method, although certain training is necessary, is also advantageous, because this method is free from radiation exposure and does not require radioisotope facilities.

The ICG fluorescence method is a newly developed technology.[7,8] It is a modification of the dye method,[9,10] in which the detection of sentinel nodes is facilitated by fluorescence navigation. Tissue penetration of near infrared (NIR) light is an important aspect of this method. Under visible light, subcutaneous lymphatic vessels and the lymph nodes in the fatty tissue are not visible to the naked eye, but fluorescence imaging makes these structures visible. High sensitivity is also beneficial. Even in cases where one can hardly tell which

Visible light   NIR Fluorescence

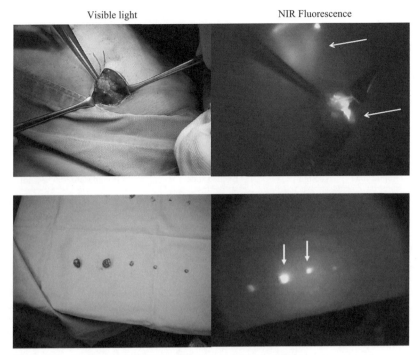

Fig. 2−B−1. Advantages of NIR fluorescence over visible light
   Tissue penetration (upper panel): Lymphatic vessels under the skin, and lymph nodes in the fatty
   tissue can be detected by fluorescence. High sensitivity (lower panel): Lymph nodes stained by ICG
   can be judged with high sensitivity. NIR−Near infrared.

nodes are stained by the ICG color, fluorescence imaging clearly shows which
nodes are sentinel (Figure 2−B−1). However, the surgical procedures are still
not easy compared with the radioisotope method, because the sentinel node
cannot be detected from the skin. The sentinel node is usually at a depth of 2
cm or more in the axilla, and the fluorescence signal from the sentinel node is
mostly lost by scattering.

Biophysical Basis of ICG Fluorescence Method

Molecular fluorescence of ICG
Molecular fluorescence of ICG consists of a two-step process of excitation and
emission (Figure 2−B−2). When light at 765 nm is emitted at ICG molecules,
they move from ground state to excited state (excitation). When the molecules
return to ground state, a part of the absorbed energy is radiated as fluorescent
emission at 830 nm. The fluorescent emission is at a longer wavelength than

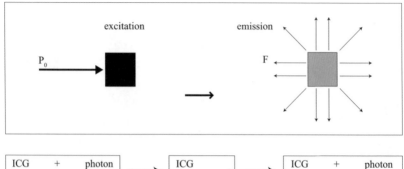

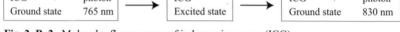

Fig. 2–B–2. Molecular fluorescence of indocyanine green (ICG)
The wavelengths of fluorescent excitation and emission are specific to ICG. High signal-to-noise
ratio can be obtained by fluorescence measurement. P_0–Excitation light. F–Fluorescent light.

the fluorescent excitation. Since the combination of these wavelengths is specific to the ICG molecule, highly sensitive measurement is possible by selecting proper wavelengths in the light source and the detector.

The general law of fluorescence spectroscopy is shown in the equation below. Only 1.2% of absorbed energy is emitted as fluorescence.[11] Fluorescence intensity has no linear relationship with ICG concentration. When the concentration of ICG is greater than 0.08 g/l, the fluorescence intensity becomes weaker[11] (quenching effect). However, the quenching effect usually does not disturb the lymphatic detection in the clinical setting.

$$F = \varphi\, P_0\, \{1 - \exp(-\varepsilon\, C\, b)\}$$

F: intensity of fluorescent light
P_0: intensity of excitation light
φ: quantum efficiency (ICG: 0.012)
exp: natural log
ε: absorption coefficient
C: ICG concentration
b: cell size

Optical properties of ICG in the living tissue

ICG has characteristic fluorescence spectra in the NIR wavelengths (Figure 2–B–3), ranging from 700 nm to 900 nm, which is called 'an optical window'. This is advantageous to clinical application, because the NIR light can penetrate deep into the tissue without being absorbed by hemoglobin or water.[12,13] However, when applied to the living tissue, light scattering becomes an important issue[14,15] (Figure 2–B–4). The fluorescent excitation and emission

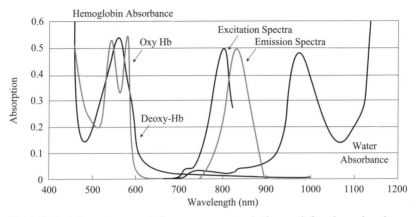

Fig. 2–B–3. Indocyanine green's fluorescence spectra in the near infrared wavelengths

The wavelengths between 700 nm and 900 nm are called the 'optical window', since the light at these wavelengths can penetrate deep into the tissue as escaped from the absorption by hemoglobin (Hb) and water.

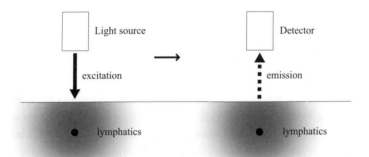

Fig. 2–B–4. The excitation and emission light is attenuated by scattering in living tissue

are attenuated by scattering when the light travels in the tissue (Figure 2–B–3). Fat droplets in the axilla are the main scatterers.[16,17] In the preliminary experiment, an ICG fluorescent signal at a depth of 1 cm in the breast phantom was detectable, but detection was difficult as the depth increased. The limit of detectable depth by fluorescence in the axilla is supposed to be 1 cm~2 cm.

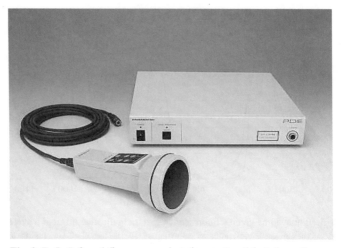

Fig. 2–B–5. Infrared fluorescence imaging system (photodynamic eye, Hamamatsu Photonics, Japan)

Clinical Presentation

Equipment

An infrared fluorescence imaging system (photodynamic eye, Hamamatsu Photonics, Japan), which consists of light emitting diodes at 760 nm as a light source, and a charge-coupled device (CCD) camera with a cut filter below 820 nm as a detector, was used to measure NIR fluorescence images[7,8] (Figure 2–B–5).

Surgical procedures

Surgical procedures of the ICG fluorescence method are principally the same as those of the dye method[7] (Figure 2–B–6). After induction of general anesthesia and sterilization of the operating site, 1 ml of ICG solution (5 mg/1 ml) is injected into the areolar skin.[18] After a few seconds, lymphatic drainage was observed with fluorescence images. Subcutaneous lymphatic channels were detected over the skin, usually in one or two minutes, towards the axilla, and disappeared beyond the lateral edge of the pectralis major muscle. This is the point where the subcutaneous lymphatic channel enters the axillary space. After a small skin incision is made at this point, the lymphatic channel is dissected towards the axilla until it reaches the sentinel nodes by the guidance of fluorescence images. The sentinel nodes can be differentiated from lymphatic channels, because the lymph nodes have a more intense fluorescent signal and

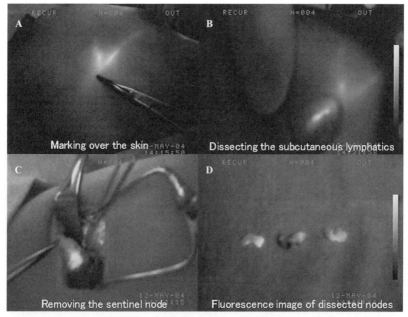

Fig. 2–B–6. Surgical procedure for the indocyanine green (ICG) fluorescence method
A: After injection of ICG around the areola, subcutaneous lymphatic drainage is marked until
it disappears before entering the axillary space. B: Skin incision is made and the subcutaneous
lymphatic channel is dissected towards the axilla. C: The sentinel node is dissected by following
the lymphatic channel. D: The removed lymph nodes are examined by fluorescence imaging, to
determine whether they are stained by ICG.

a round shape. It is important not to injure the lymphatic channels during the
dissection. Otherwise, due to the fluorescent signal of the ICG spilling into the
surgical field, further dissection becomes difficult. It is recommended that the
lymphatic channel is not exposed but dissected with surrounding fatty tissue.
Since several fluorescent spots are usually observed around the first drained
nodes, those fluorescent nodes are dissected en bloc with the surrounding fatty
tissue. Lymph nodes in the dissected specimen are isolated and investigated
under the infrared camera. All fluorescent nodes are regarded as sentinel nodes
and are examined by frozen section.

Results of validation study
A validation study of thirty-eight cases was undertaken by us in 2004–2005.
The detection rate was 96.5%, and the number of sentinel nodes was 2.7 on
average. In this method, the number of sentinel nodes is greater than in other
methods, because ICG tends to drain to farther lymph nodes than radioactive
colloid, and the detection by fluorescence is more sensitive than by ordinary

Table 2–B–1. Detection rate of lymphatic vessels and nodes by inspection and fluorescence

	Lymphatic vessels		Lymph nodes	
Inspection	24/38	(63%)	15/38	(39%)
Fluorescence	38/38	(100%)	36/38	(95%)

inspection. One false-negative case was encountered. Negative predictive value was 96.0%, and the false-negative rate was 7.1%.

The sensitivity between the green color and fluorescence was compared (Table 2–B–1), with the detection of lymphatic vessels and lymph node by fluorescence obviously more sensitive than visual perception of the green color of ICG.

Superior characteristics of the ICG fluorescence method over the conventional dye method are as follows:
1. The site of skin incision can be precisely identified.
2. Tracing the lymphatic vessels into the axillary lymph nodes is facilitated by fluorescence images.
3. Lymph nodes stained by ICG can be judged with high sensitivity.

There are some criticisms about the ICG fluorescence method:
1. Too many sentinel nodes may be detected, because ICG drains faster than with radioactive colloids. Usually, we removed one to three more fluorescent nodes around the first drained nodes, and did not pursue those beyond the central group. Although the number of nodes for pathologic examination increased, we believe that this procedure effectively reduced the false-negative rate.
2. Shadowless lights over the operating table, which contain NIR light, must be switched off during the fluorescence observation. There was no problem with room light.
3. The surgical procedures are still not easy compared with the radioisotope-guided method. The main difficulty was that during detection the sentinel nodes could not be detected from the skin. The excitation or emission light was scattered out in the axillary fatty tissue. The limit of detection depth was 1 cm~2 cm.

There are two possible solutions: improvement of hardware or reduction of light scattering. The first solution is technically difficult at present. Even if the fluorescent signal becomes strong, scattered light only illuminates the whole axilla, and the location of the sentinel nodes cannot be recognized. The second solution can be achieved by shortening the distance between the skin and the lymph node using a pressing technique, as described below.

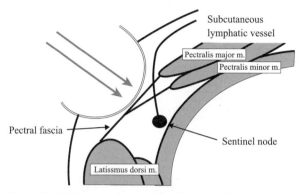

Fig. 2–B–7. Schematic drawing of axillary pressing
By reducing the depth of the lymph node through pressing, light scattering is greatly reduced. Various muscle (m) tissues are also shown.

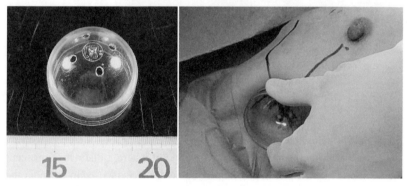

Fig. 2–B–8. Transparent hemisphere for pressing the axilla

Axillary pressing technique

Figure 2–B–7 shows a schematic drawing of the axillary pressing technique. The subcutaneous lymphatic vessels just under the skin are easily detectable. However, the excitation light attenuated by scattering cannot reach the sentinel node, and the fluorescent emission from the sentinel node is scattered out before detection. By pressing the axillary skin against the chest wall, the sentinel node is close to the skin and the fluorescent signal becomes detectable.

We used a small transparent plastic bowl for this purpose. The four small holes on the top of the bowl were for skin marking (Figure 2–B–8).

A couple of minutes after ICG injection, subcutaneous lymphatic drainage can be detected as fluorescence streams from the skin. The fluorescent signal disappears usually beyond the lateral edge of the pectralis major muscle, with

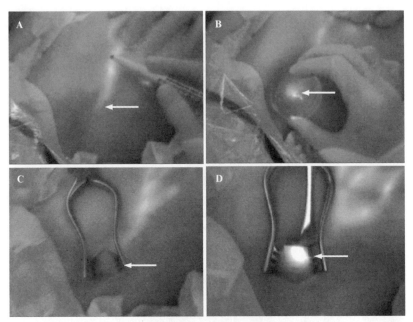

Fig. 2–B–9. Axillary pressing technique with fluorescence images

A: Subcutaneous lymphatic drainage is marked. B: Sentinel node can be detected from the skin by pressing the axilla. C: After skin incision, obscure fluorescent signal from the sentinel node can be recognized. D: After direct dissection towards the axilla, the sentinel node can be detected.

no signal in the axilla. The axillary skin is pressed against the chest wall by the transparent hemisphere to search for a point where a distinct fluorescent signal appears by the pressing. The sentinel nodes are supposed to be under the pressure-induced fluorescent point. After skin incision is made, a weak and ill-defined fluorescent signal can be observed. While dissecting the underlying fascias, the fluorescent signal becomes intense and well localized, and finally, the shining sentinel node can be pulled out of the axillary space with surrounding fatty tissue (Figure 2–B–9).

The axillary pressing technique is a convenient and effective way to improve the results. The technique necessitates caution, as it is important not to miss the sentinel nodes, and to ensure that the subcutaneous lymphatic drainage enters the dissection area.

Axillary Node Assessment and Treatment After Neoadjuvant Chemotherapy in Patients with Locally Advanced Breast Cancer

Eun Sook Lee

Summary

The proper use and optimal timing of sentinel lymph node biopsy (SLNB) within a neoadjuvant chemotherapy (NAC) setting are still being debated. SLNB is clinically useful for large tumors without neoadjuvant chemotherapy (NAC), with lymphatic mapping success rates that are very similar to those seen in patients with smaller tumors. But several key treatment disadvantages continue to hamper SLNB's wider adoption.

Introduction: Controversy about Applicability

NAC has become the standard treatment for locally advanced breast cancer, mainly to achieve breast-conserving surgery and to test in vivo chemosensitivity. It is known that NAC improves breast conservation in 20%–30% of patients after the downsizing of large tumors. After NAC, a complete remission of nodal metastasis is achieved in 20%–40% of pretreatment nodal involvement. Until recently, the removal of residual breast cancer was well accepted, but sparing axillary dissection in patients whose sentinel node becomes negative after NAC is still controversial.

The status of the axillary lymph node (ALN) is one of the most significant prognostic indicators of breast cancer. Conventional axillary lymph node dissection (ALND), however, can produce complications, such as lymphedema, nerve injury, numbness, and pain, so SLNB has been accredited as a reliable method for precisely assessing the axillary status of patients with breast cancer. With SLNB, patients with node-negative breast cancer may never need to undergo ALND. Many studies have shown SLNB to be highly predictive with a false-negative rate (FNR) of less than 5% in experienced hands. Although

45

Table 2–C–1. Assessment tools for axillary node metastasis

Assessment tools	Sensitivity	Specificity
Palpable node	Very low	High
Sono guide tissue sampling and pathologic exam	35%–95%	65%–100%
CT or MRI	70%–95%	75%–97%
FDG-PET or PET-CT	54%–67%	79%–81%
Sentinel lymph node biopsy before chemotherapy	Over 95%	Over 95%
Sentinel lymph node biopsy after chemotherapy	67%–100%	67%–100%
Meta-analysis	90%	92%

SLNB is used widely in breast cancer, its applicability in the context of NAC is controversial. Reports on the efficacy of SLNB after preoperative chemotherapy have been inconsistent, leading to suggestions that chemotherapy may interfere with the anatomy or physiology of the lymphatics and adversely affect SLNB accuracy.

NAC chemotherapy is being used more frequently in patients with stage II or stage III breast cancer, and this approach has raised a number of questions within the specialties of diagnostic imaging, surgical oncology, and radiation oncology. Here, we focus on the axillary assessment and management regarding NAC.

Assessment Tools for Axillary Node Metastasis

As shown in Table 2–C–1, there are several methods to evaluate axillary status. Ultrasonographic evaluation of axillary status without fine needle aspiration biopsy or core needle biopsy is not conclusive for node metastasis. Most studies are retrospective analyses of consecutive breast cancer series based on abnormal sonographic criteria. In the few prospective analyses, the patient numbers are too small to find meaningful evidence. These studies appropriately concluded that the indiscriminate use of sonographic examination of the axilla in all breast cancer patients, alone or in combination with fine needle aspiration or core biopsies, was not practical or cost effective. The use of chest computed tomography (CT) or breast magnetic resonance imaging (MRI) has increased in the past ten years; however, the purpose of these studies is usually not for axillary staging. MRI provides enhanced cancer detection in the cancer-affected breast and in the contralateral breast. The potential benefit of MRI includes more accurate definition of the extent of the known cancer, detection of additional foci of cancer in the affected breast, and detection of otherwise occult cancer in the contralateral breast.

There also is evidence that MRI leads to more extensive surgery without additional benefit. The routine use of bilateral MRI in women with newly diagnosed breast cancer remains controversial.

Many studies demonstrate that fluoro deoxy glucose (FDG)-positron emission tomography (PET) can find axillary node metastases in patients with breast carcinoma in a variable number and percentage of cases, with good results by some authors and less satisfactory ones by others. A good positive predictive PET value in the case of a maximal standardized uptake value index superior or equal to 1.8 was reported by Wahl et al., with a very low sensitivity. Much progress in imaging techniques has stimulated further research into refining the use of SLNB.

Though SLNB is well tolerated by patients, it still requires an invasive excision accompanied by lymphoscintigraphy and considerable pathologic examination.

In the near future, the use of FDG-PET followed by advanced techniques in ultrasound examination of axillary nodes to assist fine needle biopsy might replace SLNB in a selected group of patients, but this approach requires further investigation.

Sentinel Lymph Node Biopsy (SLNB) before Neoadjuvant Chemotherapy

ALND is usually performed after NAC. NAC may have an adverse effect on the lymph drainage pattern of the breast. Whether to perform SLNB before or after NAC is still a matter of debate. Many studies, including meta-analysis by Xing and colleagues, show that SLNB after NAC could be appropriate in terms of accuracy and FNR. However, it remains questionable, because of the wide range of FNR sensitivities, especially in cases of positive axillary metastasis.

In addition, no surgeons recommend omitting ALND when SLNB is negative after NAC, except in a clinical trial. Not all patients with large cancer of the breast have metastasis. SLNB before chemotherapy has the several advantages. The most significant advantage of performing the procedure before chemotherapy is that it assures an accurate assessment of whether the disease involves lymph nodes at the time of initial treatment. Another reason to consider SLNB before chemotherapy is that information gained about the initial extent of axillary nodes may have implications for radiation and chemotherapy decisions, especially for radiation fields and post-mastectomy radiation. However, SLNB may ultimately need two operations, and there is not strong support for the procedure (Table 2–C–2). Also, the most effective treatment for patients who have a positive SLN, but who turn out to be clinically negative

Table 2‒C‒2. Sentinel lymph node biopsy before neoadjuvant chemotherapy

Study	No. of cases	IR	FNR	AXLD	
				SNB (−)	SNB (+)
Menard, 2009	31	100%	-	No	Yes
Schrenk, 2008	45	100%	0%	Yes	Yes
Kandice, 2008	44	97.7%	-	No	Yes
Moshe, 2008	58	97%	0%	Yes	Yes
	28	100%	-	No	Yes
Grube, 2008	55	100%	0%	Yes	Yes
van Rijk, 2006	25	100%	0%	Yes	Yes
Jones, 2005	52	100%	-	No	Yes
Schrenk, 2003	21	100%	0%	Yes	Yes

after NAC, remains unclear.

SLNB after Chemotherapy

Previous studies showed that SLNB after NAC have a wide variability in identification rates (IRs) and FNRs. To date, the largest series consists of patients enrolled in the National Surgical Adjuvant Breast and Bowel Project (NSABP) B-27, in which 428 patients received NAC followed by SLNB and completion dissection. In this multicenter trial, the IR was 85%, with an FNR of 11%. These results are similar to those of the NSABP B-32 trial, in which sentinel lymph node surgery was performed before any systemic treatment. Furthermore, in meta-analysis by Xing and colleagues of SLNB after preoperative chemotherapy in patients with breast cancer, SLNB was shown to be a reliable tool for assessing the residual metastasis of axillary lymph node.

However, this technique also shows variability, as IR and FNR sensitivities were shown to range 72%‒100% and 67%‒100%, respectively (Table 2‒C‒3). Xing and colleagues reported a pooled IR of 90% and an FNR of 12%, similar to the reported rates for sentinel node biopsy before systemic therapy. It is important to remember that the clinical significance of any FNR is much greater for patients with NAC compared with that of patients with early stage breast cancer. This is because most of the early cancer patients would undergo adjuvant chemotherapy not only by axillary status but also by many other clinicopathologic parameters. Many studies reported that about 25%‒40% of patients with positive axillary lymph node status on initial examination were converted to negative status after preoperative chemotherapy. If SLNB accurately predicts axillary metastasis after chemotherapy, patients who

Table 2–C–3. Individual study characteristics and performance

Author	Year	Journal	Origin	Mean Age	Number of Patients	NPV	SIR	FNR
Aihara et al	2004	*Journal of Surgical Oncology*	Japan	62 endo, 47 chemo	16 endo, 20 chemo	0.929	0.85	0.08
Balch et al	2003	*Annals of Surgical Oncology*	USA	51	32	0.923	0.97	0.05
Brady et al	2002	*The Breast Journal*	USA	44	14	1	0.93	0.00
Cohen et al	2000	*The American Journal of Surgical Pathology*	USA	45*	38	0.813	0.82	0.20
Fernandez et al	2000	*Nuclear Medicine Communications*	Spain	55	36	0.778	0.94	0.25
Haid et al	2001	*Cancer*	Austria	53	33	1	0.88	0.00
Jones et al	2005	*American Journal of Surgery*	USA	N/A	36	0.846	0.81	0.16
Khan et al	2005	*Annals of Surgical Oncology*	USA	40*	33	0.857	0.96	0.05
Kinoshita et al	2007	*Breast Cancer*	Japan	50.2	104	0.938	0.94	0.19
Lang et al	2004	*Journal of the American College of Surgery*	USA	51*	53	0.967	0.94	0.04
Lee et al	2007	*Breast Cancer Results Treatment*	Korea	46.1	219	0.868	0.78	0.16
Mahmounas et al	2005	*Journal of Clinical Oncology*	USA	N/A	428	0.931	0.80	0.11
Miller et al	2002	*Annals of Surgical Oncology*	USA	N/A	35	1	0.86	0.00
Nason et al	2000	*Cancer*	USA	N/A	82	0.571	0.80	0.33
Patel et al	2004	*The American Surgeon*	USA	N/A	42	1	0.95	0.00
Piato et al	2002	*European Journal of Surgical Oncology*	Brazil	N/A	42	0.885	0.98	0.17
Reitsamer et al	2003	*Journal of Surgical Oncology*	Austria	31–74	41	0.917	0.63	0.07
Schwartz et al	2003	*The Breast Journal*	USA	50	21	0.909	1.00	0.09
Shimazu et al	2004	*Cancer*	Japan	51.3	47	0.733	0.94	0.12
Stearns et al	2002	*Annals of Surgical Oncology*	USA	46	34	0.875	0.85	0.06
Tafra et al	2001	*American Journal of Surgery*	USA	N/A	29	1	0.93	0.00
Tanaka et al	2006	*Oncology Reports*	Japan	N/A	70	0.958	0.90	0.03
Tausch et al	2006	*Annals of Surgical Oncology*	Austria	50*	167	0.931	0.84	0.06
Yu et al	2006	*Annals of Surgical Oncology*	Taiwan	42.6	127	0.912	0.91	0.08

would otherwise normally require an axillary dissection might be treated with sentinel node biopsy alone, thus decreasing the axillary dissection-related surgical morbidity. SLNB after chemotherapy also has several advantages and disadvantages (Table 2–C–4).

Summary of Korean National Cancer Center Study

At the National Cancer Center, we carried out a study of Korean patients to prove that SLNB produces a low IR and to determine the feasibility of replacing ALND in axillary lymph node-positive patients after chemotherapy with SLNB.

From October 2001 to July 2005, 875 consecutive patients with primary operable breast cancer underwent sentinel node biopsy and axillary dissection. Among them, 238 received NAC (Figure 2–C–1). We compared the IR, FNR, negative predictive value (NPV), and accuracy of SLNB in clinically node-positive patients with or without NAC.

The results are shown in Table 2–C–5. Our study showed a lower SLNB

Table 2–C–4. Advantages of performing sentinel lymph node surgery before and after chemotherapy

Timing of Sentinel Lymph Node Surgery	Advantage
Before chemotherapy	Provides accurate assessment of initial axillarylymph node involvement May affect decisions concerning whether to use radiation after mastectomy or whether to use radiation to treat the regional lymphatics May affect systemic treatment decisions, if a particular systemic regimen would only be used for patients with positive lymph nodes (an uncommon situation in typical candidates for preoperative chemotherapy) False-negative rates are more clearly established for patients treated with sentinel lymph node surgery before chemotherapy
After chemotherapy	Eliminates the need for doing two surgical procedures More comprehensive assessment of the ability of the preoperative chemotherapy to achieve a pathologic complete response Takes advantage of the down-staging effect of preoperative chemotherapy and as a result may decrease the number of patients that require an axillary lymph node dissection Does not delay administration of preoperative chemotherapy

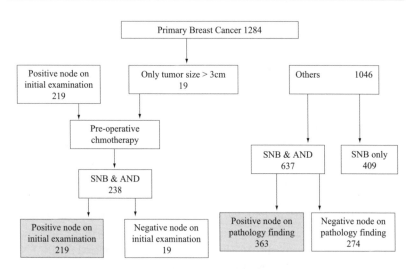

Breast Cancer Res Treat (2007) 102: 283–288

Fig. 2–C–1. Study Overview

Table 2–C–5. Results of sentinel lymph node biopsy in patients with positive lymph nodes

	%(Fraction) with pre-operative CTx (n=219)	%(Fraction) with post-operative CTx (n=363)	P-value
Identification rate	77.6 (170/219)	97.0 (352/363)	< 0.001
FNR	5.6 (7/124)	7.4 (26/352)	0.681
NPV[a]	86.8 (46/53)	0.0 (0/26)	0.181
Accuracy	95.9 (163/170)	92.6 (326/352)	

a NPV could not be calculated because the lymph nodes were all positive in patients in the non-pre-operative chemotherapy group CTx, Chemotherapy. FNR, False negative rate. NPV, Negative NAC value.

IR than for other studies. The reason may have been that the axillary node status of patients enrolled in our study was clinically or pathologically positive. We could not explain completely why a lower success rate is associated with preoperative chemotherapy, but it may be that a treatment-induced tumor necrosis alters or disrupts lymphatic drainage and leads to unsuccessful sentinel node mapping. Alternatively, if mapping is successful, it may not accurately reflect the lymphatic drainage of the original tumor. Age also influenced the IR in our study. In our study, however, the FNR did not differ significantly between the patients who had preoperative chemotherapy (5.6%) and those who did not (7.4%) (p = 0.681). Also, a current meta-analysis by Xing and colleagues shows that the FNR is accurate for early breast cancer.

Conclusion

To assess axillary nodal metastasis, the ultimate goal is to use noninvasive methods such as FDG-PET and/or ultrasonography, with or without fine needle aspiration. In future, it may be possible to adopt a wait-and-see approach, instead of SLNB or axillary dissection, especially in patients with a small primary carcinoma. Two conditions are necessary to achieve this approach. One is that the randomized trial in progress will show no differences in outcome between the axillary dissection and the wait-and-see policy. The other is that the role of axillary node mapping will lose its importance in the staging of breast cancer, and will be replaced by more sophisticated biological and biomolecular markers. So far, however, noninvasive axillary staging techniques are inaccurate and do not provide a high-enough sensitivity to be used as viable tools.

The proper use and optimal timing of sentinel node biopsy in the setting of NAC still remains controversial. The validity of SLNB has been shown for large tumors without NAC, and lymphatic mapping success rates are

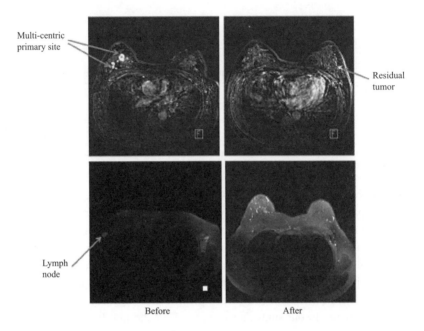

Multi-centric primary site

Residual tumor

Lymph node

Before   After

Fig. 2–C–2. MRI of locally advanced breast cancer before and after neo-adjuvant chemotherapy

very similar to those seen in patients with smaller tumors. Although SLNB performed on large tumors before NAC treatment is as accurate as SLNB performed on early breast cancer, several disadvantages including two surgical procedures, delayed administration of chemotherapeutic agent, and no additional information on axillary status after NAC, have hampered its wider adoption. Whether sentinel node biopsy after NAC is accurate in patients who present with clinically involved axillary nodes before NAC, but who convert afterward to clinically node-negative (Figure 2–C–2), remains controversial, and additional prospective data are needed before this approach can be considered as a standard of care (Figure 2–C–3).

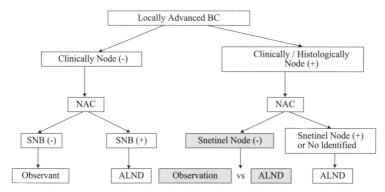

Fig. 2–C–3. Proposed algorithm of sentinel lymph node biopsy in patients with locally advanced breast cancer

Current Status of Sentinel Lymph Node Biopsy for Breast Cancer in Japan

Seigo Nakamura

Summary

An examination of the performance of several medical tracers used in sentinel lymph node biopsy (SLNB) for a large cohort of Japanese patients has confirmed overseas studies regarding the efficacy and safety of these drugs, which has implications for their future approval by health insurance authorities in Japan.

Introduction: Role of Medical Tracers in Sentinel Lymph Node Biopsy

Axillary lymph node dissection retains its important role as a prognostic factor to indicate adjuvant systemic therapy.[1] The removal of axillary nodes also may contribute to better local control of the axillae, although data of clinical trials show no survival benefit[2] (Figure 2–D–1). Until a decade ago, the standard procedure of breast cancer surgery required level I and II axillary lymph node dissection (ALND). However, the procedure sometimes risked disturbance of arm elevation or permanent lymphedema. In the early 1990s it was hypothesized that blue dye or colloidal material injected into the surroundings of the breast cancer would drain into the first node (sentinel lymph node) and remain for a while.[3,4] The agents that are widely used as a tracer are a radiolabeled sulfur colloid or in combination with a blue dye —— isosulfan blue is used in United States of America (USA), and indigo carmine or indocyanine green (ICG) in Japan. These agents are detected by a hand-held gamma probe or by visual identification of blue-stained nodes. Early confirmatory studies proved that sentinel lymph node biopsy (SLNB) was agreeably accurate, with about a 5% false-positive result through subsequent ALND.[5,6] Therefore,

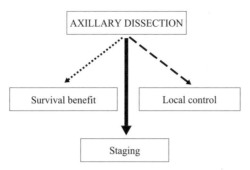

Fig. 2–D–1. The impact of axillary dissection

negative sentinel lymph node biopsy (SLNB) could be considered to avoid unnecessary ALND.

Worldwide, the accuracy and safety of SLNB is still being investigated under clinical trials. In 1999, two National Cancer Institute (NCI)-sponsored trials —— the National Surgical Adjuvant Breast and Bowel Project (NSABP) B-32 and the American College of Surgeons Oncology Group (ACOSOG) Z-0010 —— started to clarify the accuracy of SLNB and to determine whether omission of ALND in patients with a negative SLNB would affect survival or not. Increasingly, however, SLNB is being used in clinical practice.[7] This is because the technique of SLNB may allow determination of lymph node status without the use of ALND.[8–10] Moreover, SLNB is an attractive alternative to ALND, because the risks of short-term morbidity and lymphedema are markedly lower with the former technique.[11–14]

However, the SLNB procedure in Japan, which commonly uses medical tracers such as Tc-99m (a metastable nuclear isomer of technetium-99) tin colloid, Tc-99m stannous phytate, ICG, and indigo carmine, effectively is not covered under the Japanese government's health insurance schedule (Figure 2–D–2). Our study, therefore, examined the performance (efficacy and safety) surrounding the various SLNB medical tracers used in advanced medical technologies. Analysis of a large cohort of Japanese patients confirmed overseas studies on the identification rate (IR) and safety of SLNB using these drugs for their future approval by health insurance in Japan.

Method: Adverse Event and Identification Rate Comparison with Overseas Studies

The primary endpoint of this study is the safety of the two Tc-99m radioisotopic tracers, and the two tracer dyes of ICG and indigo carmine, which are used

Tc-99 m thin colloid
Tc-99 m stannous phytate

Indocyanine green(ICG)
Indigocarmine

· Frequently used in Japan

· Approved by MHLW for another purpose

Fig. 2–D–2. Radioisotope (RI) and dye for sentinel lymph node biopsy (SLNB) in Japan

commonly as tracers in Japan. The secondary endpoint is that the IRs are not inferior to those of major clinical studies previously reported in other countries.

Data about SLNB treatments in Japan were collected from patients in the 0 to IIIa stages of breast cancer. These patients were being treated at sixty-four institutions that were allowed to perform SLNB as an advanced technology. Each treatment with radioisotope (RI) or dye or in combination was evaluated separately. Each institution registered the demographic data of patients before their SLNB and reported the results of each treatment, including safety issues, within seven days of registration. If a grade 3 or grade 4 adverse event occurred, a report was sent to the data center within seventy-two hours of the finding. In previous studies, a grade 3 or grade 4 adverse event such as anaphylaxis, relating to the blue dye, was 0.5%–1.1%. Therefore, at least 1,596 cases in Japan were necessary to test the relative safety of commonly used SLNB drugs, effectively corresponding to the same number of SLNB patients trialed in the USA for blue dye treatment (event rate $<1\%$, α error 5%, β error 20%, and statistical power 80%). The minimum IR requirement was 93%, determined by other major clinical studies in the world (Figure 2–D–3). Therefore, each treatment method needed at least 292 cases (event rate 93%, α error 5%, β error 20%, and statistical power 80%)

Results: Identification Rate in Japanese Study Similar to Overseas Studies

Exactly 3,408 cases were registered for SLNB from sixty-four institutions in Japan between March 2008 and November 2008. Thirty-one cases were excluded because of cancellation or postponement of surgery. Bilateral SLNB

Medscape® www.medscape.com					
Study and reference	Study size (number of patients)	Technique	SLNidentification (%)	Accuracy (%)	False-negative rate (%)
Giuliano et al. (1996)	174	Dye	65	96	12
Veronesl et al. (1999)	376	Radioactive colloid	99	96	7
Krag et al. (1998)	443	Radioactive colloid	93	97	11
Quan et al. (2002)	152	Radioactive colloid	93	100	0
Tafra et al. (2001)	535	Both	87	96	13
Bergkvist et al. (2001)	498	Both	90	N/A	11
McMasters et al. (2001)	2,206	Both	93	97	8

Both use of radicieotope and vital blue dye labeling, SLN sentinellymphnode.
Source: *Nat Clin Pract Oncol* © 2005 Nature Publishing Group

Average FNR=8.8%. (ref. www,nci.gov)

Fig. 2–D–3. Sentinel lymph node dissection feasibility comparisons with axillary lymph node dissection (ALND)

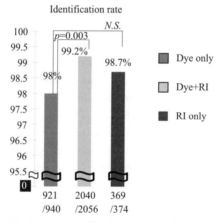

Fig. 2–D–4. Identification rate with radioisotope and dye tracer methods

was performed in fifty-three cases; therefore, safety analysis was conducted on 3,324 cases, and IR was calculated on 3,377 cases. The IR from using both RI and the dye was 99.2 % compared with 98.7% from the single RI method and 98.0% from the single dye method (Figure 2–D–4). The number of resected nodes was slightly higher in the dye-only group than in the combination group (Figure 2–D–5). There were two cases of a grade 1 (0.06%) adverse event among the single dye method and no cases of a grade 3 or grade 4 adverse event.

	Dye only	Dye+RI	RI only
Average	2.43 ± 1.54	1.90 ± 1.17	1.74 ± 1.00
Distribution	1~12	1~8	1~7

$$p=0.001$$
$$p=0.032$$
$$p<0.001$$

Fig. 2–D–5. Dissected number of sentinel nodes
by tracer methods

Discussion: Safety and Efficacy Likely in Tracer Drugs

This study was designed to clarify the safety and efficacy of SLNB with the four tracer drugs commonly used in Japan (Tc-99m tin colloid, Tc-99m stannous phytate, ICG, and indigo carmine). Our results show that SLNB using these four drugs was done safely, and that IR was higher than that of previous overseas studies.

There are however several controversies relating to SLNB. For example, Carolien van Deurzen and co-workers conducted a systematic review of the accuracy of SLNB after neoadjuvant chemotherapy in breast cancer patients.[15] They reported that twenty-seven studies out of 574 were included in this review, with a total study population of 2,148 patients. Pooled, the sentinel node (SN) IR was 90.9% (at 95% confidence interval (CI), IR = 88.0%–93.1%) and the false-negative rate was 10.5% (at 95% CI, IR = 8.1%–13.6%). Negative predictive value and accuracy after neoadjuvant chemotherapy (NAC) were 89.0% (at 95% CI, IR = 85.1%–92.1%) and 94.4% (at 95% CI, IR = 92.6%–95.8%), respectively. The reported SN success rates were heterogeneous, and several variables were reported to be associated with decreased SN accuracy, that is, initially positive clinical nodal status. Therefore, there was insufficient evidence to recommend SLNB as a standard procedure.

Further subgroup analysis using our database is required to identify whether SLNB should be done before or after chemotherapy. Figure 2–D–6 shows our protocol to clarify the significance or positioning of SLNB after neoadjuvant chemotherapy.

Another debatable issue concerns immunohistochemical (IHC) analysis of SNs, because the clinical significance of micrometastases is unknown: Should we be doing IHC on all SNs? If IHC detects micrometastasis in an SN, is lymph node dissection necessary at all? The American Society of Clinical Oncology

SNB trial in neoadjuvant setting

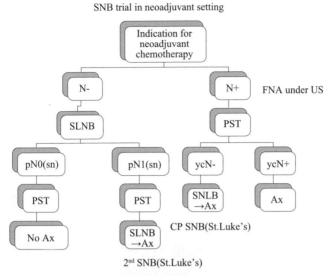

Fig. 2–D–6. Sentinel lymph node biopsy (SLNB) trial in neoadjuvant setting at St. Luke's International Hospital

(ASCO) guideline notes that the use of IHC analysis and consequential action should be decided following discussion among individual surgeons, oncologists, and pathologists, based on the best course for an individual patient.[16] Expert panels from the College of American Pathologists and the National Comprehensive Cancer Network have recommended against the routine use of IHC. Kimberly Van Zee of the Memorial Sloan-Kettering Cancer Center suggests focusing on decision making when the SN is positive. Van Zee and her co-workers developed a nomogram to help predict a patient's risk for additional disease in the axillary lymph nodes. The nomogram accounts for several factors, including tumor size, tumor type, lymphovascular invasion, multifocality, estrogen receptor status, the number of positive and negative sentinel lymph nodes, and the method of detecting sentinel lymph node metastases (that is, by frozen section analysis, routine analysis, or enhanced pathologic analysis). The recommended treatment of a woman with a positive SN includes complete axillary lymph node dissection. If a patient has an SN that is positive for micrometastatic disease, and the patient and physician are considering avoidance of dissection, a nomogram process can help in weighing the risks and benefits of dissection. The nomogram work of Van Zee can be accessed on the Memorial Sloan-Kettering Cancer Center website (www.mskcc. org) (Figure 2–D–7).

The International Breast Cancer Study Group (IBCSG) has conducted

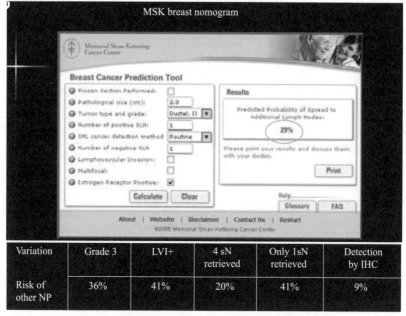

MSK breast nomogram

Variation	Grade 3	LVI+	4 sN retrieved	Only 1sN retrieved	Detection by IHC
Risk of other NP	36%	41%	20%	41%	9%

Fig. 2–D–7. Memorial Slow Kellering's (MSK) breast sentinel lymph node biopsy (SLNB) nomogram

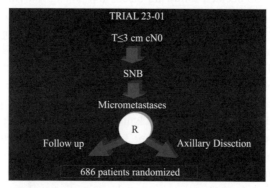

Fig. 2–D–8. International breast cancer study group (IBCSG) Trial 23–01

randomized clinical trials on micrometastases cases (Figure 2–D–8). Similarly, our large-scale data will be reviewed and analyzed for such cases.

Controversy of Axillary Diagnosis and Treatment

Tomoharu Sugie

Summary

Sentinel lymph node biopsy (SLNB) is now standard surgery to assess the stage of axillary lymph nodes. The combined method of radiotherapy and blue dye is common worldwide, but an innovative indocyanine green (ICG) fluorescence technique provides a comparable result with the radioisotope (RI) method. Timing of SLNB before or after primary systemic therapy (PST) still remains controversial. An improved algorithm is required to identify the low-risk subset of nonsentinel involvement in sentinel lymph node (SLN)-positive patients

Introduction: Challenges for Sentinel Lymph Node Biopsy (SLNB) Method

The significance of axillary lymph node dissection (ALND) has been established now for breast cancer. In the Halstedian era, breast cancer was considered to be a predominantly local disease, where cancer cells spread sequentially along the fascia and the lymphatic flows.[1] The aim of surgical treatment was en bloc mastectomy, including adjacent muscles and regional lymph nodes, which were thought to be the major route for distant metastasis. In the Fisherian era, however, breast cancer was considered to be a systemic disease with micrometastases at the time of presentation.[2] In the National Surgical Adjuvant Breast and Bowel Project (NSABP) B-04, prophylactic ALND or axillary radiation for node-negative early breast cancer (that is, nearby lymph nodes not containing cancer) had no effect on the recurrence rate and overall survival compared with subsequent ALND at the time of nodal recurrence.[3] The role of ALND therefore changed from a therapeutic method to a staging one.

SLNB is now widely accepted as an alternative to ALND. In clinical trials, the recurrence rate and the prognosis of patients with negative SLNs where the sequential ALND was spared were similar to those of patients who underwent completion ALND.[4]

However, many controversies remain regarding the SLNB method, namely, its justification and subsequent axillary management. This article discusses the current issues facing the SLNB method, based on the results of questionnaires sent to 104 breast cancer specialists and on the panel discussions at the Kyoto Breast Cancer Consensus Conference (KBCCC) 2009 in Kyoto.

Methodologies in Sentinel Lymph Node (SLN) Detection

Tracers

The first issue identified by the conference concerns the technical aspects of SLNB, including the type of tracer, site of injection, the number of the lymph nodes removed, and the handling of the sentinel node specimen. Regarding the agent for detecting SLN, 54% of surgeons prefer to use the combined method of dye and RI. No more than 20% of surgeons use the single method of dye or RI (Figure 2–E–1). Tc-99m (a metastable nuclear isomer of technetium-99) sulphur colloids and Tc-99m albumin colloids are commonly used worldwide. These radiocolloids are trapped in the SLNs to enable detection by a gamma probe. The RI and blue dye complement each other to reduce the false-negative rate. This method does not require special training but a permitted facility to handle the RI.

The most common dyes used in Western countries are patent blue and isosulphan blue. However, as these dyes are disallowed in clinical practice in Japan, indigo carmine and indocyanine green (ICG) are used as alternatives. The advantages of using a single dye are its cost effectiveness and simplicity, but the detection rate of SLN is relatively low compared with the combined method of blue dye and RI. All of these four dyes can cause hypersensitivity (1%–2%), and a lethal anaphylactic shock is also reported. Methylene blue is another dye with a relative low risk of allergy, but it can cause skin necrosis if it is injected in the skin without dilution.[5] The ICG florescence method, which is a modification of the dye method, can navigate a surgeon to the axillary lymphatic basin along subcutaneous lymphatic vessels. SLNs are identified in the basin by visual appearance of ICG's green colour and/or by fluorescence imaging on a photodynamic eye (PDE) system.[6] This method enables orderly and sequential dissection to reduce the false-negative rate.

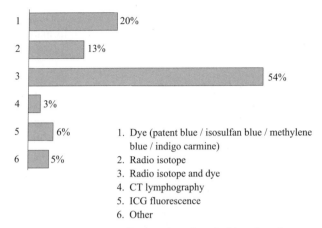

1. Dye (patent blue / isosulfan blue / methylene blue / indigo carmine)
2. Radio isotope
3. Radio isotope and dye
4. CT lymphography
5. ICG fluorescence
6. Other

Fig. 2–E–1. Agent for detection of sentinel lymph node

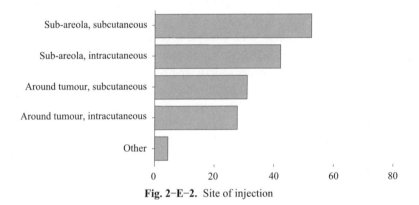

Fig. 2–E–2. Site of injection

Site of tracer injection

The second issue is where the tracer is administered. About half of the surgeons inject the tracer beneath the areola or intradermal, while about 30% of them administer the tracer around the tumor (Figure 2–E–2). Surgeons choose to inject the tracers either subareola or intradermal based on their experience. As there is a significant overlap in the subareola and peritumor lymphatic paths bound for the axillary nodes, the central injection is thought to benefit identification. As blue dye can obscure the dissection area around the lumpectomy, some surgeons avoid peritumor injection for a small tumor. Despite minor obscurities, however, the final outcome is not significantly affected by the site of injection. Drainage through the internal mammary chain could cause false-negatives for the central injection. However, all of the false-negatives were found to be in the right outer quadrant lesion, which overlap the

SLNs. As subcutaneous lymphatic channels are clearly visualized as an ICG fluorescence image, this method may provide precise information about the diffusion zone in the breast.

Adequate number of SLNs removed

The third issue is the removal of an adequate number of SLNs. There are two models of lymphatic mapping.[7] The first model is that tumor cells drain to the first single SLN before they reach the higher lymph nodes. This first SLN is definitely the 'hottest' or the most blue-stained node in the axilla. If collateral channels bypass the first SLN and reach the secondary or further lymph nodes, this may cause a false-negative study. The second model is a multiple node model. Tumor cells are trapped by a group of two or three nodes, before the cells can reach the higher lymph node. This group of lymph nodes may be defined as 'hot', blue or palpable nodes during surgery. And the collateral vessels bypass them and reach the further lymph nodes. If the actual lymphatic mapping is like the single node model, only this first node should be sufficient to predict the axillary status. In a multiple node model, however, removal of more SLNs is required to reduce the false-negative rate. In other words, it is necessary to remove these nodes orderly and sequentially to achieve a high detection rate. The number of SLNs identified in the clinical practice depends on the tracer. The average number of SLNs removed is 1.5 with RI and 2.2 with a dye alone. As the ICG fluorescence technique can identify the lymphatic basin including SLNs, the average number of SLNs identified tends to increase to 3.7 when all lymph nodes are removed from the whole basin. As M. Yi and co-workers reported, 98% or 99% of metastasis is located in the first four or five lymph nodes removed in SLNB.[8] In addition, KBCCC's panels agreed that four nodes are an adequate number of lymph nodes removed, if SLNB is unavailable. In the RI method, the decision whether more nodes should be removed is made based on the number of counts. With intraoperative injection, the counts are anywhere from 100,000 to 1,000,000. So, when one lymph node is taken out, and barely any counts are recorded in the axilla, the lymph node removed is confirmed as the first draining lymph node. When the radioactive tracer is injected sixteen to eighteen hours before surgery, the counts during operation may be only 1,000 or less. In this two-day protocol, SLNs might be removed until the tracer count drops to less than 10%

Definition of Positive SLN

The lymph node containing macrometastasis —— staged as pN1 with deposit

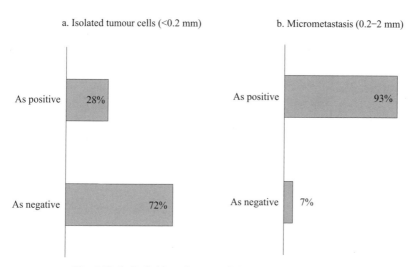

Fig. 2–E–3. Definition of metastasis in sentinel lymph node

>2 mm —— is defined as a positive. In the current American Joint Committee on Cancer (AJCC) guideline, isolated tumor cells and micrometastasis —— which are staged as pN0(i +) with deposit ≤ 0.2 mm, and pN1mi with deposit >0.2 mm to ≤ 2.0 mm —— are defined as a negative and positive, respectively. In the questionnaires, 72% of breast cancer specialists agreed that isolated metastasis is not defined as a positive, whereas 93% of them accepted that micrometastasis is a positive that requires completion ALND (Figure 2–E–3). Regarding pathologic examination, about 50% of surgeons evaluate SLNs by hematoxylin and eosin (H&E) staining only. The others, however, prefer to examine them by the combined method of H&E and immunohistochemistry (IHC). The prognostic significance of IHC has become controversial. In a recent report, adjuvant therapy was shown to improve disease-free survival in patients with isolated tumor cells or micrometastases.[9] Since patients with isolated tumor cells or micrometastases had a comparably poor five-year rate of disease-free survival, isolated tumor cells in SLNs are also a prognostic determinant.

Can Subsequent Axillary Lymph Node Dissection (ALND) Be Spared for SLN-positive Patients?

According to the conference questionnaire results, 90% of surgeons complete ALND in those patients showing a node-positive ratio of 1/1 or 1/2 for removed nodes. Even in patients with a node-positive ratio of 1/4, 81% of surgeons

a. SLNB showed metastasis as 1/1

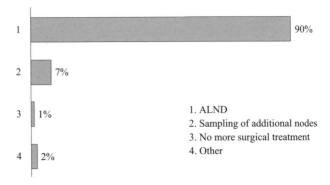

b. SLNB showed metastasis (1/2)

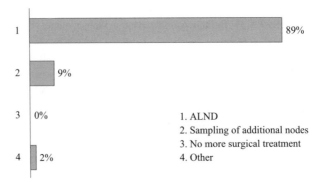

c. SLNB showed metastasis (1/4).

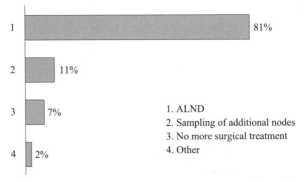

Fig. 2-E-4. What treatment do you do for patients with positive sentinel lymph node?

conduct completion ALND (Figure 2–E–4). The current consensus is that completion ALND is required for patients with involved SLNs. In our study, however, only 27% of SLN-positive patients had further nonsentinel axillary involvements (data not shown). In other word, more than two-thirds of SLN-positive patients underwent unnecessary dissection. Some nomograms are currently available to predict non-SLN involvement in patients with positive SLNs.[10,11] The predictive factors for non-SLN involvement are nuclear grade, lymphovascular invasion (LVI), multifocality, estrogen receptor status, number of negative and positive SLNs, tumor size, and method of detection. To minimize morbidity of ALND, an improved algorithm is required to identify the low-risk subset of non-SLN involvement in SLN-positive patients.

Timing of SLNB: Before or After Primary Systemic Chemotherapy?

The timing of SLNB for a patient undergoing PST still remains controversial. In the conference questionnaire (Figure 2–E–5), 67% of surgeons prefer SLNB after systemic chemotherapy. Seventy one percent of them perform SLNB in those node-negative breast cancer patients who experienced a clinical complete response (cCR) after PST, whereas 17% perform completion ALND. 70% surgeons prefer to perform completion ALND in node-positive breast cancer patients at the initial examination, despite patients experiencing a cCR after chemotherapy. SLNB before chemotherapy has several advantages, such as an accurate assessment of naive axillary status and a decision tool for choosing subsequent chemotherapy. SLNB before PST, however, does not receive any of the clinical benefits arising from a downstaging in the axillary nodes. Another disadvantage of SLNB before PST is that the surrogate marker of lymph node metastasis (probably the most important information after neoadjuvant therapy) is removed.

In conference panel discussions, the false-negative rate for SLN biosy after PST was reported to be 12%–13%. This false-negative rate is comparable to 11% at the NSABP B-27 trial[12] The timing of SLNB and PST remains controversial in patients with clinically node-positive breast cancer at presentation. SLNB after chemotherapy takes advantage of a decreasing number of completion ALND due to the nodal conversion of axillary involvement. In NSABP B-27, there was no difference in the false-negative rate of SLNB between, before, and after PST. Another study, however, reported that the false-negative rate of SLNB after chemotherapy was high (at 25%) for patients with fine needle aspiration cytology (FNAC)-proven positive nodes.[13]

a. Do you perform SLNB before PST?

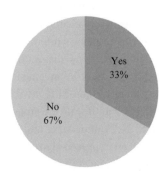

b. How do you examine the axillary status after PST?

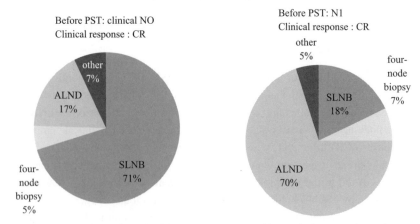

Fig. 2–E–5. Timing of sentinel lymph node (SLN) biopsy before or after primary systemic therapy (PST)

a. Do you perform SLN biopsy before PST?

b. How do you examine the axillary status after PST?

Thereafter, the 2005 American Society of Clinical Oncology (ASCO) guideline on SLNB in early-stage breast cancer concluded that insufficent data exists to recommend or to suggest appropriate timing of SLNB for patients who underwent PST.[14] A current consensus, therefore, is that SLNB before PST is acceptable and that SLNB after PST is applicable to clinical node-negative patients at presentation.

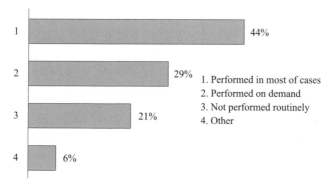

Fig. 2–E–6. Do you conduct SLN biopsy for ductal carcinoma in situ diagnosed by core needle biopsy?

Is SLNB Applicable to Ductal Carcinoma In Situ (DCIS)?

Ductal carcinoma in situ (DCIS) cells are localized in the ductal lumen, and have not crossed through the basement membrane into the surrounding tissue. Given that DCIS should seldom cause axillary involvement, the practice of evaluating nodal status in the axilla is an unnecessary routine. In the conference questionnaires, 44% of surgeons usually conduct SLNB for core needle biopsy (CNB)-proven DCIS, whereas 21% think that SLNB for DCIS can be omitted. However, 29% perform SLNB based on patient demand (Figure 2–E–6). Because the final pathologic diagnosis of 'a definite DCIS' is made on the whole tumor specimen, an eventual microinvasion may be missed by a mammotome or an CNB. This underestimation can reach 30%. P. Veronesi and co-workers reported that the rate of axillary metastasis in DCIS is about 2%, and the predictive factors for the invasive components are a high nuclear grade and a mass formation in mammograpy.[15] In questionnaires, the common predictive factors for the invasive component are tumor size, grade, mass formation, and age. The ASCO guideline recommends that SLNB for DCIS is applicable to the patients with >5 cm or larger mass, a comedonecrosis, and a scheduled total mastectomy.[14] As the morbidity of SLNB is not 0%, we need to identify high-risk DCIS patients to undergo SLNB, and to conduct a second operation when a final pathology diagnosis identifies invasive breast cancer

Future Perspectives

SLNB procedures in patients is currently accepted as a surrogate for the selection of clinical node-negative breast cancer patients, who do not need completion ALND. The high identification rate in SLNB is essential if the tailored therapy is to obtain the best clinical benefit with the lowest morbidity. To improve axillary staging and management, the following issues need to be considered.

Who should be treated: patients with DCIS, local advanced cancer for DCIS, micrometastasis, versus isolated tumor cells?
For SLNB to be applicable, patients must have early breast cancer at stages I–II with clinically negative nodes. Local advanced breast cancer with nodal conversion after chemotherapy may be subject to SLNB, but insufficient data exists to recommend it. DCIS, which seldom gives rise to metastasis, eventually results in microinvasion as high as 40%. All DCISs, of course, should not be subject to SLNB, but the prediction of a high risk of invasive cancer may help surgeons to reduce the number of unnecessary SLNB. Most surgeons carry out the subsequent completion ALND when SLNs contain micrometastasis. If isolated tumor cells have a prognostic impact comparable to that of micrometastasis, pathologic examination with H&E and IHC might become the standard method to avoid missing them.

Improving the technical aspects of SLNB
The combined method of Tc-99m colloid and blue dye is common worldwide. Single use of the dye is efficacious and cost effective, but provides a relatively lower identification rate and higher false-negative rate than the combined method. The ICG fluorescence method makes the lymphatic flows and draining SLNs visualized as a fluorescent signal, and enables orderly and sequential dissection. The adequate number of SLNs for removal remains unclear. The discussion panels at the KBCCC reported that the average number of SLNs removed increased as follows: 1.5 for the combined method of RI and dye, 2.2 for dye alone, and 3.7 for the ICG fluorescence method. Four nodes, however, are an acceptable number of lymph nodes to predict the axillary status when the SLNB method is unavailable. The number and order of SLN removal needs to be addressed in future clinical studies. The morbidity of SLN biopsy is not 0%, and axillary reverse mapping is a novel method to minimize lymphedema due to SLNB.[16]

Is SLNB better before or after preoperative systemic therapy, and which patients can be spared completion ALND?
SLNB before PST has the advantage for assessing naive axillary status, but does not account for the benefit of nodal conversion after chemotherapy. Most

surgeons (67%) prefer SLNB after PST, because the response of axillary node to chemotherapy is thought to be the most important surrogate factor to predict the responsiveness and the prognosis of breast cancer. However, the detection rate and the false-negative rate of SLNB after PST remain controversial in node-positive breast cancer at initial examination.

Can subsequent ALND be spared in SLN-positive breast cancer?

Two-thirds of SLN-negative patients receive unnecessary completion. As SLNB potentially has a therapeutic impact like completion ALND, an improved algorithm may determine subsequent treatments based on individual demands.

The site of injection

As there almost is a significant overlap of both subareola and peritumor lymphatic paths bound for the sentinel node, the subareola is widely accepted as the site for a single injection. Whether a subareola or intradermal location, the surgeon may choose either site based on his or her experience.

Chapter 3

Optimum Breast Surgery

Optimum Breast Surgery

John R. Benson

Summary

Until recently, the Fisherian concept of biological predeterminism appeared preeminent and a worthy successor to the Halstedian doctrine of centrifugal spread of cancer. However, evidence has now emerged from clinical trials, which casts doubt on the universal application of this concept to breast tumors. Prevention of local recurrence (LR) can save lives, local control does matter, and rates of LR should be minimized in the first five years. Up to one-quarter of cases of LR will be a determinant and not simply a marker of risk for distant relapse and death. Both types of LR are manifestations of the same biological processes and reflect intrinsic behavior of the tumor. This principle applies to a reduction in local relapse from both adjuvant RT and surgical modalities.

Introduction: Is Local Recurrence (LR), a Determinant or an Indicator of Distant Cancer?

The significance of ipsilateral breast tumor recurrence (IBTR) following breast-conserving surgery (BCS) remains controversial.[1,2] Of principal concern is the relationship to distant relapse and whether LR represents a determinant of distant metastases or indicates a risk for development of distant disease and a de facto poor prognosis. Should LR have a determinant role, then inadequate primary loco-regional treatment may compromise overall survival. To quote Umberto Veronesi, 'it is important to distinguish local recurrences linked to increased risk of distant spread from those due to inadequate local treatment'.[3] In the latter case, patients could develop disseminated disease as a result of failure to remove residual but viable cancer cells at the time of primary treatment. Strategies for loco-regional and systemic treatment of breast cancer have been guided by two dominant paradigms of tumor pathogenesis over the past century, but an intermediate paradigm may be emerging, which reflects the biological heterogeneity of this disease. These two paradigms (Halstedian and Fisherian) will be discussed within the context of the natural history of breast cancer and whether they can be merged into an 'intermediate' paradigm that can better inform current management of breast cancer.[4]

Halstedian Paradigm

According to the Halstedian paradigm, breast cancer is a localized disease at inception, which commences as a single focus and spreads in a centrifugal manner, encroaching upon ever more distant structures, with progressive and sequential spread along fascial planes and lymphatics.[5] Metastatic spread to distant organs by hematogenous dissemination is preceded by infiltration of lymph nodes, which provide a circumferential line of defense and initially serve as barriers but subsequently permit access of tumor cells into the circulation when nodal filtration capacity is exhausted (Figure 3–A–1). This hypothesis was based on the observation that LR was a common antecedent to death from breast cancer following initial surgical excision. The focus of LR was considered to be the cause of distant metastases, and the chances of a patient being cured were related to the extent of surgery. Thus, treatments that allowed en bloc resection of tumor and adjacent loco-regional tissues offered the best chance of 'cure' and minimized the chance of LR. Halstedian radical mastectomy resulted in a dramatic reduction in rates of LR (from 60% to 6%), with up to three-quarters of patients remaining free of loco-regional relapse at the time of death from distant disease. However, long-term survival was unaffected following radical mastectomy, and the procedure incurred significant disfigurement. Nonetheless, though Halstedian radical mastectomy failed to cure most patients of breast cancer, it provided excellent local control of the disease.

Just over forty years ago, George Crile proposed that breast cancer was a systemic disease at an early stage in its natural history.[6] This alternative hypothesis led to early forays into local tumor excision, which tampered with tradition and presaged clinical trials of conservative forms of surgery for breast cancer. These trials have confirmed that breast conservation techniques yield rates of survival comparable to those from mastectomy. Rates of local relapse are inversely related to the extent of surgical resection and irradiation, but local management appears to have little, if any, impact on survival. Trials of systemic therapies have demonstrated only modest absolute gains

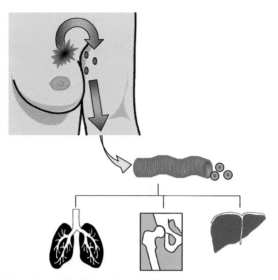

Fig. 3–A–1. The Halstedian paradigm
Sequential spread of breast cancer is from a single focus within
the breast. Lymph node involvement precedes hematogenous
dissemination, and according to this paradigm, bloodstream
spread cannot occur without obligate nodal disease.

in survival in the range 5%–10%.[7,8] Though systemic treatment has been
shown to be effective in prolonging overall survival of breast cancer patients,
other modalities of treatment, such as surgery and radiotherapy (RT), until
recently have shown no proven benefit on long-term survival. Nonetheless,
though more extensive surgery does not improve survival in patients studied
hitherto, there may be a subgroup of patients with truly localized disease. For
these patients, local therapy involving surgical excision plus (+) RT might be
curative and thus influence the natural course of the disease. Analysis of long-
term survival of patients treated for stage I disease before the widespread use
of adjuvant systemic therapy suggests that breast cancer is a loco-regional
process in up to 75%–80% of node-negative cases, who statistically may be
considered 'cured'.[4] In a series of patients from New York's Memorial Sloan-
Kettering Cancer Center with node-negative and node-positive tumors less
than or equal to 2 cm (T1N0 and T1N1), comparison of observed-to-expected
survival at a median follow-up of eighteen years revealed that 89% of patients
with node-negative tumors less than or equal to 1 cm were estimated to be
cured, with survival curves becoming parallel or congruent during the second
decade of follow-up, that is, an odds ratio (OR) of 0.89 at a 95% confidence
interval (CI) of 0.80–0.98.[9] For tumors between 1 cm–2 cm, the figure was
slightly lower at 77% (OR, 0.77; 95% CI, 0.70–0.85). Though the time taken to

attain parallelism was thirteen years for tumors less than 1 cm, and 18 years for tumors between 1 cm and 2 cm, there was no statistically significant difference between the observed and expected curves after ten years. Any divergence of the curves beyond twenty years is unlikely to detract from the conclusion that a substantial proportion of patients will not die of breast cancer, and are likely to have achieved a 'personal cure' and to succumb to nonbreast cancer-related causes.

An absolute survival benefit of 8%–10% is associated with adjuvant chemoendocrine treatment (five-year disease specific survival rate increased from 67% to 75%) and complete pathologic response rates ranging 10%–20% with neoadjuvant chemotherapy are documented. Therefore, in the absence of any form of local therapy, 90% of patients theoretically would die from breast cancer. However, following standard loco-regional treatment, 50%–60% of patients with breast cancer will survive for at least ten years, implying that either local treatments are effective or that some tumors possess low innate biological aggressiveness.

Fisherian Paradigm

Bernard Fisher formulated an alternative hypothesis in biological predeterminism, which challenged the existing paradigm based on the concept of progressive centrifugal spread according to anatomical, mechanical, and temporal criteria. The fundamental tenets of this alternative paradigm are embodied in the following two statements pertaining to the clinical behavior and pathobiology of breast cancer:[10,11]

> As far as survival is concerned there is no difference between local excision, local excision plus radiotherapy and modified radical mastectomy; there is however a progressive decrease in local recurrence with the more aggressive treatments. Local recurrence is associated with worse survival, but survival is the same with the various types of treatment; local recurrence is not the cause of, but simply an indicator of poor prognosis.

Clinical trials conducted by Fisher and others demonstrated that mastectomy and BCS were equivalent in terms of survival, but it is the significance attributed to LR that is perhaps of greater interest and has until now been underestimated. An update of the largest breast conservation trial (National Surgical Adjuvant Breast and Bowel Project, or NSABP, B-06) with twenty-year follow-up confirms that post-operative irradiation improves LR-free

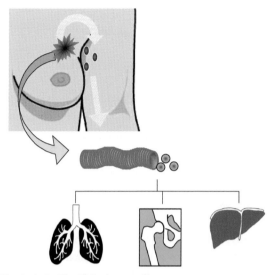

Fig. 3–A–2. The Fisherian paradigm
Spread of tumor cells into the bloodstream occurs early in tumorigenesis and precedes lymph node infiltration. The lymphatic and hematogenous systems are not independent routes of dissemination.

survival and, in particular, rates of early LR.[12] Of note, distant disease-free and overall survival are similar in the three arms of the trial, namely, wide local excision (WLE), WLE and RT, and modified radical mastectomy (MRM). The results suggest that residual cancer cells are a determinant of local failure but not of distant disease.

According to the Fisherian paradigm, breast cancer is considered to be a predominantly systemic disease at the outset, with cancer cells entering the bloodstream at an early stage of tumor development via the leaky vessels of the neovasculature and lymphatico-venous communications. Initially circulating cells may be destroyed by the immune system and fail to establish viable foci of micrometastases (Figure 3–A–2). A corollary of Fisher's conclusions is that current forms of treatment have modest effects on reduction of mortality from breast cancer. Though a primary tumor can be excised surgically or may regress completely with chemotherapy and/or RT, it is the presence of micrometastases at the time of presentation that will determine a patient's clinical fate. LR is viewed as an indicator of poor prognosis and reflects a host-tumor relationship, which favors development of distant disease or activation of processes, leading to 'kick start' of micrometastases.[13] The biological potential of residual tumor cells within the breast is resonant with this more aggressive phenotype. Distant disease and mortality are governed by innate pathobiological features of the disease and not by the extent of loco-regional treatments.

Factors Determining Local Recurrence (LR)

A proportion of relapses within the ipsilateral breast following BCS represents new primary tumors and not cases of true recurrence. These are biologically unrelated to the original tumor and have independent prognostic significance. Two factors emerge as principal determinants of true LR within the ipsilateral breast: first, margin status; and second, the presence or absence of an extensive intraduct component (EIC).[14,15] The presence or absence of an EIC is correlated with margin status and indeed EIC is probably a predictor for positive margins. It predicts for residual disease at re-excision and reflects a greater tumor burden locally. Other factors have been implicated in determining risk of local relapse, but correlations generally are much weaker than for margin status and EIC. Among these, lymphatic invasion, young age (35 years) and absence of chemohormonal therapy have been shown to be primary predictors for increased risk of LR.[16] Consistent associations have been found for larger tumor size (>2 cm) and higher histologic grade, but not for tumor subtype or nodal status. These findings are consistent with the notion that LR develops from regrowth of residual cancer cells in peritumoral tissue. Increased rates of LR associated with positive margins and EIC suggest that incomplete removal of tumor may contribute to LR. Rates of LR are more than three times greater for tumorectomy (where about 1 cm of surrounding normal tissue is removed) compared with quadrantectomy, in which a larger volume of tissue is excised (typically 2 cm–3 cm). Furthermore true recurrences occur within the index quadrant and are of the same histologic type and grade as the primary tumor. In the NSABP B-06 trial, the annual LR rate was 8.5% in the first three years of follow-up for patients undergoing WLE only, compared with a constant rate of 1.4% for patients receiving adjuvant RT.[12]

Significance of LR

The surgical dogma that mandates a finite degree of surgical excision in order to minimize LR may be misguided: if LR does not affect survival, why strive to prevent LR and risk overtreating patients? In the B-06 trial, 39.2% of patients undergoing only WLE had developed LR at 20 years follow-up compared with only 14.3% for those receiving RT post-lumpectomy. Despite great variation in the incidence of IBTR, this does not translate into survival differences, and

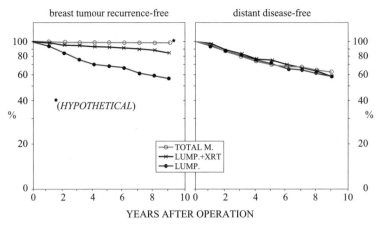

Fig. 3–A–3. Relationship of ipsilateral breast tumor recurrence (IBTR) to distant disease-free survival (DDFS)

Despite variation in rates of IBTR, overall rates of survival are equivalent irrespective of the extent of loco-regional treatment (wide excision only, wide excision and radiotherapy, or mastectomy).

Fisher concluded that no causal relationship exists between IBTR and distant disease (Figure 3–A–3). He subsequently examined differences in distant disease-free survival (DDFS) between patients with and without IBTR using a Cox regression model based on the fixed covariates of age, nodal status, tumor size, and grade, together with the time-varying covariate of IBTR. IBTR was found to be the strongest predictor of distant disease and was considered to be a marker for increased risk, but not a cause of distant metastases (3.41-fold increased risk; 95% CI, 2.70–4.30).[17] Early LR was associated with a shorter distant disease-free interval, and IBTR was better correlated with distant disease than tumor size, which has been reported to be highly predictive of the development of distant metastases. IBTR is an independent predictor of distant disease and a marker of risk, but not an instigator of distant metastases. Though loco-regional treatment in the form of surgery or RT may prevent or reduce chance of expression of the marker, such therapy does not alter the intrinsic risk of developing distant disease. Fisherian precepts would dictate that breast cancer be managed by simple surgical excision of the primary lesion in conjunction with systemic therapy. Though rates of LR would be greater, overall survival would be unaffected. Moreover, such a strategy is less likely to eliminate a marker of risk for the development of distant disease, and IBTR under these circumstances would indicate the need for systemic therapy to maximize survival.

Bruce Haffty and colleagues examined the prognostic significance of IBTR among a group of almost 1,000 patients with invasive breast cancer treated with BCS and RT.[18] Overall rates of distant metastasis (50%) were higher in patients with IBTR than those without local breast relapse at 17% (p<0.01). In particular, early IBTR was a significant predictor for distant metastases. However, the authors were unable to conclude whether IBTR was a marker of risk or a determinant of distant disease. Similar conclusions were reached more recently by a Japanese group evaluating outcomes in 1,901 patients who underwent BCS (with or without irradiation) for invasive tumors measuring less than or equal to 3 cm.[19] They also used a Cox proportional hazards model to estimate the risk of distant metastases following IBTR. Though IBTR strongly correlated with subsequent development of distant metastases (hazard rate, 3.93; p<0.0001), it was unclear whether IBTR was an indicator or a cause of distant disease relapse.

Can Loco-Regional Recurrence Influence Survival?

There is limited evidence that not all cases of breast cancer are systemic at the outset and that a subgroup of patients with early breast cancer exists for whom micrometastatic spread has not occurred before clinical (or mammographic) detection. Two randomized studies of post-mastectomy RT have shown a survival benefit of about 10%) in a subgroup of premenopausal node-positive patients receiving chemotherapy, suggesting that persistence of local or regional disease can lead to distant metastases and impaired survival.[20,21] Vincent Vinh-Hung and colleagues performed a meta-analysis of fourteen randomized trials of breast-conserving therapy (BCT) and showed that omission of RT after WLE was associated with a relative risk of LR of 3.0. This translated into a marginal increase in mortality (relative risk, or RR, 1.086; 95% CI, 1.003–1.175).[22] A more definitive meta-analysis by the Early Breast Cancer Trialists' Collaborative Group (EBCTCG) suggested an overall survival benefit of fifteen years from local radiation treatment to either the breast following BCT or the chest wall after mastectomy.[23] For those treatment comparisons where the difference in LR rates at five years was less than 10%, survival was unaffected (Figure 3–A–4). Among the 25,000 women where differences in local relapse were substantial (>10%), there were moderate reductions in breast cancer specific and overall mortality (Figure 3–A–5). It can be seen that where there were minimal differences in LR, survival curves were parallel. Where differences in LR were more substantial, survival differences become apparent. The absolute reduction in LR at five years was 19%, and the absolute reduction in breast cancer mortality at fifteen years was 5%. This represents one life saved for every four loco-regional recurrences prevented by RT at five years.

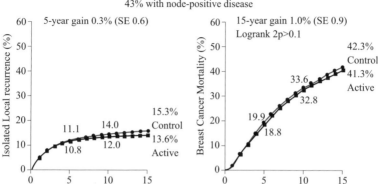

12 comparisons with <10% local recurrence risk: 16,804 women,
43% with node-positive disease

Fig. 3–A–4. Treatment comparisons with minimal (<10%) differences in rates of local recurrence

Where there are minimal differences in local recurrence, survival curves are parallel. SE = 0.9. Logrank 2p>0.1 (not significant).

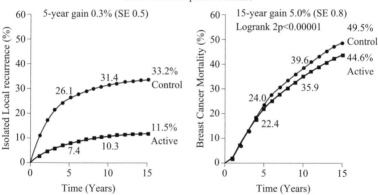

12 comparisons with >10% local recurrence risk: 25,276 women,
51% with node-positive disease

Fig. 3–A–5. Treatment comparisons with substantial (>10%) differences in rates of local recurrence

Where differences in local recurrence are more substantial, survival differences become apparent. SE = 1.9. Logrank 2p = 0.006.

However, the precise proportional contribution of local versus regional reductions is unclear, as absolute nodal recurrence rates were very low in the two studies. There is some evidence that LR might be a cause of distant metastases, arising from analysis of hazard rates for distant metastases in patients who underwent BCS with and without local control.[24] Those patients with local control demonstrated a peak in the hazard rate at about two years,

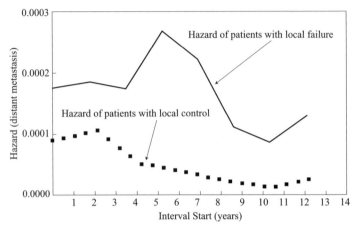

Fig. 3–A–6. The hazard rate for distant metastasis illustrated for patients with and without local control.

Those patients with local control demonstrate a peak in the hazard rate for distant metastases at about two years, after which there is a steady decline (dotted curve). By contrast, patients with local failure have a second hazard peak, which is seen at or beyond five years, and which is absent in those with local control (continuous curve). Note: Hazard rate for metastases is always higher in patients with local failure than those with local control.

after which there was a continual decline in the rate of distant metastases. By contrast, for those patients with local failure, a second hazard peak was seen at or beyond five years, which was absent in those patients without LR (Figure 3–A–6). It should be noted that the hazard rate for metastases is always higher in patients with local failure than those with local control. The first peak, which is seen in patients with or without local control, represents micrometastases present at the time of diagnosis. When patients with local failure are excluded from the analysis, the late mortality peak is reduced in amplitude, and actually disappears when patients with local failure and positive margins are excluded (Figure 3–A–7). It therefore appears that local failure has a causative relationship to this late mortality peak, and this second peak is evidence that local failure can be a source of new distant metastases and subsequent mortality; when this occurs, patients are more likely to have suffered early loco-regional or contra-lateral recurrence.

These results support the Halstedian paradigm as does the reduction in mortality from breast cancer screening, which aims to detect cancers during the preclinical phase when they remain localized without micrometastatic dissemination. Breast cancer is a heterogeneous disease, for which '"small" if rapid may mean "late", and "large" if slow may still be early'.[25] Some tumors behave in a relatively indolent, 'benign' manner, while others are inherently

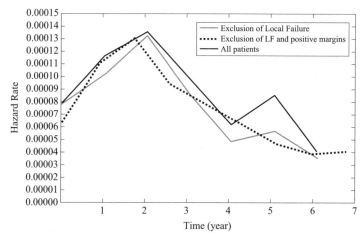

Fig. 3–A–7. Effect of exclusion of patients with local failure on late mortality peak

The late mortality peak is reduced in amplitude when patients with local failure are excluded from the analysis (heavy continuous line), and disappears when patients with local failure and positive margins are excluded (dotted line).

more biologically aggressive and lethal despite intensive therapies at both a local and systemic level. As micrometastases can never be excluded, any irrefutable declaration that a tumor remains genuinely localized at the time of diagnosis is impossible. The propensity to metastasize can be estimated using prognostic indices, and current attempts at genetic fingerprinting may increase predictive capacity.

LR as Determinant or Indicator of Metastasis

Loco-regional treatments, such as surgery or RT, are potentially curative in the absence of micrometastases when the disease is confined to the breast and lymph nodes. Under these circumstances, when local management is incomplete, viable cells persist within loco-regional tissues and can develop into distant metastases at a later date. Therefore, where micrometastases are either absent at presentation or have been obliterated by systemic therapy, LR is a determinant of distant disease and assumes a different significance from Fisher's postulate of LR being a marker for distant disease. By contrast, where micrometastases exist and have not been ablated with systemic therapy, LR would be an indicator of poor prognosis. LR predicts, and is a marker for, distant disease whether breast conservation treatment precedes or follows systemic therapy, and timing of recurrence is important (the earlier the recurrence, the greater the chance of distant disease). Both events are manifestations of the same biological process, which reflects the intrinsic behavior of any particular breast tumor. The foci of residual tumor and distant occult disease are maintained in a state of dynamic equilibrium, until some event triggers recurrence.[1]

However, studies have revealed partial independence among prognostic factors in determining the potential for local and distant relapse. In their study of IBTR in more than 2,000 patients undergoing BCS with quadrantic resection, Veronesi and colleagues found that tumor size and nodal status are correlated with distant, but not local, disease recurrence, while young age and peritumoral invasion predict both local, and to a lesser extent distant, disease relapse.[3] LR conferred an overall increased risk of distant relapse of 4.62 fold (95% CI, 3.34–6.39). There actually was evidence of an inverse relationship between nodal status and LR, which may be due to the confounding effects of concomitant chemotherapy. Furthermore, EIC predicts for LR only, which under these circumstances, represents inadequate local treatment and is not a marker for inherently increased risk of distant metastases.

Of interest, the benefits of chemotherapy may be compromised when loco-regional control is inadequate due to the reduced efficacy of chemotherapy in the presence of a greater burden of tumor cells in loco-regional tissues. Any persistent loco-regional disease could represent oligometastases and become a source of distant metastases.[26] Within the trials of breast conservation, most of the cases of LR occur against a background of micrometastatic disease and therefore represent a marker of distant relapse. Those patients without micrometastases at presentation and who undergo adequate loco-regional treatment have the same outcome irrespective of type of surgery. However, where there is inadequate or incomplete loco-regional therapy, survival differences may emerge, because LR is a determinant of distant disease and may render systemic therapy less effective. It is perhaps not surprising that no survival difference is detectable in BCT trials, because the majority of patients have received adequate primary loco-regional treatment (with or without mastectomy at time of relapse) and LR is not a cause of distant disease. Those cases where LR is a determinant of distant failure are probably too few, and follow up too short, to have any statistical impact.

Implications for Management

It would be provocative to suggest that all patients should be managed in line with Fisherian principles, if LR is an effect of aggressive tumor biology and not worth preventing. Thus, cases of early breast cancers amenable to conservative surgery would undergo lumpectomy only, without axillary dissection or post-operative RT. Those tumors with an innate risk of dissemination subsequently would declare themselves with the manifestation of LR, which would be an indicator and not an instigator of distant relapse and poor prognosis. A higher rate of LR would be the price of avoiding unnecessary adjuvant treatment in those patients (40%–50%) who do not relapse either locally or systemically after simple lumpectomy. RT and systemic (chemohormonal) therapy would be administered at the time of local relapse (unless this mandated mastectomy). However, local relapse can be psychologically devastating for a patient, even when informed that long-term survival is unaffected.[27] Moreover, there is a doubling of the psychiatric intervention rate at the time of LR. Though randomized clinical trials have previously failed to identify any group of patients for whom LR produces a decrement in survival, these trials may not have possessed the statistical power to detect any effect of attenuated loco-regional treatment on overall survival. The number of events are relatively small and some cases of distant recurrence may not yet have occurred at the time of analysis. The overview by the EBCTCG implies that survival and LR are related, but not in a simple one-to-one manner. Interestingly, in the EBCTCG overview, those patients in whom the difference in local relapse rates was less than 10% had presumably received adequate loco-regional treatment from surgery alone, with little further reduction from more surgery or RT.[23] These latest clinical results accord with the intuitive assumption that viable cancer cells remaining in the peritumoral tissue of the breast following conservation surgery could ultimately proliferate and metastasize to distant sites.

Adequacy of Breast-conserving Surgery

Results of the EBCTCG overview have reinforced the link between local control and mortality, leading to greater emphasis on adequacy of surgical excision and other treatment-related variables such as RT. BCS is now an established surgical modality and is the preferred standard of care for women with early-stage breast cancer. Introduction of BCS has coincided with instigation of widespread mammographic screening over the past twenty-five years. With a smaller average tumor size at presentation, the majority of patients are eligible for BCS, though rates of mastectomy vary at both institutional and geographical levels.[28] These variations in patterns of surgical management are likely to reflect differences in philosophy and training among surgeons, together with an element of fear and concern about recurrence. Selection of patients for BCS is of crucial importance, with an inverse relationship between the oncological demands for surgical radicality on the one hand and cosmesis on the other hand. There is a balance between the risk of LR and the cosmetic results. Most patients deemed eligible for BCS will have a favorable tumor-to-breast size ratio and will be suitable for conventional forms of WLE, in which the tumor is excised with a 2 cm–3 cm margin of surrounding breast tissue without any formal breast remodeling. It is no longer acceptable to merely attain gross macroscopic clearance of the tumor at operation; all radial margins should be clear of tumor at the microscopic level. The NSABP and others have reported higher rates of LR with microscopically positive margins, with rates increasing significantly with duration of follow-up, than in negative margin tumors, with regression coefficients of 0.75 (p = 0.008) and minus (−) 0.31 (p = 0.35), respectively.[15,29–32] However, some studies have found no correlation between LR and positive resection margins,[33,34] although relapse rates may have been influenced by modification of RT regimens with a proportionate increase in booster dose to 'compensate' for positive margins.

Margin Width

There has been a lack of uniformity in the definition of positive resection margin, and this in turn has compounded issues relating to microscopically negative margins and degrees of surgical clearance - how wide must a negative margin be to result in acceptable rates of LR (<1.0%–1.5% per year).[14] Some authors have defined a further category of 'close margins' and have found correlations between margin status and LR based on strict and consistent criteria.[15] Several studies have examined the impact of close margins (≤ 2 mm) on rates of LR. Although these are relatively small studies —— with some variability in other factors, such as age, EIC, and systemic therapies —— they all reveal a statistically significant increase in rates of LR for 'close' compared with negative margins.[35–38]

Many surgeons consider a margin clearance of 2 mm–3 mm to be appropriate, though up to 45% of American radiation oncologists consider a margin as negative provided there are no tumor cells at the inked edge. The Cambridge Breast Unit (CBU), along with about 30% of breast units in continental Europe and a mere 10% in the United States of America, strives for a radial margin clearance of 5 mm. Such a policy can be associated with very low rates of IBTR (actuarial rate of 1.1% at five years for invasive breast cancer),[39] which compares favorably with contemporary rates of 3.5%–10%

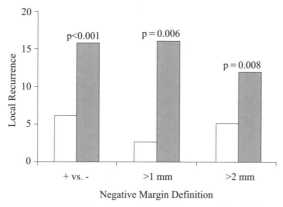

Fig. 3–A–8. Local recurrence in relation to margin widths

When studies of local recurrence are grouped according to how a 'negative' margin is defined, there is a consistent and statistically significant difference between 'positive' and 'negative' margins.

at ten years.[40] However, a wider-margin mandate can lead to re-excision rates varying up to 50%. It is unusual to find further tumor when re-excision is performed to achieve a wider margin rather than a negative margin per se. An analysis of data from the CBU has shown that residual disease is found in 60% of patients with involved margins, 40% of those with negative margins up to 2 mm, and only 6% for patients with a margin of 2 mm–5 mm, with the OR for 2 mm–5 mm margin versus involved margin at 0.05 ($p = 0.004$).[41]

Eva Singletary has provided a useful analysis which shows median rates of IBTR of 3%, 6%, and 2% when margins of clearance were 1 mm, 2 mm, and just clear (no tumor cells at inked margin), respectively.[42] Thus patients with no tumor cells within one microscopic field of the cut edge had the lowest rates of recurrence, ranging 2%–4%. When studies of LR are grouped according to how a negative margin is defined, there is a consistent and statistically significant difference between positive and negative margins (Figure 3–A–8). Thus, although rates of recurrence are determined by negative margin status, no direct relationship exists between margin width and rates of LR. When the first re-excision fails to achieve surgical clearance, mastectomy is often indicated and becomes necessary if margins remain positive after a 'reasonable' number of surgical attempts.[43]

Oncoplastic Surgery

The newer techniques of oncoplastic surgery ⎯ for example, therapeutic mammoplasty —— are advancing the limits of surgical resection, which may be associated with an increased chance of tumor-free margins though not necessarily with lower rates of IBTR. Furthermore, positive margins under these circumstances usually reflect extensive disease, for which mastectomy (rather than re-excision) is indicated. It has been suggested that the chance of local relapse could be reduced by more aggressive approaches to BCS,[44] but there currently are no data on longer term follow-up of these oncoplastic procedures. Moreover, there is no information from clinical trials on the safety of BCS for invasive tumors in excess of 4 cm.[45] Though margin status and the presence or absence of an extensive in situ component are the principal determinants of LR, consistent associations have been found for tumors greater than 2 cm.[46] For node-positive patients, tumor size exceeding 5 cm was the only risk factor for LR on a multivariate analysis.[47] Therefore, it is likely that the risk of relapse would remain high for larger tumors, despite adequate surgical clearance. Nonetheless, it may be possible to excise large areas of nonhigh-grade ductal carcinoma in situ (>4 cm) with clear margins and to partially reconstruct the breast with autologous tissue replacement.

The patient's age (<35 years) and family history of breast cancer are additional factors that must be considered when selecting patients for either oncoplastic surgery with a high percentage of breast volume excised or skin-sparing mastectomy with whole breast reconstruction (there is a higher risk of LR or de novo cancer risk after breast conservation). Though it may not be feasible in routine clinical practice to formally estimate the percentage excision from radiological measurements of tumor and breast size, consideration of magnetic resonance imaging, or MRI, assessment of the breast is advisable. This can confirm unifocality or exclude multifocal disease involving different quadrants. Where imaging is equivocal and tumor parameters are borderline for BCS, it may be preferable to undertake a two-stage procedure; initial 'wide' local excision of tumor permits full histopathologic evaluation and assessment of margins. A definitive oncoplastic procedure can be carried out subsequently, either two to three weeks later or following RT to the breast. A one-stage procedure is optimal and avoids any technical difficulties relating to the sequelae of previous surgery and RT (such as scarring and fibrosis). There are less likely to be problems with skin viability when completion mastectomy is undertaken after simple excision of tumor, compared with a more complex oncoplastic procedure with parenchymal undermining and transposition.

The biological consequence of these residual foci of tumor cells depends on whether they represent a 'determinant' or an 'indicator' of distant disease. In the absence of micrometastases, adequate loco-regional management theoretically can cure patients, and LR in this group represents persistent disease and failure to eradicate all tumor cells by primary treatment. In this case, LR is a determinant of distant disease, the probability of which depends on both temporal and innate biological factors. So IBTR is worth preventing.

Maximal Treatment at Initial Diagnosis Versus Relapse

Where LR is a determinant of distant disease, treatment at relapse may prevent distant dissemination, and the timing of diagnosis and initiation of treatment would be critical. However, where LR develops against a background of preexisting micrometastatic disease, LR represents a marker for distant disease, which would have developed whatever the extent of primary loco-regional treatment. In the former group, it is important to administer maximal loco-regional therapy at the time of initial diagnosis with curative intent. In the latter group, minimal early loco-regional treatment would suffice, as any LR that develops secondary to 'inadequate' loco-regional treatment would not impact on survival, but be an indicator of a relationship between tumor and host, which favored distant relapse. This would be an indication for maximal treatment at the time of LR, including systemic therapy. Clearly, distinguishing between these two groups is difficult, but may be aided in the future by microarray techniques, which better characterize the biology of individual tumors and provide a molecular 'portrait'. The latter group can potentially yield recurrence scores, which can be incorporated into clinical decision-making processes after rigorous clinicopathologic correlation.

Conclusions

Can we justify continuing to follow Fisherian principles on the basis that the current evidence is premature and inadequate to modify practice? Alternatively, should we revert to Halstedian principles of more thorough loco-regional management at the time of presentation? An 'intermediate', or 'spectrum', paradigm may be relevant, which encompasses elements of both Fisher and Halsted but which is less restrictive than either of these paradigms in pure form. However, this is difficult to translate into practice, as differentiation between the basic groupings is problematic.

A compromise solution may be to select those patients for whom more aggressive loco-regional treatment at the outset may confer a survival advantage. This is likely to include younger patients, for whom the risk of LR in the conserved breast is almost twice as high compared with that of older women. Rates of LR at five years are 5.5% for women 50 years of age and above compared with 18% for women under 50 years of age. Avoidance of death from breast cancer gains more additional years of life expectancy for younger women. With the stage shift witnessed in recent years, fewer women will have micrometastases at presentation, and LR assumes a greater significance and consequence as a source of distant metastases.

Local Management of Primary Breast Cancer

Nasim Ahmadiyeh and Mehra Golshan

Summary

Overall, breast surgery - particularly for early-stage breast cancer - is safe and highly rewarding for the surgeon as well as the patient. Breast surgery attempts to eliminate tumor burden in an effort to minimize spread of disease, with due attention to the optimal cosmetic outcome potential for each patient. Axillary lymph node staging by sentinel lymph node biopsy (SLNB) is the best prognostic indicator for a breast cancer patient, and guides postoperative therapy. The breast surgeon works within an interdisciplinary team to guide the patient toward a treatment option that is best suited for that patient.

Introduction: Burden of Disease

Breast cancer represents a primary source of global disease burden for women, and is a leading cancer for women in Europe, North America, Australia, many countries in Asia, as well as various countries in the developing world.[1-4]

The surgeon is often the first and primary member of the multidisciplinary team to evaluate, triage, and treat a breast cancer patient. Breast surgical oncologists focus exclusively on the surgical treatment of breast disease, while general surgeons still find that 14%–25% of their practice volume is devoted to treating diseases of the breast.[5-6] Mounting evidence suggests that patient outcome is linked to surgical volume, institution expertise,[7] and surgical technique.[8] We review the current standard of surgical care for local management of breast cancer, including the indications for surgery, surgical treatment options, surgical technique and relevant anatomy, and surgical complications.

Indications for Surgery

Elimination of tumor burden

Mortality from breast cancer occurs due to the effects of distant metastases. The primary surgical aim in the treatment of breast cancer is to eliminate tumor burden before detectable distant metastasis and thus reduce the chance of distant breast cancer recurrence. Therefore, breast surgery is indicated in any patient with breast cancer whose tumor is confined to the breast tissue and axillary nodes (stages 0-III). Controversy currently exists in the primary extirpation of tumor in the stage IV setting. There is some suggestion in retrospective cohorts that debulking surgery in stage IV breast cancer improves survival,[9,10] but this is not the current standard of care.

Surgical technique attempts to minimize the chances of local recurrence. Radiation therapy is a critical component of the treatment plan in those choosing breast-conserving therapy (BCT) and for certain patients who require or choose a mastectomy.

Staging

In addition to removing tumor burden to decrease the chance of distant spread of disease, surgery is the primary staging modality for breast cancer. Stage of disease is a principal prognostic indicator of breast cancer and helps to determine the patient's treatment course. Careful surgical staging is critical to optimal patient outcome.

Surgical Treatment Options

The surgical treatment options available to breast cancer patients today are vastly different from those available even one generation ago. Before the turn of the 20th century, breast cancer was considered uniformly fatal, and few surgical interventions were attempted. In a major medical advance, radical surgical treatment of breast cancer was described independently by William Halsted and Willy Meyer in 1894. With the procedure of radical mastectomy —— where overlying skin, breast, pectoralis muscles, and axillary lymph nodes at level I, II, and III are all removed —— patients experienced a 40% survival rate at five years, double the survival rate of untreated patients.[11] This form of therapy remained the mainstay of breast cancer surgery for nearly 80 years. In the mid-1970s, a series of randomized controlled clinical trials conducted by the National Surgical Adjuvant Breast Project (NSABP) in the United States of America (USA) and the Institute Tumori in Milan in Italy were initiated.[12] The Auchincloss modified radical mastectomy —— which left the pectoral muscles intact —— and the simple mastectomy —— which additionally left the axilla intact —— were found to have survival rates equivalent to the radical mastectomy, but with much improved quality-of-life outcomes. The equivalence of survival for various forms of mastectomy was followed by studies comparing BCT with mastectomies, ushering in the era of breast-conserving surgery. In 1990 a panel of the National Institutes of Health Consensus Development Conference indicated BCT and irradiation combined as an appropriate and preferred treatment option for women with early-stage breast cancer.

Toward the mid-1990s, another revolution in surgical management of breast cancer took place. The adoption of lymphatic mapping of the sentinel lymph node (SLN) —— a technique first used widely in melanoma staging —— became the new gold standard in surgical staging, eliminating the need for axillary lymph node dissection (ALND) in a large subset of women. The codification of sentinel node biopsy as appropriate staging for a clinically node-negative patient has been confirmed by a randomized trial and a wealth of retrospective literature. With SLNB, many women recovered much faster due to less extensive surgery, shorter exposure to anesthesia, and foregone drain placement. In most cases, they were spared future disability and complications more commonly seen with ALND, such as lymphedema, paresthesias, decreased mobility, and brachial plexus injury.

The repertoire of skills and techniques available to the surgeon in treating breast cancer is more specialized and more varied than before. This requires even more attention and sensitivity, to ensure the establishment of a sound relationship between surgeon and patient, whereby the surgeon is able to guide the individual patient through the various aspects of the decision-making process in choosing the optimal surgical therapy. The choice of optimal surgical treatment for breast cancer then becomes a task where attention to excellent surgical technique is equal to the task of sound judgment in the face of varied patient and tumor characteristics.

Breast conserving surgery

Breast-conserving surgery —— also known as lumpectomy or partial mastectomy —— confers the same survival advantage when coupled with postoperative irradiation as does mastectomy alone. In a twenty-year follow-up study to the NSABP-B06, lumpectomy with or without radiation, compared with mastectomy, was found to be equivalent regarding disease-free survival, distant disease-free survival, and overall survival. The incidence of recurrent tumor in the ipsilateral breast, however, was significantly increased for those women who underwent lumpectomy without radiation (39.2%), as opposed to the women who underwent lumpectomy with radiation (14.3%).[13] In reality, the rate of local recurrence today for women undergoing lumpectomy with radiation is even smaller, with rates ranging from 0.3% at thirty-nine month follow-up to 5.8% at ten years.[14,15] This decreased incidence in local recurrence is due to increased attention to clear margins, use of radiation with boost, and three-dimensional planning, as well as use of adjuvant therapies that are based on the molecular features of tumor pathology.

In a study of more than 16,000 stage I and stage II breast cancer patients, Monica Morrow and colleagues studied predictive factors in patients receiving BCT versus mastectomy. The likelihood of receiving BCT decreased for every decade of increase in age. Regional variations in care also have been reported, with those living in the northeast region of the USA more likely to be offered BCT over mastectomy, after accounting for other variables such as insurance status and age. Furthermore, radiotherapy post-BCT, which is the standard of care, was far less likely to be offered to women over the age of seventy years and to non-Whites.[16] Others also have documented a higher likelihood of performing BCT versus mastectomy in academic versus community settings,[17] and by breast surgeons versus general surgeons,[18] respectively.

Contra-indications to breast conservation for breast cancer fall into two main categories: first, anatomic; second, inability to tolerate or complete radiation therapy. Anatomic reasons for choosing mastectomy over breast conservation include tumor size —— the larger the tumor, the more tissue will need to be removed for clear margins. Hence, large tumor size relative to size of breast, diffuse disease, persistently positive margins after reasonable attempts at breast conservation, and multicentric disease are anatomic reasons to choose mastectomy. For similar reasons, the standard of care for male breast cancers is usually a mastectomy. Contra-indications to radiation therapy include prior mantle radiation, active connective tissue disease (making tolerance to radiation difficult), and radiation during pregnancy. In a patient for whom completion of radiation therapy or clinical follow-up with annual mammograms will be difficult, a mastectomy might offer the best treatment option in the long term. Last, a patient whose primary breast cancer was treated by lumpectomy and radiation, and whose cancer recurs in the ipsilateral breast, cannot undergo radiation a second time and must therefore undergo a mastectomy for treatment of a local recurrence.

Mastectomy

Any of the contra-indications (listed above) to breast-conserving surgery would be indications for a mastectomy. Prophylactic mastectomy is the treatment of choice in women with strong genetic risk, namely, mutations of the breast cancer 1 and 2 susceptibility genes, or BRCA1/2. Such women have a 50%– 85% lifetime risk of developing breast cancer. In these patients, prospective studies have shown prophylactic mastectomies to reduce the risk of breast cancer by 90%.[20] Referral to a genetic counselor in high-risk cases or extensive discussion with their surgeon, to ensure that patients adequately grasp their own risk, is the best practice to ensure that patients feel comfortable with their surgical treatment decisions over the long term.

Another emerging category of patients choosing mastectomy over breast conservation are those patients without a gene mutation, who are contemplating contralateral mastectomy as a prophylaxis. Sometimes, a patient diagnosed with breast cancer in one breast will choose at that same time to have bilateral mastectomies with reconstruction. This is often driven by the desire to be 'done with' the disease, to never have another mammogram or follow-up, or because they believe bilateral reconstruction would confer a better cosmetic outcome. Patients treated with mastectomy for early-stage breast cancer should be cautioned that an approximate 3%–5% chance still exists for chest wall or local recurrence.[19] Also, to date, there is no survival benefit associated with prophylactic mastectomy for patients outside of documented gene mutation carriers.

If mastectomy becomes the preferred surgical treatment for breast cancer in a given patient, the option of reconstruction should be presented to the patient, and referral to a reconstruction surgeon be made available.

Staging axillary lymph nodes

Axillary nodal status is the most accurate prognostic indicator in breast cancer staging and helps to determine the type of adjuvant therapy. ALND, which consists of removing all of the level I and level II nodes of the axilla, has been the gold standard of treatment. However, it is associated with substantial risk of adverse long-term sequelae, such as paresthesia, restricted range of motions, pain, and lymphedema.[21,22] Since about 70% of T1–T2 breast cancer patients will have negative axillary nodes,[23] the need for a less invasive test of nodal status is clear. Thus, when SLNB —— a technique previously used in staging melanoma —— was shown by Armando Giuliano,[24] David Krag,[25] and their colleagues to be a highly sensitive mode of detecting nodal metastases in breast cancer, it steadily has replaced ALND as the staging modality of choice.

When SLNB was first described, surgeons had to demonstrate their ability with the technique at special training sessions, where they would document their skill in conducting SLNB followed by completion ALND. A study by

Kelly McMasters and colleagues[23] tried to define this learning curve in 226 surgeons by prospectively enrolling 2,148 patients to undergo SLNB followed by completion axillary dissection. Improvement in the SLN identification and false-negative rates was found after twenty cases were performed. Since SLNB has now replaced ALND as the primary modality for axillary staging in clinically node-negative women in many places around the world, new trainees and young surgeons often no longer need to demonstrate their competence in SLNB compared with the gold standard of ALND. For young general surgeons without further breast specialization, the majority of breast cancer surgeries would have been performed, while still at junior levels of training. No regulations governing training or accreditation for surgeons carrying out SLNB exist apart from those required for board certification in general surgery, but surgeons need to be mindful that the learning curve for SLNB appears to be real.

Despite some of these uncertainties, SLNB is a definite advance in the field of breast cancer surgery, avoiding the need for ALND for many patients. Furthermore, with a little over a decade of worldwide experience with SLNB, data concerning axillary node recurrence rates in negative sentinel nodes are encouraging. A recent meta-analysis of four-eight studies, involving 14,959 sentinel node-negative breast cancer patients followed for a median of thirty-four months, demonstrated an axillary recurrence rate of 0.3%, which closely mirrors those who underwent axillary node dissection.[27]

Surgical Techniques

The primary principles of surgical technique in breast surgery are to maximize tumor removal with adequate margins while aiming for the best possible cosmetic outcome, and to minimize complications by maintaining excellent hemostasis, avoiding critical structures, and administering appropriate preoperative antibiotic treatment and adequate pain control.

A sound understanding of breast anatomy and surrounding structures and planes is critical to a well-planned surgery. Before incision, a review of imaging modalities, such as mammograms, ultrasound, and magnetic resonance imaging, or MRI, is imperative to confirm the spatial orientation of the lesion. This is particularly important in wire-guided lumpectomies where the lesion is not clinically palpable. A physical examination is also imperative to determine any new symptoms, including the presence of clinically palpable nodes, which would warrant a full ALND. A well-planned incision is key to both successful surgery and optimal cosmesis.

Lumpectomy

In general, a curvilinear incision along the natural creases, or Langer's lines, of the skin is preferred for most lumpectomies. This allows the scar to form along natural lines of tension and to be less visible. The surgeon must then create an artificial three-dimensional plane of dissection around the tumor, often in the form of a cube, cylinder, or quadrant, which pays attention to the margins on all sides of the dissected tissue. Care must be taken to maintain the orientation of the specimen for proper pathologic assessment of margins. Clips may be left in the tumor cavity to aid with radiation planning and in the event re-excision is required.[28] In general, margins of 3 mm are considered adequate; however, this is a point of discussion around the world. In wire-guided excisions, gentle handling of the wire is required, since movement of the wire's hook from the center of the abnormality may result in inadequate tumor removal. Wire-guided excisions are sent for radiographic confirmation before the end of surgery.

Attention to homeostasis is important, and the skin is often closed in two layers with absorbable suture. In some oncoplastic procedures, where the amount of tissue removed is relatively large, healthy surrounding breast tissue may be mobilized and approximated with sutures, so as to fill in the dead space created by tumor removal. Care must be taken in these cases to appropriately mark the site of the original tumor with clips to help aid planning of post-BCT radiation. In general, however, minimal tissue manipulation is required. In a lumpectomy, generous doses of long-acting anesthetic to skin incision after closure will aid in postoperative recovery. Bulky dressings should be avoided in favor of minimal well-placed dressings, as this too affects the patient's sense of wellbeing postoperatively. Patients are typically able to return home after a few hours in the recovery room, with minimal need for narcotics.

Mastectomy

In skin-sparing mastectomies, a circumareolar incision often is used, with or without lateral extension, where reconstruction will follow. In cases of mastectomy without reconstruction, elliptical incisions incorporating the nipple areolar complex and allowing for minimal skin redundancy are planned. Dissection follows the anatomic boundaries of the breast superiorly to the clavicle, inferiorly to the rectus sheath insertion, medially to the sternum, laterally to the latissimus, and posteriorly to the chest wall, with removal of the pectoralis major fascia. Whether dissection occurs with scalpel, electrocautery, harmonic scalpel, or tumescence (a combination of lactated ringers with lidocaine and epinephrine), patient outcome seems more likely to result from the surgeon's comfort and familiarity with a particular technique than from the technique itself.

While traditionally, the pectoral fascia is removed in a mastectomy (as is common practice in the USA), some surgeons will keep this intact as long as they appear to have an otherwise clean dissection. There does not appear to be a difference in local recurrence rate from leaving the pectoral fascia intact.[29]

Closure of mastectomy will depend on plans for reconstruction. Drains are usually placed to decrease seroma formation. Patients undergoing a mastectomy with reconstruction generally should have an overnight hospital stay, although in the USA increasingly the procedure of mastectomy without reconstruction is on a day surgical basis. The need for systemic narcotics may be minimized by the use of pain pumps, which deliver measured doses of local anesthetic to the wound through a narrow tube that is easily pulled upon discharge. If immediate reconstruction is not planned, a snug dressing applying moderate pressure to the chest wall at the site of surgery is often beneficial, both to minimize discomfort for the patient and to potentially prevent seroma formation.

Complications

The more common complications of breast and axillary surgery include skin infection, abscess formation, seroma, lymphedema and hematoma formation, arm numbness, and chronic pain at incision.[31] Postoperative skin infections are most commonly caused by staphylococcal species, and in a meta-analysis are reported to be 3.8%.[32] A single dose of a cephalosporin about 0.5 hr–1 hr before incision has been found to decrease the rate of infection by 38%–40%.[33] Abscess formation is rarer, but if present, must be opened and drained, and allowed to heal secondarily. Seroma formation in the lumpectomy cavity is expected, and helps restore the contour of the breast, being replaced over time by scar tissue. Generally, needle aspiration of seromas is useless, as the fluid simply reaccumulates. The skin flaps of mastectomies and axillary dissections tolerate seromas less well, in which case drains placed at the site of the operation are used to decrease the incidence of seromas. Fastidious hemostasis, coupled with avoidance of medications that affect hemostasis, are the best preventative measures against hematoma formation.

Numbness over a small aspect of the arm can occur, given sacrifice of branches of the intercostobrachial nerve during axillary dissection. More severe consequences are damage to the long thoracic nerve of the serratus anterior, which results in winged scapula (a protruding scapula), or damage to the thoracodorsal nerve of the latissimus dorsi, which results in weak internal rotation or shoulder abduction. Chronic intermittent burning or searing sensation is frequently described in patients who have undergone lumpectomy or mastectomy. These are likely due to damage to peripheral nerve endings in the skin of the breast, and usually can be tolerated. However, long-term sequelae have been described, and pharmacologic intervention may be necessary.

One of the most feared complications of ALND is chronic upper extremity lymphedema. Sometimes taking ten years or more to present itself, lymphedema occurs in about 13%–27% of patients with ALND.[31] A recent study looking at the five-year outcomes of SLNB versus SLNB and ALND found a 5% prevalence of lymphedema at five years in the patients who had SLNB compared with 16% prevalence of lymphedema in the patients who had SLNB followed by completion ALND.[34] Main factors for increased risk of lymphedema include number of lymph nodes removed, number of lymph nodes containing metastatic disease, and the use of axillary field radiation. Infection and obesity seem to be associated with increased risk of lymphedema. A rare but serious complication of longstanding lymphedema is angiosarcoma, or Stewart-Treves syndrome, identified as blue-red macules or nodules on the skin of the affected arm. Most patients with Stewart-Treves have metasases at the time of diagnosis.

Rarer complications that can occur as a result of surgical treatment for breast cancer include pneumothorax, particularly in thin patients. This can occur during wire placement for wire-localized excisions or during injection of blue dye if the angle of the needle is too steep. A variety of allergic reactions including anaphylaxis have been reported with isosulfan blue dye (1%–2%).[35] Some have suggested that methylene blue is less allergic, while others choose not to use blue dye for fear of adverse reaction, and use the radioactive isotope instead. The downside of radioactive isotope use includes cost and often time for migration of the tracer.

Preferred Surgery for Breast Cancer: Is There an Optimal Technique?

Michail Shafir

Summary

Surgery remains one of the mainstays of treatment of breast cancer. At present, resection of the primary tumor, with or without preservation of the breast and staging with lymphadenectomy (sentinel or more extensive), continues to be the crucial therapeutic modality, in combination with different permutations of chemoherapy, hormonal therapy, and radiation.

Introduction: Operative Approach Dependent on Clinical Presentation

The history of medicine and surgery has taught us that that knowledge is an evolving concept: what was considered to be true in the past may not be true today, and what is true today will probably not be so in the future. In this respect, is there an optimal surgery that is universally accepted for breast cancer treatment? I do not believe so.

Instead, a variety of operative approaches exist, from ultra-radical to minimally invasive breast-conserving surgery, which may all be acceptable depending on the clinical presentation of each patient. There is an abundance of data, based on randomized clinical trials, which need to be presented to each patient before a surgical procedure is agreed on. A frank discussion, based on the patient's age, risk factors, histology, comorbidities, and staging, needs to take place every time. When alternative surgical techniques are similar in tumor control, the patient's choice needs to be considered; similarly, if a clinical trial is available to answer alternative approaches, the patient should be informed in detail and offered participation in the trial.

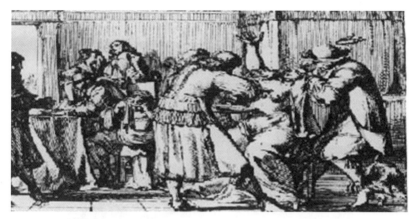

Fig. 3–C–1. Renaissance era mastectomy
Source: Reproduced in Michael B Shimkin (1979), *Contrary to Nature,* National Institutes of Health, US Department of Health, Education and Welfare: 65.

History

Breast cancer has been recognized since ancient times, and even though the biology of the disease was poorly understood by today's criteria, the concept of 'local disease' has prevailed throughout the centuries (Figures 3–C–1 and 3–C–2), and only the surgical techniques have changed.

Since George Crile and Bernard Fischer introduced the concept of safety of breast-conserving surgery,[1] several landmark clinical trials demonstrated the equivalence in cure rate and survival for women with small tumors, compared with mastectomy.[2,3] Donald Morton pioneered the concept of sentinel node biopsy in melanoma, in an attempt to minimize the need for extensive lymphadenectomy.[4] Armando Giuliano extended the technique for breast cancer,[5] and sentinel lymph node biopsy is currently an accepted technique to 'stage' the axilla when no suspicious lymphadenopathy is found. Multiple clinical trials have validated this technique.[5] At present, new clinical trials are being conducted, and novel ideas proposed in cancer cooperative groups, to determine the best timing of sentinel node biopsy with adjuvant/neoadjuvant chemotherapy and/or hormonal therapy.[6,7]

A further issue is that there are patients, who after what is considered to be 'optimal surgery' —— with negative sentinel and/or axillary dissection nodes and adequate resection of the primary tumor —— will develop recurrent disease in the ipsilateral breast and/or metastatic disease. The significance of this observation is that, in order to improve cure rates and patient survival, other therapies have to be combined with surgery, namely chemotherapy, hormonal

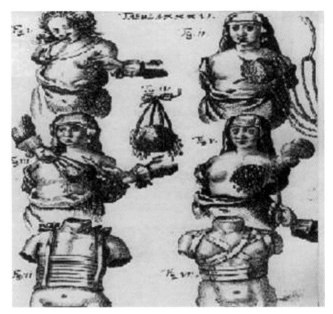

Fig. 3–C–2. Halsted radical mastectomy
Source: Reproduced in Michael B Shimkin (1979), *Contrary to Nature,*
National Institutes of Health, US Department of Health, Education and
Welfare: 66, 154.

therapy, and radiation therapy. For the implementation of this concept, once again a variety of controlled randomized clinical trials have demonstrated the validity of combined therapies with multiple permutations.

Between 9% and 40% of mastectomy specimens have additional cancer cells beyond the margins of the primary tumor, implying that 'lumpectomy' per se may not be sufficient.[8] Consequently, the National Surgical Adjuvant Breast and Bowel Project (NSABP) and others conducted conceptually important trials:

1. In the NSAPB-04 trial, mastectomy with/without postoperative radiation demonstrated reduced loco-regional recurrence, but no difference in survival was evident after twenty-five years of follow-up.[9]
2. In the NSABPB-06 trial, modified radical mastectomy was carried out versus lumpectomy plus (+) axillary dissection +/minus (?) radiation. Radiotherapy significantly reduced local recurrence, but no difference in survival was observed at twenty years follow-up. The addition of systemic therapy further reduced the incidence of local recurrence.[10]
3. In the Danish Breast Cancer Cooperative Group 82 b and c studies, post-mastectomy radiation was shown to decrease local recurrence and also to improve overall survival with the addition of adjuvant systemic therapy.[11]

4. In the NSABP B-14, trial, the effectiveness of tamoxifen —— added to radiation —— was demonstrated to lower the rate of local recurrence in breast-conserving surgery (10.3% with radiation alone versus 3.4% with addition of tamoxifen to radiation, at ten-year follow-up).[12]

5. In the Early Breast Cancer Trialists' Collaborative Group study (also known as the 'Oxford' meta-analysis), 42,000 patients encompasing seventy-eight randomized controlled trials, aiming to study outcomes of local treatment of breast cancer, mastectomy and breast conserving surgery were analyzed, as well as extent of surgery and use or not of radiation therapy. There was an 18.6% reduction in local recurrence with postoperative radiation after breast-conserving surgery at five years and a 5.4% decrease in mortality at fifteen years. After mastectomy, radiation decreased local recurrence by 17.1% and showed a 4.4% decrease in mortality at fifteen years.[13]

Surgery for Ductal Carcinoma In-situ

Ductal carcinoma in situ is a spectrum of different tumors. Currently, the majority of DCIS patients are diagnosed by mammographic screening, are often nonpalpable, and thus are amenable to limited surgical excision by localizing with different techniques (Kopans' wire $+/-$ methylene blue $+/-$ isotopic injections). In small foci of DCIS, there is rarely an invasive component, and consequently also, a sentinel lymph node biopsy is indicated rarely. Conversely, larger areas of DCIS, particularly associated with palpable tumor, are often accompanied by a microinvasive component, and thus benefit from a sentinel node biopsy at the time of the resection.

However, the extent of DCIS often is underestimated by radiological and pathological criteria. B. Doyle and colleagues recently have reported on 145 patients diagnosed with DCIS by core biopsies: fifty-five resected specimens (37.9%) contained invasive carcinoma and seven (4.8%) had a positive sentinel node biopsy.[14] A. Grin and colleagues emphasized the need to utilize several methods to accurately stage DCIS, as there is not one standardized modality to estimate the extent of DCIS, based on a retrospective analysis of seventy-eight excisions.[15]

Furthermore, a recent report by Udo Rudloff and colleagues reported an increased risk of ipsilateral breast recurrence in patients with DCIS undergoing breast-conserving surgery when a concurrent lobular neoplasia is present. Two hundred and ninety-four patients operated on at Memorial Sloan-Kettering Cancer Center in New York were analyzed —— 14% were found to have concurrent lobular carcinoma in situ (LCIS), atypical ductal hyperplasia in 13%, and columnar cell changes in 24%. After a median follow-up of eleven years, the local recurrence in the ipsilateral breast was twice as high in patients with DCIS + LCIS compared with DCIS alone (p = 0.002).[16] The NSABP B-17 trial demonstrated a highly significant decrease in ipsilateral local recurrence, when radiation was added to lumpectomy (32% vs. 16%, p = 0.001 for noninvasive recurrence and p = 0.00001 for invasive recurrence). However, at twelve-year follow-up, the survival was similar in both groups.[17] The European Organisation for Research and Treatment of Cancer (EORTC) performed a similar trial, involving 1,010 patients, with similar conclusions.[18]

The relationship between atypical ductal hyperplasia (ADH), LCIS, and DCIS remains a subject of high interest. M. J. Wagoner and colleagues reported on 123 patients who underwent core biopsies; when more than two foci of ADH were present, DCIS was found more frequently (16/41 vs. 6/82 with less than three foci, p = 0.0001), thus suggesting a clear relationship between these entitities.[19] Ben Arora and colleagues analyzed forty-four patients with resected ADH involving the margins and re-examination after re-excision. Almost 29% of patients had associated DCIS, and only two patients had an invasive cancer; therefore, again a continuum of malignancy was demonstrated.[20]

An intriguing recent report by M. Hu and colleagues describes up-regulation of cyclo-oxygenase-2 (COX-2) in DCIS xenografts and the relationship of the tumor cells with fibroblasts, promoting their growth and transformation into invasive cancer; the administration of celecoxib, a selective COX-2 inhibitor, decreased the tumor weight and inhibited progression to invasion, suggesting that it may be used for the treatment and prevention of breast cancer.[21]

Breast-conserving surgery is the norm for DCIS. However, because in the majority of cases no palpable lesion exists, there is a significant number of patients who will have positive margins after the first resection. B. Dunne and colleagues analyzed 4,660 patients from Memorial Sloan-Kettering Cancer Center in New York and University Hospital in Dublin: margins of 2 mm were as good as 5 mm; margins less than 2 mm yielded a high risk of recurrence, but wider margins often had poor cosmetic results.[22]

Sentinel Node Biopsy

Since Morton introduced the concept of sentinel node biopsy in melanoma and Giuliano extended the concept to breast cancer, an important clinical trial was conducted by the NSABP (the B-32 randomized phase III trial) assessing the accuracy of the technique in 5,611 women, comparing sentinel node biopsy with conventional axillary lymph node dissection, in patients with clinically negative nodes. In the sentinel node group that was histologicly negative, no further intervention was done; if the histology was positive, an axillary dissection was performed. The accuracy of the technique was outstanding, at 97%.[23] Helen Mabry and Giuliano stated that sentinel node biopsy has become the standard of care for clinically node-negative patients and that the future revolves around optimal timing when neoadjuvant chemo and/or hormonal therapy are considered.[24] In a series of 129 patients who underwent neoadjuvant chemotherapy, P. Gimbergues and colleagues achieved successful identification of the sentinel node in 93.8% of the patients utilizing the isotopic method.

The question still remains as to whether sonography and fine-needle aspiration play a role before and after neoadjuvant chemotherapy.[25] The issue of age remains controversial, and many studies have determined that physiologic rather than chronologic age is more important. In a recently published study by Anees Chagpar and colleagues of 700 patients with a median age of seventy-six years and a median tumor size of 1.4 cm, 16% had positive sentinel node; and age, tumor size, and lymphovascular invasion were prognostic of the risk of recurrent disease.[26]

A further controversial issue is the value of frozen section $+/-$ touch-prep analysis intraoperatively versus conventional histopathology. K. M. Vanderveen and colleagues in a prospective randomized study of 118 patients, with 233 lymphnodes analyzed, concluded that the intraoperative evaluation results were similar to the conventional histopathology, thus sparing a second surgery for metastatic sentinel node; and the only false-negative results occurred in micrometastatic lymph nodes, for which the value of completion of axillary dissection is still an unresolved issue.[27]

The risk of recurrence in the axilla after a negative sentinel node has been studied by Umberto Veronesi and colleagues: 3,548 patients at the Milan Cancer Center were followed for a median of forty-eight months, with thirty-one patients developing overt metastasis in the axilla, of whom twenty-seven patients are alive and well after their axillary dissection. The five-year overall survival was of 98%.[28] The value of sentinel prediction was studied by R. Ramjeesingh and colleagues: 400 sentinel nodes were analyzed in 397 patients, of which ninety patients had positive sentinel nodes and underwent axillary dissection, and of these, 29% has metastatic nonsentinel nodes. In patients with DCIS, multifocality and lymphovascular invasion were predictors of metastasis to lymphnodes.[29]

Various techniques have been proposed and studied, to optimize the detection of a sentinel node. Borys Krinicky and colleagues have reported a "triangulation" imaging technique of lymphoscintigraphy with technetium-99

(Tc-99) isotope injection. Localization, without blue dye, was 98%, and allowed visualization of internal mammary and or/supraclavicular nodes when the lymphoscintigraphy so indicated.[30,31] More recently, S. Bines and colleagues reported equivalent rate of identification of sentinel node with isotope alone versus isotope + blue dye injection, thus 'optimizing' the surgery and minimizing the risks (the blue dye has been reported to produce allergic reactions in 2% of patients).[32]

Indications for Mastectomy

For many years, different types of mastectomy have been proposed and performed as the 'optimal' surgery for breast cancer:
1. 'Halstedian radical mastectomy', with resection of pectoralis major and minor muscles + 'complete' axillary lymph node dissection;
2. 'Extended radical mastectomy', including resection of part of the chest wall, internal mammary, and supraclavicular lymph nodes, as proposed by Jerome Urban; and
3. 'Modified radical mastectomy', a less mutilating mastectomy proposed by D. Patey, with preservation of the pectoralis major muscle, but resecting the pectoralis minor and a complete axillary dissection.

The tendency today is towards less extensive and less mutilating surgery, with less functional and cosmetic morbidity, achieving similar survival rates. So, the question arises: why are so many mastectomies still performed in the 21st century? Is there a rationale? Why are bilateral mastectomies part of the surgical options? The following are possible indications for mastectomy in the modern era:
1. The presence of a large tumor in a small breast, which would not allow an adequate margin and/or an acceptable cosmetic result if a breast-conserving surgery were to be performed.
2. Uncontrollable ulcerated and/or bleeding tumor, after failure of medical and radiation treatments.
3. Prophylactic bilateral mastectomies in high-risk patients, with mutations of breast cancer 1 and 2 susceptibility genes (BRCA 1/2) and/or significant family history. L. C. Hartmann and colleagues reported on 214 women at high risk, with 176 testing for BRCA mutations, of which twenty-six were positive, and none had cancer in bilateral prophylactic mastectomy specimens.[33] A more recent study of 540 women at the MD Anderson Cancer Center revealed that of those with mutations, 70% chose bilateral mastectomy as their best option, and in addition, the majority also

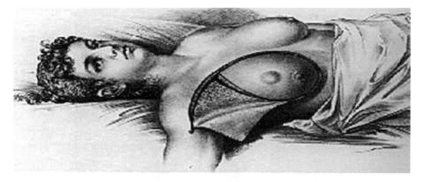

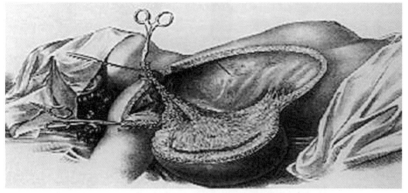

Fig. 3–C–3. BRCA 1/2 mutations ⸺ Risk of breast and ovarian cancer

Source: Reproduced from MYRIAD Genetic Laboratories Inc (2006), Informational card.

considered bilateral oophorectomy[34] (Figure 3–C–3).

4. Patient preference for a 'peace of mind' surgery, namely, prophylactic mastectomy. T. M. Tuttle reported on 51,000 women with unilateral DCIS from 1998 and 2005, and emphasized the increase in number of patients undergoing prophylactic mastectomies from 4.1% to 13.5%. There is no evidence that contralateral mastectomy improves survival, and the decision often is made by the patient to have a greater 'peace of mind'. Whether this is 'optimal' surgery, the debate continues.[35]

5. The evolution of plastic surgery repair after a mastectomy renders this operation much more acceptable to patients who opt for this alternative. In fact, often the cosmetic result frequently approaches that of breast-conserving surgery. (Figures 3–C–4, 3–C–5, and 3–C–6). The simplest approach is the insertion of breast saline/silicone implants, and the more complex repairs are performed with autologous tissues with myo-cutaneous flaps. So, which is the 'optimal' plastic repair? All alternatives have advantages and drawbacks: the implants are technically simpler, with fewer

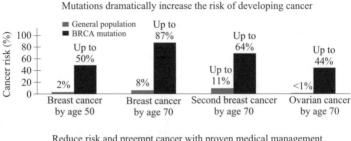

Mutations dramatically increase the risk of developing cancer

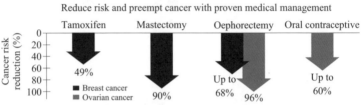

Reduce risk and preempt cancer with proven medical management

Fig. 3–C–4. Happy patient after bilateral mastectomy without reconstruction

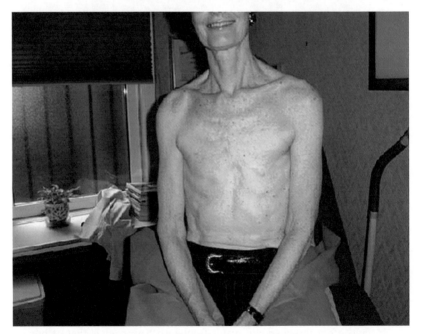

Fig. 3–C–5. A patient 17 years after right mastectomy, implant, and nipple tattoo

complications, but involve the insertion of a foreign body. The flaps are more complex, longer to perform, and may even require microvascular anastomosis to assure viability of the mobilized flaps; when complications occur, they are more difficult to manage, and adjuvant treatment may be

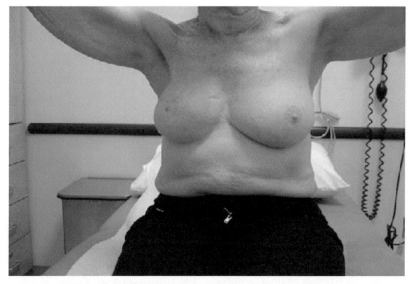

Fig. 3–C–6. A patient 20 years after breast-conserving surgery

significantly delayed. Therefore, the decision is jointly made between the surgeons and the patient. There are patients who will forego reconstruction and are perfectly satisfied with a double 'butterfly' scar of bilateral mastectome (Figure 3–C–4). Furthermore, less invasive techniques —— such as skin-sparing endoscopic mastectomy have been developed —— allowing also a sentinel node biopsy and insertion of an implant. Ken-ichi Ito reported a series of thirty-three patients with endoscopically assisted skin-sparing mastectomy (21 had DCIS or LCIS, and 12 had invasive carcinomas). After a follow-up of fifty-one months, there were no local recurrences and no distant metastatic disease.[36] For women who elect to have breast-conserving surgery but where a large defect is created, the 'oncoplastic' technique —— a mastopexy with volume displacement of the remaining breast tissue —— is performed to minimize deformity.[37]

New Techniques

The established method for 'spot-localization' for nonpalpable lesions is the Kopans' hooked wire with or without methylene blue at the time of the wire insertion. Several new techniques have been devised in attempts to increase precision and decrease the volume of the excised specimen. S. Sahoo and colleagues have reported on six cases of sonographically inserted cryoprobe

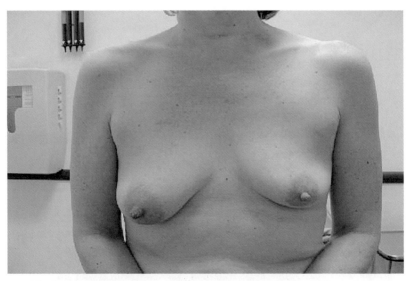

Fig. 3–C–7. Spot localization specimen, with technetium-99 and Kopans' wire

and resection of the previously biopsied tumors, where resecting by a sonographically guided "ice-ball" encompasses the tumor and surrounding normal tissue. The drawback of this technique is that tumor histology was altered, as well as expression of estrogen/progesterone receptors.[38] S. Harlow and colleagues compared spot localization with Kopans' wire versus intraoperative ultrasound for excision of DCIS: ninety-six patients were localized with ultrasound: 10% had positive margins and 23% had a margin of less than 1 mm; and fifty-nine patients were localized with Kopans wire: 12% had a positive margin and 27% had a margin of less than 1 mm. The re-excision rate was 21% versus 31%. They concluded that ultrasound guidance is simpler, but not always possible.[39] B. Krynickyi and colleagues reported on improved spot localization with injection of Tc-99 labeled macroaggregated albumin on thirty-eight patients, in addition to the Kopans' wire (Figure 3–C–7). The radioisotopic localization was accurate in all patients, and all margins were clear. This technique allowed a more direct incision, guided by a hand-help probe, and made assessment of margins intraoperatively easier, and the Kopans' wire was not the primary guiding tool.[40]

The same group has developed a 'double isotope' technique, utilizing Indium-111 labeled macroaggregated albumin for the primary breast tumor and Tc-99 injected periareolarly for the sentinel node biopsy; this combination permits a precise localization of both the primary tumor and the sentinel node without necessitating wire localization nor injection of blue dye, thus simplifying the process and decreasing morbidity (unpublished data).

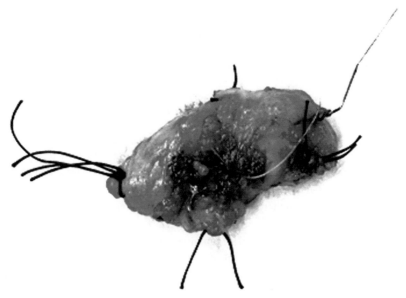

Fig. 3–C–8. Spot localization specimen with 99TC and Kopans' wire

A different and simpler method of spot localization utilizes intraoperative sonography to localize the hematoma created by the core, vacuum-assisted biopsies. This technique was compared with the established wire localization. The precision of the excision and patient comfort were emphasized, and margin positivity was significantly higher in the needle group.[41]

H. G. Hughes and colleagues reported the Mayo Clinic experience, comparing wire localization with iodine (I)-123 radioactive seed localization. There was a higher percentage of negative margins in the seed group (73% vs. 54%), and consequently a smaller percentage of reoperations for margins (8% vs. 25%). This technique was found to be simpler, more convenient, and facilitated operating room schedule, as the seed implant could be performed up to five days before surgery This technique also allows surgeons to perform a sentinel node biopsy with injection of Tc-99.[42]

Surgical management of breast distant metastases remains anecdotal and controversial. In search of new approaches, C. T. Sofocleus and colleagues have published a series of radio-frequency ablation of predominantly liver metastatic breast cancer in twelve patients. The median overall survival was sixty months, with a three-year survival at 70% and a five-year survival at 30%. Of course, thepatients were highly selected, and the validity of this exciting new surgical tool needs to be proven by randomized series.[43]   R. Adam and colleagues emphasized the concept of surgical treatment of breast cancer metastatic to the liver and other sites when stability had been obtained with medical treatment. In a series of eighty-five patients with resectable liver metastases, a thirty-two months median survival and a 37% five-year survival were achieved.[44]

What Is in the Future?

Should surgery be performed on the primary tumor of a patient who presents initially with distant metastases? The accepted practice is to treat such a patient with systemic chemotherapy and limit surgical resection for palliative reasons only. Khan has shown that resection of the primary tumor (breast lumpectomy or mastectomy) significantly increases survival by 40%–50%, validating the concept that surgery on the primary tumor is beneficial due to debulking and/or eliminating the primary source of further metastatic foci.[45] Should loco-regional radiation be performed on the primary tumor in such patients? R. LeScodan analyzed 581 patients with distant metastatic disease treated with aggressive loco-regional radiotherapy, and there was a significant survival advantage compared with patients treated only with systemic therapy.[46]

As breast cancer is a heterogeneous disease, each patient can be characterized as low/intermediate/high risk, considering tumor type, size, lymph node involvement, luminal type, oncotype, hormonal receptors, and expression of growth factors, is it conceivable that the ultimate treatment will not require major surgery? Maybe.

Is breast cancer a viral disease? J. F. Holland and colleagues , in ongoing research, have found evidence that a high proportion of human breast cancers contain sequences of the murine breast cancer virus. If this discovery is confirmed in larger studies, it is conceivable that the 'optimal' surgical treatment for breast cancer will be reduced to tissue procurement and treatment with antiviral vaccines.

Concluding Remarks

Breast surgery has become more precise, and personalized, on the basis of our progressive knowledge of the biology of the disease and the availability of a larger number of chemotherapeutic and hormonal agents, as well as more refined radiation techniques. All these aspects have prompted multiple clinical trials that have demonstrated the value of a combination of therapeutic modalities in varied permutations.

The earlier diagnosis of breast cancer, extending to nonpalpable tumors, DCIS, and small invasive cancers, has allowed the development of multiple breast-conserving surgical techniques, as well as sentinel node biopsies, rather than systematic axillary dissection, thus reducing the morbidity and mutilation of more extensive surgery. However, mastectomy, including bilateral therapeutic and prophylactic, remain forever present in the surgical panorama. Why? How can one explain the need for mastectomy — except in very specific circumstances — when a less drastic irreversible procedure yields similar cure and survival rates. A possible explanation resides in the fact that patients are progressively more informed and are participants in therapeutic decisions. Today, many a woman decides that a mastectomy gives her 'peace of mind', and this emotional/rational decision becomes a better option with sophisticated plastic surgical techniques to reconstruct the resected defect.

Therefore, the question. Is there an optimal surgical technique for breast cancer? The answer is no. There are many techniques, and for each patient, a different one is preferable, including participation in clinical trials that study different modalities for sentinel node identification, control of the margins after lumpectomy, and so on.

Furthermore, surgical alternatives can vary depending on the patient's geographical location, age, and comorbidities. For example, an elderly lady in a rural environment may not have easy access to radiation therapy or prolonged medical treatment, and for such a patient, a mastectomy is often the simplest and most efficient solution. The Cancer and Leukemia Group B (CALGB) has conducted a trial in women over the age of seventy years, with or without radiation therapy after breast-conserving surgery. The cure rate and survival were similar in both groups, emphasizing the need to parsonalize the decision making.

Surgery remains one of the mainstays of treatment of breast cancer. At present, resection of the primary tumor, with or without preservation of the breast and staging with lymphadenectomy (sentinel or more extensive), continues to be the crucial therapeutic modality, in combination with different permutations of chemoherapy, hormonal therapy, and radiation.

As biological, biochemical, and genetic knowledge evolve, it is conceivable that surgery in the future will be confined to establishing the diagnosis with biopsies only. For now, surgery is still a fundamental pillar in the treatment of breast cancer.

Results of Questionnaire Survey of Breast Cancer Specialists about Optimal Surgery for Patients with Breast Cancer

Takashi Inamoto, Masahiro Takada, and Masakazu Toi

Summary

As part of the Kyoto Breast Cancer Consensus Conference in April 2009, an international survey of breast cancer specialists found that a variety of opinions existed about the optimal local management of surgery for early breast cancer. The results assisted conference participants to frame several critical research questions in the ongoing pursuit and development of a medical consensus.

Introduction: Paradigm of Breast-conserving Surgery (BCS)

Breast-conserving surgery (BCS), introduced under the paradigm that breast cancer is a systemic disease at an early stage,[1,2] has imparted great cosmetic advantage to early breast cancer patients over that of radical mastectomy without comparative losses of a cure.[3]

When deciding whether to perform BCS as an adequate local treatment, as breast cancer specialists we have to consider factors that intimately link to local failure. Distance from surgical margin to tumor, cut margin status, and histologic characters of main tumors may be important factors related to local failure. Moreover, biological markers, such as estrogen receptor (ER) status and age of patients, may also be factors related to local failure after BCS. The importance of these factors will be different for invasive ductal carcinoma and ductal carcinoma in situ (DCIS). Hereditary breast cancer carrying the breast cancer 1 and 2 susceptibility genes (BRCA1/2) abnormality is another important decision-making factor in BCS.[4]

We therefore decided to survey breast cancer specialists about the local management for early breast cancer, to establish the extent or otherwise of

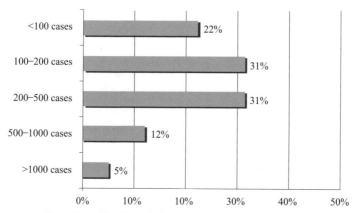

Fig. 3–D–1. Number of primary breast cancer cases per year

consensus among respondents. The survey was conducted just before the Kyoto Breast Cancer Consensus Conference held in April 2009 in Kyoto. In this paper, we present the results of part of the survey, concerning optimum breast surgery for the local management of the disease.

Background Characteristics of the Respondents

The online questionnaire was sent to about 1,000 breast cancer specialists and we obtained 104 replies (response rate: 10.4%). The respondents were from twenty-six countries, although more than a half were Japanese. Almost 77% of the respondents had more than ten years of clinical experience in breast cancer. The number of primary breast cancer cases per year varied between institutes, but 17% of cases belonged to high-volume institutes, where the number of primary breast cancer cases was more than 500 per year (Figure 3–D–1).

The primary breast cancer cases of DCIS was less than 15% in 62% of the institutes (Figure 3–D–2a), and cases of lobular carcinoma, including noninvasive and invasive carcinoma, were less than 10% in 81% of the institutes. Stage I was 20%–40% of invasive ductal carcinoma in 60% of the institutes, stage II was 20%–40% in 73% of institutes, and stage III was less than 20% in 82% of institutes (Figure 3–D–2b, Figure 3–D–2c, and Figure 3–D–2d).

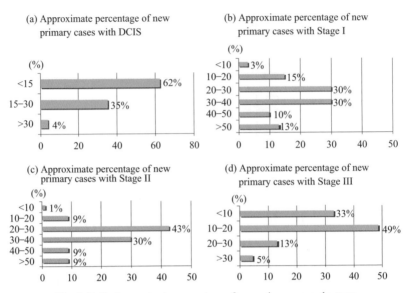

Fig. 3–D–2. Approximate percentage of new primary cases by type

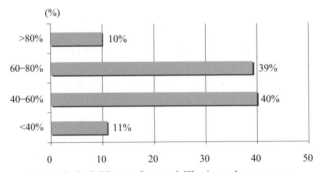

Fig. 3–D–3. BCS rate of stages 0-III primary breast cancer

BCS in Stages 0 to III Primary Breast Cancer

The BCS rate in stages 0 to III primary breast cancer patients of the institutes also varied. In half of the institutes, BCS rate was less than 60%, and in the other half, it was more than 60% (Figure 3–D–3). In 10% of the institutes, BCS was performed in more than 80% of stage 0 to III primary breast cancer; and in 11% of the institutes, BCS was performed in less than 40%.

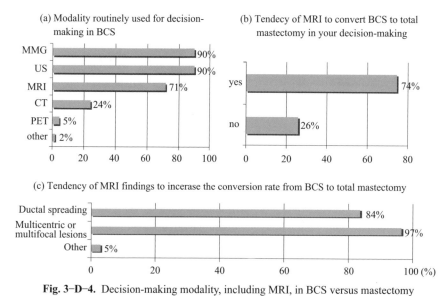

(a) Modality routinely used for decision-making in BCS

(b) Tendecy of MRI to convert BCS to total mastectomy in your decision-making

(c) Tendency of MRI findings to incerase the conversion rate from BCS to total mastectomy

Fig. 3–D–4. Decision-making modality, including MRI, in BCS versus mastectomy

Modality Used for Decision Making in BCS

Most of the respondents routinely used mammography and ultrasonography for decision making in BCS (Figure 3–D–4a). Contrast-enhanced magnetic resonance imaging (MRI) was used by 71% of the respondents. Computed tomography and positron emission tomography generally were not used for decision making in BCS. Almost 74% of the respondents thought that MRI tended to convert BCS to total mastectomy (Figure 3–D–4b). The major reasons for this conversion were multicentric or multifocal lesions and ductal spreading found in MRI (Figure 3–D–4c).

Safety Cut Margin and Definition of Margin Involvement

The safety cut margin commonly used in BCS for invasive ductal carcinoma was diverse among the respondents, with 19% of the respondents using less than 5 mm for the safety cut margin in BCS, 34% using 5 mm–10 mm, and 38% with 10 mm–20 mm (Figure 3–D–5a). Only 9% of the respondents chose more than 20 mm as the safety cut margin.

Definition of margin involvement also was diverse among the respondents to this questionnaire, with 35% of the respondents defining tumor as extending

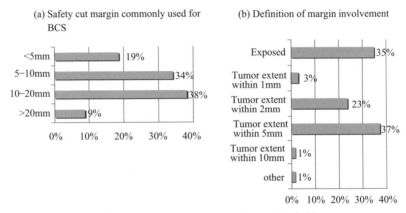

(a) Safety cut margin commonly used for BCS

(b) Definition of margin involvement

Fig. 3‒D‒5. Safety cut margin —— Use and definition

to the margin of the tissue (tumor on ink), 24% of them defining tumor extent within 2 mm, and 37% within 5 mm, as margin involvement (Figure 3‒D‒5b).

Risk Factors for Local Recurrence after BCS in Invasive Ductal Carcinoma

In this questionnaire, we picked up seven factors, which might relate to risk of local recurrence after BCS in invasive ductal carcinoma: young age (for example, less than 40 years old), histologic high grade, lymphatic invasion, margin status, presence of lobular carcinoma in situ (LCIS), ER negativity, and extended intraductal spread. Most of the respondents thought that margin status was one of the risk factors for local recurrence after BSC in invasive duct carcinoma, and about 60% of respondents thought lymphatic invasion, extended intraductal spread, young age, and histologic high grade as risk factors for local recurrence (Figure 3‒D‒6a). Presence of LCIS and ER negativity were not regarded as significant risk factors for local recurrence in invasive ductal carcinoma.

Risk Factors for Local Recurrence After BCS in Ductal Carcinoma in Situ

For DCIS, we picked up six risk factors in this questionnaire; young age (for example, less than forty years old), histologic high grade, margin status, presence of LCIS, ER negativity, and tumor size. Almost all of the respondents

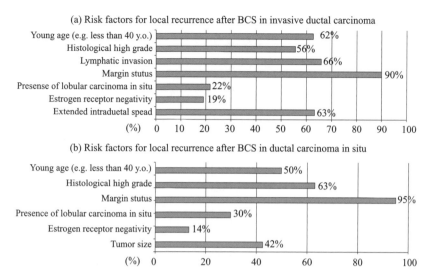

Fig. 3–D–6. Local recurrence risk factors after breast-conserving surgery (BCS)

chose margin status as a risk factor for local recurrence after BCS in DCIS (Figure 3–D–6b). Histologic grade, young age, and tumor size were also considered as risk factors for local recurrence in DCIS. However, presence of LCIS, and ER negativity were not regarded as significant risk factors for local recurrence in DCIS.

Type of Surgery Recommended for Primary Breast Cancer with BRCA1/2 Abnormality

Of all the risk factors, hereditary breast cancer carrying the BRCA1/2 abnormality is an independent risk factor because of its significantly high incidence in contralateral breast cancer and ipsilateral recurrence compared with its incidence in sporadic cancer.[5,6] However, the availability of BRCA testing in the institutes of the respondents was relatively low. More than 60% of the respondents cannot perform BRCA testing in their own institutes (Figure 3–D–7a). Under this constraint, the opinions of the respondents about the types of surgery recommended to the breast cancer patients with BRCA1/2 abnormality were completely concordant (Figure 3–D–7b).

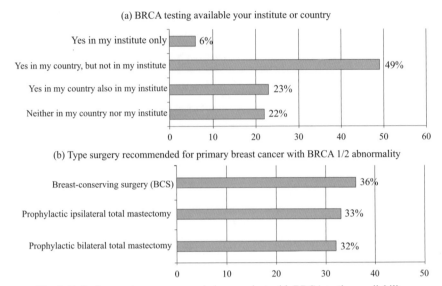

(a) BRCA testing available your institute or country

(b) Type surgery recommended for primary breast cancer with BRCA 1/2 abnormality

Fig. 3–D–7. Surgery type recommended concordant with BRCA testing availability

Future Studies for Consensus on Optimal Breast Surgery

According to the questionnaire results, a variety of opinions exists about the optimal local management of breast cancer surgery. Several critical research questions on a range of issues therefore emerged at the conference, the eventual answers to which will assist in the ongoing pursuit and development of a medical consensus. These questions included:

1. What is the optimal safety cut margin for BCS either for invasive ductal carcinoma or for DCIS?
2. Is MRI necessary for decision making for BCS?
3. Is it necessary to change safety cut margin for BCS according to risk factors for local recurrence after BCS?
4. Which treatment, re-excision, or boost irradiation is necessary according margin status?
5. Is it necessary to change treatment according to risk factors, except for margin status of local recurrence after BCS?
6. Is prophylactic mastectomy inevitable for the patients with BRCA1/2 abnormality?

To answer these questions, large-scale outcome studies with long-term follow-up are necessary. Surgery for breast cancer started with the paradigm that scientists and physician viewed breast cancer as a local disease that could be surgically treated, and it then shifted to another paradigm that viewed breast cancer as a systemic disease requiring systemic treatment.

In 1993 an editorial in *The Lancet* posed the question about breast cancer: 'Have we lost our way?',[4] to which it answered, 'yes'. The journal's response was based on breast cancer mortality figures that were holding steady, instead of dropping significantly. The editorial challenged researchers to submit abstracts of innovative research for an April 1994 conference in Belgium, titled 'The Challenge of Breast Cancer'.[5] Since then, a new paradigm has emerged that considers breast cancer as a biological process, inducing biomarker and molecular targeting therapy. The use of anti-angiogenesis drugs is one of the strategies in this new paradigm. The relationship between local management and systemic treatment should be considered in this new paradigm.

Chapter 4

Pathology

Histopathologic Prognostic Factors of Early Breast Cancer

Yoshiki Mikami and Hironobu Sasano

Summary

A review of histopathologic prognostic and predictive factors in breast cancer reveals problems and debates surrounding evaluation of these factors in a practical clinical setting. Optimal combination of factors, such as node status, tumor size, histologic grade and type, lymphovascular invasion, morphologic features, hormone receptor status, gene status of the human epidermal growth factor receptor 2 (HER2), Ki-67 labeling index, basal-like phenotype, and response to neoadjuvant chemotherapy, may help to identify high and low risks determining breast cancers. But for cancers with an intermediate risk, novel approaches such as molecular grading based on multiple gene assays will be needed.

Introduction: Reviewing the Factors

About 20%–30% of patients with node-negative breast carcinoma will have a recurrence or die of the disease.[1,2] Indications by clinicians for adjuvant chemotherapy are therefore based on prognostic and predictive factors provided by histopathologic examination of tumors. On the one hand, the prognostic factor represents information for assessing probability of patient outcome. On the other hand, the predictive factor provides information on the likelihood of the patient's response to therapeutic modalities. There are a variety of tumor-related prognostic and predictive factors identified in the literature.[3] At present, traditional histopathologic features that include axillary lymph node status, tumor size, histologic grade, histologic type, and peritumoral vascular invasion are widely accepted for assessment of prognosis and likelihood of therapeutic response (Table 4–1).[3] In addition, status of hormone receptors and human

Table 4-1. Tumor-related prognostic factors of breast carcinomas*

Essential	• Nodal status • Tumor size • Histologic grade • Histologic type • Mitotic figure count • Hormone receptor (ER/PR) status • Effect of tumor recurrence or metastatsis after primary therapy
Additional	• HER2-neu (c-erbB2) • Peritumoral vascular invasion • Ki-67 labeling index • S-phase fraction by flow cytometry • P53 gene expression
New & promising factors	• Cytokeratin staining of histologicly negative axillary lymph nodes • DNA ploidy • Angiogenesis • EGFR/TGFα • bcl-2 • pS2 • Apoptosis

*This table is modified from: International Union Against Cancer [UICC], *Prognostic Factors in Cancer,* 2nd ed.[3]

epidermal growth factor receptor 2 (HER2) are considered to be important predictive factors. In this section, representative histopathologic prognostic and predictive factors are reviewed, with emphasis on problems and controversies regarding evaluation of these factors in a practical setting.

Node Status

Axillary lymph node metastasis is the single most important prognostic factor in patients with breast cancer.[4-7] Accumulated data indicate that the absolute number of positive nodes has an impact on patient outcome. Relapse-free survival and overall survival are lowered for patients with four or more involved nodes, compared with those with one to three involved nodes. The prognosis is substantially worse for those with ten or more axillary nodal metastasis. About 70% of patients with axillary node metastases will develop recurrence within ten years, compared with 20%–30% of those with negative nodes, in the absence of adjuvant systemic therapy. In node-positive cases, the pathology report should include number of nodal metastasis, size of metastatic deposits, and presence or absence of perinodal fat invasion.[7] The perinodal fat invasion has been shown to indicate an increased risk for recurrence,[8] but some studies of cases controlled for extent of axillary involvement,[9] including microscopic extranodal extension,[10] does not necessarily support this view.

Following the current American Joint Committee on Cancer (AJCC)/Union Internationale Contre le Cancer (UICC) staging classification,[11,12] presence of isolated tumor cells (ITC) — measuring 0.2 mm or less — is regarded as node negative and designated as pN0(i +), while metastasis measuring 0.2 to 2 mm is micrometastasis and designated as pN1mi. Micrometastasis and ITC are found in 10%–20%, and 1%–2%, respectively,[13] of apparently 'node-negative' cases by serial tissue section and/or cytokeratin immunohistochemistry (IHC). The significance of such microscopic metastasis remains undetermined,[14–16] and recent studies have shown conflicting results regarding its impact on disease-free survival and/or overall survival. Based on a study of a cohort of 214 consecutive histologically node-negative cases with a median follow-up of eight years, Harriette J. Kahn and colleagues demonstrated that cytokeratin-positive occult micrometastases, as defined by the AJCC/UICC system, were identified in 14% of cases, and were not significantly associated with disease-free interval or disease-specific survival.[13] In this particular study, 95% of patients did not receive adjuvant chemotherapy. However, Steven L. Chen and colleagues, analyzing data retrieved from the surveillance, epidemiology, and end-results (SEER) database, reported that nodal micrometastasis of breast cancer carries an intermediate prognosis between N0 and N1 disease, even after adjusting for tumor- and patient-related factors.[17] Based on a cohort study of 856 patients with ITC or micrometastases, who had not received systemic adjuvant therapy, and 995 patients with ITC or micrometastases, who had received such treatment, with a median follow-up of 5.1 years, Maaike de Boer and colleagues recently demonstrated that ITC or micrometastases in regional lymph nodes were associated with a reduced five-year disease-free survival among women with favorable early-stage breast cancer in the absence of adjuvant therapy, and that in patients with ITC or micrometastases, who received adjuvant therapy, disease-free survival was improved.[18]

The presence of more than one focus of ITC may also provoke a diagnostic problem. The substantial number of ITC throughout one lymph nodes might be regarded as pN1, rather than ITC or micrometastasis, by some pathologists,[19] although the definition of 'substantial' is arbitrary. Therefore, the definition and significance of micrometastasis and ITC are still matters of controversy. From a practical viewpoint, routine use of cytokeratin immunohistochemistry and/or serial section may not be justified, and the College of American Pathologists (CAP) notes that a single microscopic hematoxylin and eosin (H&E) stained section from each lymph node block is considered sufficient for evaluation of both sentinel and nonsentinel lymph node status.[7] The significance of ITC identified by molecular study using reverse transcription-polymerase chain reaction (RT-PCR), which detects messenger ribonucleic acid (m-RNA) for cytokeratins, mucin 1 (MUC1), mammoglobin, or carcinoembryonic antigen, is still limited. Although the technique appears highly sensitive, further studies are awaiting to confirm the clinical impact of these sophisticated, but expensive, analyses.

Tumor Size

Tumor size is a powerful independent prognostic factor among both node-negative and node-positive patients. In cases of tumor measuring 1 cm or less (pT1a and pT1b), incidence of axillary node metastasis is 10%–20%,[20,21] ten-year disease-free survival is up to 90%,[21–23] and death occurs in less than 2% of node-negative cases. Significant relationship between tumor size, node status, and prognosis even among pT1 patients also has been reported.[24] Melvin J. Silverstein and colleagues reported that in cases of pT1a tumors measuring 5 mm or less, incidence of axillary lymph node metastasis is 3%, whereas in cases of pT1b tumors measuring 6 mm–10 mm, the incidence is 17%.[25] Therefore, they concluded that axillary lymph node dissection may be avoided in cases of grade I or II and pT1a tumors. According to a 1990 National Institutes of Health (NIH) consensus recommendation,[26] neoadjuvant chemotherapy (NAC) is avoided in node-negative patients with tumors measuring less than 1 cm, and is considered in cases of tumors exceeding 3 cm. Indication for NAC is controversial in the case of node-negative tumors measuring 1 cm–3 cm.

Precise assessment of tumor size is mandatory to properly stratify patients for treatment purposes, particularly in cases of pT1 cancer. However, gross examination more frequently underestimates tumor size in pT1 tumors than in tumors larger than 2 cm. Highly infiltrating carcinoma, such as invasive lobular carcinoma, is a problem, because the extent of invasion cannot be well appreciated on both gross inspection and imaging studies. Results of gross and microscopic examination should be combined together to evaluate the exact size of a tumor. The tumor should be submitted intact for examination to get the largest dimension.[7] Confirmation by microscopic examination is mandatory, because the macroscopic tumor size is equal to the microscopic size in only 22% of cases.[27] The pathologic T (pT) factor should be determined by the largest diameter of an invasive component, excluding ductal carcinoma in situ (DCIS) or lobular carcinoma in situ (LCIS).[7,11] In the case of a multiple foci of invasion, independent foci should be measured separately,[7] with the largest size determining the pT factor. However, some studies have shown that the aggregate size of multiple invasive foci more accurately predicts the number

Table 4–2. Modified Scarff-Bloom-Richardson system, or Nottingham combined histologic score*

Microscopic features	DOES THIS NEED HEAD ING??	??	Score
Tubular formation			
• Majority of tumor (>75%)			1
• Moderate degree (10%–75%)			2
• Little or none (<10%)			3
Nuclear pleomorphism			
• Small, regular uniform cells			1
• Moderate increase in size and variability			2
• Marked variation			3
Mitotic counts			
• Dependent on microscope field area (x40, Nikon)	0–5		1
	6–10		2
	>11		3
Score, category of grade, and definition			
3-5 points, grade I: Well differentiated			
6-7 points, grade II: Moderately differentiated			
8-9 points, grade III: Poorly differentiated			

*The Nottingham combined histologic score was developed by Elston and Ellis, who modified and improved the Scarff-Bloom-Richardson system.

of positive nodes,[28] and that presence of multiple invasive foci is associated with higher frequency of lymph node metastasis.[29]

Histologic Grade

Histologic grade is an important determinant of prognosis, allowing risk stratification.[30–37] It correlates with disease-free survival, overall survival, and recurrence, even among patients with pT1a/1b carcinoma. In addition, higher grade indicates likelihood of response to chemotherapy. Some special types are partially defined by grade. For example, tubular carcinoma and medullary carcinoma are by definition grade I and grade III, respectively.

Currently, the most widespread and clinically used grading scheme is the modified Scarff-Bloom-Richardson (SBR) system (Table 4–2),[33] also called the Nottingham combined histologic score, which employs tubular formation, nuclear pleomorphism, and mitotic count for grading (Figure 4–1). In this system, when tubules are present in more than 75% of areas, the

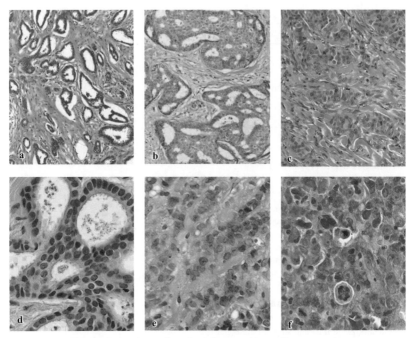

Fig. 4–1. Tubular formation and nuclear pleomorphism of breast carcinomas

(a) Well-formed tubules occupying more than 75% is assigned a value of 1.

(b) In case of 10%–75% showing tubular formation, a value of 2 is assigned.

(c) At less than 10%, a value of 3 is assigned.

(d) Nuclear score 1 indicates small and regular uniform nuclei without prominent nucleoli.

(e) Nuclear score 2 indicates intermediate degree of heterogeneity in nuclear size and shape.

(f) Nuclear score 3 indicates marked nuclear pleomorphism with conpicuous eosinophilic nuclei.

tubular formation is assigned a value of 1, and when it is less than 10%, the value is 3. When nuclei are small, regular, and uniform in appearance, the nuclear pleomorphism is assigned a value of 1, and when nuclei show marked heterogeneity in shape and size, and the nucleoli is conspicuous, the value is 3. The two values of tubular formation and nuclear pleomorphism are then added to the mitotic count value ranging from 1 to 3, and together produce numerical scores ranging 3 to 9, to determine the final grade. Tumors with total scores of 3 to 5 are categorized as grade I, those with scores of 6 and 7 are grade II, and those with scores of 8 and 9 are grade III. It should be noted that mitotic count value must be adjusted, based on the field diameter of the microscope's objective lens.

The modified SBR system has been confirmed to be valid by a couple of follow-up outcome studies. The assigned grade accurately predicts the prognosis outcome for the patient. Overall survival is significantly decreased among patients with grade III carcinomas compared with those with grade I

Table 4–3. Ten-year survival and histologic type and grade (MSBR system)

	Overall (%)	Grade I (%)	Grade II (%)	Grade -III (%)
Invasive ductal carcinoma, NST	46	76	55	39
Classical lobular carcinoma	53	71	55	38
Mucinous carcinoma	81	86	75	NONE*
Tubular carcinoma	90	90	NONE**	NONE**
Medullary carcinoma	51	NONE***	NONE***	51

MSBR – Modified Scarff-Bloom-Richardson. NST – Nonspecific type. *Mucinous carcinoma is not by definition grade III. **Tubular carcinoma is by definition grade I. ***Mudullar carcinoma is by definition grade III.
Source: Pereira, H., Pinder, S. E., Sibbering, D. M., et al. (1995).[38]

tumors.[37] Importantly, the grade can be a determinant of prognosis in some special-type carcinomas (Table 4–3).[38] Ten-year survival among patients with grade I, II, and III invasive ductal carcinoma of nonspecific type is 76%, 55%, and 39%, respectively, and grade I, II, and III classical invasive lobular carcinoma shows the same trend. Mucinous carcinoma, although generally considered to be low grade, can be grade II with a decreased survival rate, compared with grade I mucinous carcinomas. Tubular carcinoma is by definition grade I and thus survival is about 90%, better than grade I nonspecific-type invasive ductal carcinomas. However, medullary carcinoma is by definition grade III, but the ten-year survival rate is 51%, still better than grade III nonspecific-type invasive ductal carcinoma, indicating that grade and histologic type are 'good friends'. A problem with grading is interobserver variation, in other word, reproducibility. Although the kappa value in assigning tubular formation is 0.64 (substantial), kappa for nuclear grade and mitotic count is 0.40 (near moderate) and 0.52 (moderate), respectively.[39] Agreement on mitotic count is moderate.[39] Agreement on overall modified Scarff-Bloom-Richardson grade appears generally good. The reported kappa is 0.70[40] and 0.73,[41] but one study demonstrated a kappa of 0.43,[42] indicating moderate agreement. Therefore, the grading appears to have some limitations. In fact, the grade II category is still a heterogeneous group of neoplasms in terms of prognosis.

Recent studies have demonstrated a significance of 'molecular grading'. Expression profile of genes involved in cell-cycle regulation and proliferation may well divide patients with grade II tumor into high-risk and low-risk groups showing different outcome.[43] A variety of molecular assays, such as the 21-gene recurrence score (Oncotype DX™) and the 70-gene prognostic signature (MammaPrint®), are currently available, with some promising usefulness in determining an indication for chemotherapy.[44]

Table 4–4. Diagnostic group by histologic type and grade

Excellent prognostic group (10-year survival, >80%)	• Tubular carcinoma (grade 1) • Mixed tubular carcinoma (grade 1) • Invasive cribriform carcinoma (grade 1) • Mixed ductal NST/special type (grade 1) • Mixed ductal NST/lobular carcinoma (grade 1) • Mucinous carcinoma (grade 1) • Tubulolobular carcinoma (grade 1)
Good prognostic group (10-year survival, 60%–80%)	• Ductal carcinoma, NST (grade 1) • Classical lobular carcinoma (grade 1) • Mixed lobular carcinoma (grade 1) • Alveolar lobular carcinoma (grade 2) • Solid lobular carcinoma (grade 2) • Mucinous carcinoma (grade 2) • Tubular carcinoma, mixed (grade 1) • Atypical medullary carcinoma (grade 2)
Moderate prognostic group (10-year survival, 50%–60%)	Mixed ductal NST/special type (grade 2, grade 3) Ductal carcinoma, NST (grade 2) Mixed ductal NST/special type (grade 2) Classical lobular carcinoma (grade 2) Mixed lobular carcinoma (grade 2) Medullary carcinoma (grade 3) Invasive papillary carcinoma (NA)
Poor prognostic group (10-year survival, <50%)	Ductal carcinoma,NST (grade 3) Classical lobular carcinoma (grade 3) Mixed lobular carcinoma (grade 3) Mixed ductal NST/lobular carcinoma (grade 3) Solid lobular carcinoma (grade 3) Mixed tubular carcinoma (grade 3)

NST – Nonspecific type.
Source: Pereira, H., Pinder, S. E., Sibbering, D. M., et al. (1995).[38]

Histologic Type

Histologic tumor type is also a vital factor, although grade and tumor size are more important in cases of infiltrating ductal carcinoma of nonspecific type. Special-type carcinomas are of a mostly favorable histology, with a lower frequency of lymph node metastasis (resulting in overall improved survival of the patient), but may be combined with grade. A strict criteria should be used when making the diagnosis, so as to keep the clinical significance of each special type. In general, defining histology should occupy more than 90% of tumor area (the '90% rule'). Representative favorable histology includes tubular carcinoma, invasive cribriform carcinoma, mucinous carcinoma, and adenoid cystic carcinoma.[21,38,45,46] Marked nuclear pleomorphism, if present in these histologic types, does not justify the diagnosis. Table 4–4 summarizes a prognostic group by histologic type.[38] Nonspecific infiltrating ductal carcinoma is included in the 'poor' prognostic group showing ten-year survival at less than 50%, whereas classical invasive lobular carcinoma is included in the 'moderate' prognostic group with ten-year survival ranging 50%–60%. However, grade I nonspecific infiltrating ductal carcinoma is included in the 'good' prognostic group, with ten-year survival at 60%–80%. Grade I classical invasive lobular carcinoma is included in the 'good' prognostic group, whereas at grade III, the prognosis for patients with this carcinoma is 'poor'. However, grade II alveolar variant of invasive lobular carcinoma and grade II solid variant of lobular carcinoma also are included in the 'good' prognostic group. Therefore, all invasive carcinomas, except tubular carcinoma and medullary carcinoma, should be graded.[7]

Lymphovascular Invasion

Some studies have demonstrated that peritumoral vascular invasion correlates with loco-regional lymph node status,[47,48] early recurrence in N0 patients,[49] local recurrence after breast-conserving therapy,[50] and distant metastasis.[51] Overall survival also is lowered in the presence of peritumoral lymphovascular invasion.[24,48,52] The distinction between lymphatic vessels and blood vessels is occasionally difficult, but is not necessarily needed, because its clinical significance is shown to be negligible.[7] Therefore, just the term lymphovascular invasion (LVI) is acceptable. It is actually rather rare to see tumor emboli in blood vessels with muscular wall, and LVI mostly represents lymphatic invasion.[47] Retraction artifact —— that is, formation of spaces surrounding tumor nests due to tissue processing —— should be distinguished from LVI using strict criteria. The different criteria may explain considerable variation in the frequency of LVI reported in the literature, ranging 20%–54%. Ancillary techniques such as D2-40 immunostaining for podoplanin, which decorates lymphatic endothelial cells, may be helpful in recognizing lymphatic invasion,[53] but its routine use is not necessarily recommended, and there is no consensus on the need for special staining. LVI in the skin should be specifically reported because of increased risk of skin recurrence and metastasis.

Miscellaneous Morphologic Features

There are some other morphologic features indicating aggressiveness of invasive breast carcinomas. Some studies showed that coagulative tumor necrosis is a predictor of time to recurrence, and has impact on overall survival.[54] However, there is controversy on how we define and quantify the necrosis. Essentially, the necrosis may reflect estrogen receptor (ER)/ progesterone receptor (PR)/human epidermal growth factor receptor 2 (HER2) status, histologic grade, and growth rate. In fact, a substantial number of high-grade triple-negative carcinomas with basal-like phenotype show extensive coagulative tumor necrosis.

Fibrotic focus was first described by Takahiro Hasebe and co-workers in Japan in 1996.[55] It is characterized by a central acellular zone composed of hyalinized collagen in cases of invasive ductal carcinoma. They showed that overall survival rate is lowered in the presence of a fibrotic focus among patients with node-negative ER-positive invasive ductal carcinoma.

Significance of tumor-infiltrating lymphocytes has been investigated, with conflicting results,[56–59] although intensity of infiltrating T-cells appears to correlate with prognosis,[56,58,59] particularly among younger patients at less than 40 years of age.[60]

Hormone Receptor Status

ER and PR status represents a weak prognostic factor, but is the strongest predictive factor for the response of patients to hormonal therapy.[42,61–63] Therefore, ER and PR assays, mostly IHC performed on paraffin sections, are an essential component in the current standard of practice.[7] However, there has been controversy on assessment of the receptor status.[64] In many institutions, rate of positive cells has been noted in the pathology report, but H-score evaluating both distribution and intensity also has been used.[65] The Allred score, also evaluating both distribution and intensity of positive cells, may be a solution, because it is rather simple and user friendly, and has validation data based on patient outcome.[42] Cutoff for positivity has been a problem. One study showed significant difference in criteria for positivity among institutions, and there is a concern that a substantial minority of tumors are erroneously regarded as ER-negative.

The Allred score is determined by proportion and staining intensity of positive cells.[61] Based on reference illustration, proportion is graded as 0, 1, 2, 3, 4, or 5, and staining intensity is graded as 0, 1, 2, or 3. These values are added together to produce the score, ranging from 0 to 8.[61] Follow-up study of patients treated with adjuvant endocrine therapy has demonstrated that the score 3 is considered to be minimal cutoff for positivity, indicating the view that only more than 1% of weakly positive cells, that is with a score of 2(proportion score) + 1(intensity score) = 3, are considered to be positive.[42,61] This fact supports the NIH consensus conference recommendation that any ER staining in a tumor should be sufficient to consider a patient eligible for endocrine therapy.[66] Regarding an indication for chemotherapy, however, different cutoffs might be required in women with ER-positive tumors.[67]

Human Epidermal Growth Factor Receptor 2 Gene Status

HER2-neu is the gene encoding for the transmembrane protein p185, which is HER2, or human epidermal growth factor receptor 2. Previously, overexpression of HER2, identified in 15%–20% of breast cancers, was recognized as a prognostic factor in both node-negative and node-positive patients, but is now widely accepted as a predictive factor for the response of patients to chemotherapy, anti-endocrine agents, and more importantly, anti-HER2 agents, such as trastuzumab (Herceptin®). In the current standard, IHC is the first-line test to assess HER2 status of patients in most institutions, and in cases of equivocal IHC results, evaluation of gene amplification using fluorescence in situ hybridization (FISH) is recommended. American Society of Clinical Oncology (ASCO) and CAP recently have established a guideline recommendation regarding standardized assessment of HER2 status.[68] In this guideline, positive immunoreactivity is defined as uniform intense membranous staining of more than 30% of invasive tumor cells. Intermediate staining intensity is regarded as equivocal and needs confirmation by tests with validated assay for gene amplification. Uniform intense membranous staining in 10%–30% of tumor cells, previously regarded as positive, also is regarded as equivocal to minimize false-positive cases. In addition, the importance of specimen handling and tissue processing, including type of fixative and fixation time, is emphasized in this guideline.

Despite the concordance rate between FISH and IHC assays, reaching to about 90%, accumulated data indicate gene amplification, rather than protein expression, better determines a patient's response to trastuzumab with or without chemotherapy. Up to 10% of patients may have false-negative or false-positive IHC results, and miss receiving the therapy or are erroneously classified as candidates for the treatment, which is associated with increased risk of cardiotoxicity and unnecessary substantial treatment costs.[69] Therefore, the primary FISH might be justified, based on the balance of costs for FISH and trastuzumab.[69]

Ki-67 Labeling Index

Ki-67 is a protein expressed in the gap1 (G1), DNA synthesis (S), gap2 (G2), and mitosis (M) phases of the cell cycle. Therefore, IHC using anti-Ki-67 antibody can be used to assess cell proliferation. Ki-67 measurement, combined with a variety of factors such as hormone receptor status, has prognostic value for patients with node-negative cancer,[70,71] and those treated with preoperative chemotherapy (PCT) or endocrine therapy.[72–75] In addition, Ki-67 labeling index may predict a better response to PCT[76–78] and aromatase inhibitor.[79,80] Russell Burcombe and colleagues demonstrated that tumors displaying more than 75% reduction in Ki-67 index after chemotherapy were more likely to achieve a pathologic response.[81] Valentina Guarneri and colleagues reported that PCT induced a significant reduction in the expression of Ki-67, and that by multivariable model, Ki-67 index greater than or equal to 15% and nodal positivity after PCT were significant predictors of worse disease-free survival.[72] Cecilia Ahlin and colleagues also demonstrated that the optimal cutoff value average was 15% and the maximum value was 22%.[71] J. Lee and colleagues demonstrated that the post-treatment ER status and Ki-67 proliferation index were prognostic of overall survival following neoadjuvant adriamycin/docetaxel chemotherapy.[73] Mitch Dowsett and colleagues found that higher Ki-67 expression after two weeks of endocrine therapy was statistically significantly associated with lower recurrence-free survival, whereas higher Ki-67 expression before PCT was not.[75]

However, some studies failed to demonstrate utility of the Ki-67 labeling index,[82–84] and thus the issue is still controversial. Robin L Jones and colleagues showed that the Ki-67 level, ER status, HER2 status, and histologic grade of the tumor before PCT were associated with a complete pathologic response, but in a multivariable model, HER2 was the only significant predictor, and no significant relationship was demonstrated between pre-therapy Ki-67 and relapse-free survival and overall survival.[82] Therefore, Ki-67 does not appear to be an independent predictor of complete response. Giuseppe Viale and colleagues also showed that a high Ki-67 labeling index was associated with factors that predict poor prognosis, but that the index failed to predict the relative efficacy of chemoendocrine therapy compared with endocrine therapy alone. They concluded that the Ki-67 labeling index is an independent prognostic factor, but is not predictive of a patient's better response to adjuvant chemotherapy.[83] Ander Urruticoechea and colleagues suggested that high Ki-67 level indicates an ominous prognosis and simultaneously a good chance of clinical response to chemotherapy, but the impact of Ki-67 index appears to be

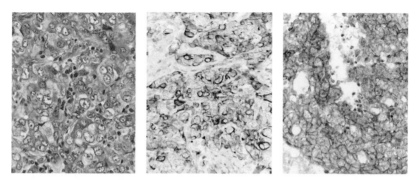

Fig. 4–2. Triple negative carcinoma with basal-like phenotype
(a) Solid growth of cells with marked nuclear pleomorphism and increased mitotic figures.
(b) Mitotic figures showing immunoreactivity for cytokeratin (CK) 5/6.
(c) Mitotic figures showing immunoreactivity for epidermal growth factor receptor (EGFR).

rather modest, and thus does not merit routine use as an indicator.[85]

There are some problems to be solved regarding Ki-67 measurements, including standardization of methodology for staining, and interobserver variability. Although the index is expected to be used as a means of eligibility for PCT or chemoendocrine therapy, absence of consensus regarding method of evaluation, reporting, and more importantly, cutoff preclude the incorporation of Ki-67 staining in a routine histopathologic evaluation.[44]

Basal-like Phenotype

Gene expression profiling has provided molecular classification and has demonstrated the existence of basal-like breast carcinomas.[86] Although concordance between molecular classification and conventional assessment of morphology and ER/PR/HER2 status is not complete, some surrogate markers appear promising. Basal-like carcinomas can be well recognized using cytokeratin 5/6 (CK5/6) and epidermal growth factor receptor (EGFR) staining among triple negative cancers (Figure 4–2).[87] Some studies have demonstrated that the basal-like phenotype has prognostic impact,[88,89] and that this phenotype significantly predicts decreased survival within the moderate Nottingham prognostic index group.[90] Interestingly, earlier studies before the era of gene profiling suggested an aggressive nature of vimentin-positive breast carcinomas, which is considered to represent basal-like breast carcinomas.[91] Therefore, a battery of markers evaluated by the IHC technique is considered to be useful to stratify breast carcinomas.

Histopathologic Evaluation of Response to Neoadjuvant Chemotherapy

Response to PCT has been considered to be a prognostic indicator, and thus various methods have been proposed for this purpose,[92-99] although each has advantages and disadvantages. In fact, there are some difficulties in evaluating therapeutic effects after NAC. Information obtained by image studies is important, but assessment of microscopic features is a gold standard. From a pathologic point of view, cellularity, which is the ratio of carcinoma cells to stromal cells, is a vital component for precise evaluation. Therefore, pathologists are encouraged to evaluate both pre- and post-NAC specimen.

Two tumors with a similar decrease in tumor size may show markedly different changes in cellularity after NAC.[100] For example, One tumor decreased from 2.0 cm to 1.8 cm and showed an increase in cellularity from 70% on the pretreatment core needle biopsy to 80% on the post-treatment excision specimen. However, another tumor decreased from 1.7 cm to 1.5 cm and showed a decrease in cellularity from 90% on core needle biopsy to 5% on the post-treatment excision specimen. In this example, the latter is considered to be more chemosensitive, compared with the former. This particular example well illustrates the importance of evaluating cellularity.

The Miller-Pane grading system defines a patient's response to NAC, based on a decrease in overall cellularity, ranging from grade 1 and grade 5.[95] Grade 1 indicates no change or some alteration of neoplastic cells without reduction in cellularity, whereas grade 5 indicates no residual invasive carcinoma. These assigned grades correlate well with disease-free and overall survivals. Another eye-catching scheme is the residual cancer burden (RCB) system proposed by Fraser W. Symmans at MD Anderson Cancer Center (MDACC).[96] In this scheme, primary tumor bed area, overall cancer cellularity, percentage of DCIS, number of positive nodes, and diameter of largest metastasis provide a continuous parameter of response, which determines the RCB class, ranging from RCB-0 to RCB-III. RCB-0 and RCB-III indicate pathologic complete response (pCR) and chemoresistance, respectively, and RCB-I and II correspond to pathologic partial response (pPR). On the website at MDACC, a calculator is available for determining the RCB class. The MDACC researchers demonstrated that RCB scores and categories correlate well with patient outcomes after therapy. There is a significant likelihood of distant relapse in cases of RCB-III, compared with RCB-0, I, and II. The differences are much more substantial without additional adjuvant hormone treatment.

Conclusion

Conventional histopathologic prognostic and predictive factors, combined with biomarkers, are informative for recognizing low-risk and high-risk breast carcinomas. Optimal combination of traditional factors, evaluated in a standardized manner, may accurately predict patient outcome and therapeutic response. In fact, the Nottingham prognostic index, determined by tumor size, node status, and histologic grade (modified Scarff-Bloom-Richardson score), has been used to stratify patients into good, moderate, and poor prognostic groups.[101] However, uncertainty in the subset of carcinomas with intermediate-risk necessitates a more novel approach. In this context, molecular grading based on multiple gene assays, such as 21-gene recurrence score (Oncotype DX™) and 70-gene prognostic signature (MammaPrint®), appears promising.

Chapter 5

Genetics - Personal Genomics Data

Personalized Treatment of Breast Cancer: Challenges and Expectations

Dimitrios H. Roukos and Dimosthenis Ziogas

Summary

Advances in molecular oncology and genetics are starting to impact on surgical practice in breast cancer treatment. Despite medical compliance with current guidelines on breast-conserving surgery (BCS) in early breast cancer and for multimodal treatment, a subgroup of patients continues to develop ipsilateral breast cancer (IBC) recurrence and/or contralateral breast cancer (CBC).

In this paper we critique the bio-medical literature on the role and utility of genetic testing for high-risk patients. The objective of this review is to identify the high-risk patients for local failure (IBC and/or CBC), based on genetics and genomics, to assess the impact of chemoradiotherapy and targeted therapy on the risk of IBC/CBC, and to find out which patients might benefit from aggressive surgery such as bilateral mastectomy (BM).

Our methodology involved looking at all published data on these topics from 1995 to 2009 in PubMed at United States of America's (USA) National Library of Medicine, from which data we identified about eighty key references.

Our literature survey reveals that for long-term follow-up of results after breast-conserving multimodal treatment, the rate of IBC/CBC as an isolated event without any evidence of distant metastasis is substantial in a specific subgroup. Preclinical and clinical data reveal that at the highest risk of IBC/CBC are patients with inherited mutations of the breast cancer 1 and 2 susceptibility genes (BRCA1/2). Patients with cancer-causing BRCA1/2 mutations particularly may benefit from BM rather than BCS in survival rates.

For the vast majority of patients, namely those with familial non-BRCA1/2 (BRCA-test negative) cancer or sporadic breast cancer, prediction of local failure risk is currently unfeasible.

It appears that trastuzumab in patients with the human epidermal growth factor receptor 2 (HER2) reduces IBC/CBC rates, but longer follow-up data are

145

required for definitive conclusions.

Extensive genetic studies, including sequencing techniques and, more currently, genome-wide association studies (GWASs), already have identified novel risk alleles with a series of tumor-initiating single-nucleotide polymorphisms (SNPs). The genetic catalogue of genetic alterations contributing to breast carcinogenesis is nearly complete, but next challenges include understanding the functional role of 'cancer' genes and the prediction of biological networks outcomes.

From our review, we conclude that genetic testing of patients with a family history of breast cancer can guide decision making on BCS and BM. In patients testing positive to BRCA1/2 mutations, BM should be considered and discussed with the individual patient. Rapid technological advances provide promises for an accurate identification of high-risk patients, but multiple challenges remain to predict IBC/CBC risk among familial non-BRCA1/2 or sporadic breast cancer and on the application of such predictions to BM.

Introduction: Improving Survival Rates with Genetic Testing

The most common cancer among females worldwide is breast cancer. In the USA, 182,460 women were expected to have a new diagnosis of invasive breast cancer, with 67,770 in situ breast cancers, during 2008.[1] In recent years there has been an incidence decrease in that country, which likely is related to a reduction in the prescribing of estrogen-progesterone agents as hormone replacement therapy (HRT) in postmenopausal women in the general population. A woman's mean lifetime risk for breast cancer ranges 10%–14% in Europe and the USA,[1] but it reaches up to 85% for the small subpopulation of women with inherited BRCA1 and BRCA2 mutations.[2] Genetic testing increasingly is being incorporated into a diagnostic workup of patients with breast cancer and family history, because genetic testing may affect surgical decisions.[3]

Complete resection of the tumor is a standard approach in breast cancer treatment, but the extent to which surgery should be performed in patients with nonmetastatic breast cancer is a hot topic of debate. Limited surgery, like lumpectomy, followed by irradiation not only is a safe oncological procedure, but also improves quality of life, and the patients prefer it. However, despite adherence by hospitals to recent patient guidelines on the selection of candidates for BCS and adjuvant treatment, a substantial proportion of these patients develop a recurrence or a new tumor in the affected or unaffected breast. Apparently, established clinicopathologic risk factors are suboptimal in identifying high-risk patients who might benefit from an aggressive surgery, including BM. Genetic predisposition may play an important role in local failures.

The Importance of Local and Nodal Control

Most research has focused on reducing distant recurrence. Single randomized controlled trials (RCTs) have shown that loco-regional recurrence does not affect overall survival, supporting the theory that breast cancer even at its early stage is a systemic disease.[4] However, a recent meta-analysis conducted by the Early Breast Cancer Trialists' Collaborative Group of seventy-eight RCTs involving about 42,000 patients showed that improved local surgical control at five years resulted in a marked improvement in both breast cancer survival and overall survival at fifteen years.[5] Although current standard adjuvant treatment may further decrease loco-regional recurrence, every effort should be taken to prevent local events without resorting to surgical overtreatment.[9]

It is not surprising therefore that there currently is renewed interest and debate on the optimal extent of surgery for operable breast cancer. The endpoint of a first surgery should be to isolate loco-regional recurrence, as a way of avoiding distant recurrence. Based on their first short-term survival results, most RCTs reveal the importance of using surgery in reducing local events after modern adjuvant treatment, including targeted agents.[7-9] This importance is highlighted by a new trial —— an international collaboration —— by the Breast International Group (BIG), the International Breast Cancer Study Group (IBCSG), and the National Surgical Adjuvant Breast and Bowel Project (NSABP).[10] The accrual goal is 977 patients, suggesting also the degree of the problem. Accordingly, patients with locally recurrent isolated breast cancer undergoing complete surgical resection are randomly assigned to receive chemotherapy or no chemotherapy. Radiation, hormonal therapy, and trastuzumab are given as appropriate, namely according to the patient's hormonal status —— estrogen receptor (ER) and progesterone receptor (PR) —— and HER2 status. The collaborative study will provide important research and clinical information on loco-regional failure.

To prevent these local failures in the affected breast as IBC recurrence or a new tumor and in the unaffected breast as CBC, a rapidly growing number of breast cancer patients in the USA choose a more aggressive surgery than the current preferred BCS. The Surveillance, Epidemiology and End Results (SEER) Program database shows that the rate of contralateral prophylactic mastectomy (CPM) has increased by 150% in five years[11] (Table 5–1).

Table 5–1. Current change in extent of surgery for localized breast cancer toward more aggressive surgery in USA-SEER Program data

Surgery	1998 (%)	2003 (%)
BCS	56.1	59.7
UM	42.0	35.9
CPM	4.2	11.0

SEER–Surveillance, Epidemiology and End Results. BCS–Breast-conserving surgery. UM–Unilateral mastectomy. CPM–Contralateral prophylactic mastectomy.
Source: Data is from Tuttle, T. M., Habermann, E. B., Grund, E. H., et al.[11]

However, this apparent surgical overtreatment may be contrary to the evidence-based approach of health professionals, and may harm patients, society, and health insurances.[12]

Stratifying breast cancer patients before surgery into high, moderate, and low risk for local failure would have important and beneficial implications. For example, patients with a high risk of local failure may benefit from an extensive surgery, such as BM. However, this risk assessment is currently difficult or, for most patients, unfeasible. Multiple variables, including conventional clinicopathologic factors, biological genetic tumor profile, and current adjuvant systemic treatment, may affect local failure.[5–9,13] Thus, there is an urgent need for markers to predict both local failure and response, so as to tailor the best treatment for preventing local events.

Personalized oncology is a major goal for maximizing the benefits and minimizing the adverse effects in each individual patient.[17] The completion of the Human Genome Project in 2001, cheaper high-throughput deoxyribonucleic acid (DNA) sequencing techniques, and microarray technology allow simultaneous examination of thousands of genes and proteins. Genetic variants can now be identified more effectively, but the clinical utility of the discoveries has not been determined yet. Differences in genetic variation in both the coding and noncoding portions of our DNA make each of us unique, and also can contribute to our personalized susceptibility to the disease. The catalogue, or atlas, of genes involved in the initiation of breast cancer is nearing completion, but this is only the first step in the personalized management of breast cancer, and much more research work, including functional studies, is needed.[15] The recent completion of the HapMap II project, which characterizes more than 3.1 million SNPs,[16] allows for the searching of SNPs involved in human disorders. Over the past year, a series of GWASs correlating human genetic variation with various complex diseases provide exciting findings for a person's genome profile and the risk of developing a disease. Human genetic variants are separated into qualitative differences in the genome (in the form of SNPs) and quantitative differences, such as structural genomic variants (deletions and duplications), which result in copy number variants (CNVs).[17-19] Most recently, GWASs have identified low-penetrance genes with novel genetic variation, or SNPs, associated with increased risk of breast cancer[20-22] and other common cancer types.[23,24]

Local Recurrence and Contralateral Breast Cancer: Factors and Mechanisms

Several host-related factors, tumor characteristics, and treatment regimen affect local failures. The degree to which these parameters increase or decrease the rate of IBC/CBC varies. Several classic factors, including patient's age, family history, histologic features, surgical margins, and adjuvant treatment, have been reported to affect local recurrence or CBC.[6-9] Lately, new data on the impact of cancer genetics,[2,12] breast cancer subtypes based on gene-expression profiles[28,29], and current targeted agents[6-9] on local failures have become available and should all be considered in patient treatment regimen. For example, it seems that the current standard agents — trastuzumab, and tamoxifen or aromatase, inhibitors for HER2-positive and hormone receptor (HR)-positive disease, respectively — reduce local failures.[7-9,13] However, longer follow-up data are needed for robust conclusions, but the nonresponders to these agents likely remain at higher risk to IBC/CBC, compared with responder patients. This discrimination between responders and nonresponders is currently unfeasible and represents a major research goal.

Surgery for localized unilateral breast cancer includes BCS, unilateral mastectomy (UM) of the affected breast, and possibly CPM of the unaffected breast as a means of BM. Key research questions remain. Is it possible to tailor design optimal surgery, so as to achieve the best oncological outcome and quality of life for each patient? Is currently a risk stratification-based surgery for individual patients feasible? The answers are probably 'yes', but any tailored treatments will require consideration of host-related factors.

Adjuvant breast irradiation
Whole-breast irradiation of 50 gray (Gy) over five to six weeks, with or without a boost of 16 Gy, is the standard adjuvant treatment following BCS.[13] This treatment strategy significantly reduces the risk of loco-regional recurrence and also may improve overall survival.[5,6] However, whole-breast irradiation may be associated with late toxicity impacts on lung, heart, and contralateral breast, including a possible contribution to carcinogenesis in the contralateral breast. Indeed, a current large (n = 7,221) study from the Netherlands found an

increased risk of CBC among those young patients with both family history and tangential irradiation treatment.[27] To reduce these irradiation-related adverse effects on the whole breast, partial breast irradiation has been developed. However, until data from the current randomized trials become available, partial breast irradiation cannot be applied in routine clinical practice.[28] Aggressive surgery, such as BM, can avoid irradiation's adverse effects, but with the risks associated with more surgery and frequently reconstruction.

Impact of molecular-targeting therapy on loco-regional control
Recent RCTs provide accumulating evidence supporting the efficacy of modern adjuvant treatment to reduce loco-regional failures. Endocrine therapy for HR-positive (ER and/or PR) tumors with tamoxifen reduces local failures. Further reduction is observed when the therapy is switched from tamoxifen to an aromatase inhibitor (AI),[29,30] and even higher efficacy with direct treatment using AIs. Indeed, the 'Arimidex, and Tamoxifen Alone or in Combination' trial provides evidence for the higher efficacy of AI versus tamoxifen alone or of tamoxifen followed by AI, in reducing IBC/CBC.[7] However, this treatment is limited to postmenopausal women only, and thus younger patients treated with tamoxifen potentially have a higher risk of local failure.[7]

Current guidelines consider HER2 status as one of the key factors in treatment decisions.[13] Given that HER2-positive disease accounts for 25% (15%–20%) of all cases, with a response rate to trastuzumab of 40% (generally lower as a single agent, but far greater when given with chemotherapy), only 10% or more of all patients would benefit from such a personalized treatment. It appears that HER2 status-guided adjuvant treatment, beyond the reduction of distant metastasis, also decreases the local failures of IBC/CBC. However, data are still limited.

Table 5–2 summarizes loco-regional recurrence and CBC as first events after treatment. Trastuzumab, a monoclonal antibody against HER2-positive disease, reduced such local failures in the two largest RCTs.[8,9] However, longer follow-up results and new trials with IBC/CBC as endpoints are required to assess accurately the oncological outcomes.

Markers for Personalized Systemic and Local Control

The advent of high-throughput technologies allows basic sciences to focus on the development and validation of prognostic and predictive markers to achieve the major goal of personalized medicine. Research on individual tumor's molecular profiling, pharmacogenomics, and whole-genome scans provide

Table 5–2. Ipsilateral loco-regional recurrence and contralateral breast cancer as isolated first events after treatment for nonmetastatic breast cancer

Study	No. of patients	Follow-up (years)	Local or regional recurrence		Contralateral breast cancer		Ref.
			Control group	Trastuzumab	Control group	Trastuzumab	
HERA trial	3,387	1	3.0%	1.6%	7 (0.4%)	6 (0.4%)	8
B-31 trial	1,736	2.4	35/872 (4%)	15/864 (1.7%)	6 (0.7%)	2 (0.2%)	9
N9831 trial	1,615	1.5	22/807 (2.7%)	12/808 (1.5%)	0	1 (0.12%)	9
Nyuyen et al.* HER2 negative	109	5	8.4%*	NA	NA	NA	25
(HER2/ER/PR−)	684	5	7.1%*	NA	NA	NA	25

*Retrospective study in 792 patients with invasive breast cancer who received breast-conserving treatment approximating gene-expression profiling-based molecular classification (luminal, HER2-like, and basal-like subtypes, with ER/PR and HER2 status). No patient with HER2-positive disease received trastuzumab.

exciting findings, but at present, there is limited clinical success.

Microarray technology has enabled the simultaneous investigation into the expression of thousands of genes. Gene-expression profiling studies have identified new molecular classification and also prognostic gene signatures. Breast cancer can be grouped into at least four subtypes: luminal A and luminal B (HR-positive), HER2-like (HR-negative/HER2-positive), and basal-like (HR/HER2-negative) subtypes.[31,32] This grouping is thought to have distinct clinical outcomes and response to therapy,[33] but in an absence of randomized evidence, this new classification has not been in clinical use.

Most recently, two large retrospective studies have evaluated the potential utility of this molecular classification to predict risks of loco-regional recurrence. P. L. Nguyen and colleagues[26] reported on gene-expression data from 793 patients in the USA, and M. Kyndi and colleagues[26] looked at 1,000 patients as part of the Danish 82b/c randomized trials. In these studies, both HER2 and basal subtypes were significantly associated, on multivariable analysis, with an increased risk of loco-regional recurrence, compared with luminal subtypes. After a mean patient follow-up of five years following breast-conserving treatment, the local recurrence rates were 8.4% for HER2 and 7.1% for basal subtypes.[25]

Despite these higher rates in loco-regional recurrence, there currently is no evidence that such patients with HER2-positive or basal subtypes would benefit from a more aggressive surgery, like UM, for two main reasons. First, the HER2-positive patients in these previous studies did not receive the current standard agent trastuzumab, which reduces loco-regional recurrence.

Therefore, it is likely that the loco-regional recurrence rates may be lower when trastuzumab is added.[34] Second, the prognosis of basal subtype is poor.[35] Whether better local control therefore would improve overall survival of such patients is unknown, given that most of these patients die early from systemic disease before they develop local failures, which usually require a long-term process to be clinically evident.

Gene-expression profiling studies have developed several gene signatures, two of which already have been commercialized ⸺ the 70-gene signature test for tailoring chemotherapy in early-stage node-negative patients,[36] and the 21-gene assay (Oncotype DX™) for decision making regarding adding chemotherapy or not to hormonal therapy in the early-stage, node-negative, estrogen receptor positive disease.[37] Two large phase III randomized trials, the Microarray In Node-Negative Disease May Avoid ChemoTherapy (MINDACT) trial and the Trial Assigning Individualized Options for Treatment (TAILORx) trial, are underway to test the clinical utility of these two genetic assays, respectively.

Following initial enthusiasm for gene signature-based decisions for personalized treatment, there is now suggestion that in an attempt to tailor risk estimation for distant or loco-regional recurrence, research should focus on genes with mechanistic implication in breast cancer rather than on gene-expression data, for developing robust predictors of outcomes.[38,39]

Furthermore, pharmacogenomic studies genotyping cytochrome P450 2D6 (CYP2D6, a member of the cytochrome P450 mixed-function oxidase system) and other enzymes involved in tamoxifen metabolism genotype may guide the selection of endocrine therapy for personalized treatment of breast cancer.[40]

Despite advances with trastuzumab and AIs in loco-regional tumor control, the research question remains how to identify the nonresponders to these agents and which patients are likely to be at higher risk of IBC/CBC. HER2-negative and HR-negative patients, who do not benefit from such treatment, potentially are at higher risk of local failure. Another question is whether these targeted agents are effective in patients who are carriers of inherited BRCA1/2 mutations.

Analysis of Breast Cancer Genetic Mutations

Overall, local failure rates five years after treatment are low. Indeed, most recent studies indicate that the incidence of IBC and CBC, as a first event at five years after appropriate local and adjuvant systemic treatment, is low overall, at about 5% each. However, longer follow-up from previous studies showed higher relapse rates ranging 10%–20%.[18,41] Previous reports not considering genetic testing have reported young age of patient, family history, and lack of systemic treatment as risk factors for IBC and CBC, and surgery-related positive or close resection margins as risk factors for local recurrence[6]. Although the overall risk is low, specific subsets of patients are at high risk of local failures and may benefit from aggressive surgery.

Genetic testing identifies the subgroup with the highest risk of IBC and CBC as women with a family history of breast cancer. Such women are grouped into carriers of BRCA1/2 mutations (testing positive) who have a known high risk of IBC/CBC, and non-BRCA carriers (testing negative) for whom no accurate risk estimation can be made. The genes responsible for this familial susceptibility to breast cancer are unknown. Patients with a BRCA1/2 mutation face the highest risk of both IBC and CBC after treatment of the unilateral breast cancer.[2,42–44] The risk of CBC among BRCA1/2 mutation carriers in the study by K. Metcalfe and colleagues was 3% annually or 29.5% at ten years after unilateral breast surgery; and CPM was very effective at reducing this risk by up to 97%.[42] In another recent study, L. J. Pierce and colleagues found significantly higher rates of CBC after treatment of breast cancer among BRCA1/2 mutation carriers than noncarriers.[43] Rates of IBC were similarly higher when BRCA1/2 carriers who had undergone prophylactic bilateral salpingo-oophorectomy (PBSO) were excluded from the analysis.[43] These data support a guided CPM for patients who are BRCA1/2 carriers, as shown by the high 49.3% rate among patients with BRCA1/2 mutations in the USA.[44]

However, there still is no universal agreement about the extent of surgery among women who are both patients and BRCA1/2 mutation carriers. For example, the rate of CPM in Norway was 0%.[42] In the absence of RCTs comparing the efficacy of BM versus BCS for breast cancer patients stratified into BRCA1/2 and non-BRCA1/2 mutation carriers, and lack of awareness by patients and physicians to the genetic testing's clinical utility, this variety in the extent of surgery is not surprising.

Despite the absence of a randomized validation trial, accumulating preclinical and clinical evidence suggests the clinical utility of more aggressive surgery. Patients with BRCA1/2-associated breast cancer benefit from BM rather than BCS.[45] How can the IBC/CBC risk among BRCA1/2 carriers be explained biologically? Healthy women with germ-line BRCA1/2 mutations face a high lifetime risk of cancer, where up to 85% of women with breast cancer have BRCA1 or BRCA2 mutations, and up to 25% with BRCA2 mutations, while 60% of women with ovarian cancer have BRCA1 mutations.[2,46] Both BRCA1 and BRCA2 genes have an important role in the repair of a double-strand DNA break, activation of cell-cycle checkpoints, and maintenance of chromosome stability.[47,48] Not surprisingly, the loss of these functions leads to cancer in either intact or residual breast and in ovarian tissues after surgery.

Prophylactic surgery as either prophylactic BM or PBSO has long been considered the most effective intervention for the primary prevention of breast cancer in healthy patients with BRCA1/2 mutation carriers.[2,46,49] This inherited susceptibility to cancer, which currently cannot be repaired by genetic intervention, causes transformation of normal epithelial cells —— in residual breast tissue, the transformation occurs after therapy —— into cancer cells and IBC/CBC development.

Inherited BRCA1/2 susceptibility explains only a fraction of all local failures after breast cancer treatment. At present, prediction of IBC/CBC based on standard clinicopathologic factors and treatment is inaccurate. It is generally accepted that new robust markers are needed to identify patients at high risk of IBC/CBC among those with BRCA-negative testing or sporadic cancer.

Genome-wide Association Studies (GWASs) and DNA Variation

Cancer is the result of interactions between genetic and environmental factors. Breast cancer is a highly complex disease thought to be caused by multiple gene variants, gene-gene interactions, and interactions between genetic and environmental factors. Some of the established lifestyle and environmental risk factors for breast cancer, including variables relating to pregnancy, menarche and menopause, use of exogenous hormones, height, weight, body mass index (BMI), and alcohol intake, might influence the course of the disease and patient survival.[50] According to a recently proposed polygenic model, a large number of low-penetrance genes are involved in breast carcinogenesis, but that only a few of the genes have been identified.[51] Thus, a full account of disease susceptibility awaits the identification of these multiple variants and their interactions in well-designed studies.

Following the discovery of high-penetrance BRCA1 and BRCA2 genes in the 1990s,[52,53] BRCA1/2 testing has identified only 5%–10% of breast cancer cases caused by BRCA1/2 mutations. So far, the research has focused on the identification of genetic risk factors to explain the remaining 90% of cancer risk. Candidate gene studies in multiplex kindreds affected by breast cancer have implicated rare variants of CHEK2, ATM, BRIP1 and PALB2 in the subset of families lacking BRCA1/2 mutations, but in most cases, the rarity and small effect sizes of these associations have precluded clinical application.[54]

GWASs now provide great promise for the unbiased identification of gene variants involved in breast cancer initiation for the remaining 20% of familial BRCA-negative cases and 70% of sporadic breast cancer cases. The identified variants can also be evaluated to assess whether they modify the risk of breast cancer among BRCA1/2 mutation carriers. Table 5−3 lists the results of most recent GWASs and case-control studies on three breast cancer populations: familial BRCA1/2 carriers, familial non-BRCA1/2 cases, and sporadic cases. Several research groups have carried out GWASs for selected familial breast cancer cases lacking BRCA1/2 mutations: in the first study, 227,876 SNPs were genotyped in 390 European patients;[20] in the second study, 249 Ashkenazi Jews were screened using 150,080 SNPs;[21] and in the third study, 1,145 postmenopausal sporadic breast cancer cases of European ancestry were screened with 528,173 SNPs.[22] These studies identified at least seven novel genes with several SNPs. Three of these SNPs, FGFR2 (rs2981482), TNRC9 (rs3803662) and MAP3K1 (rs889312), and another SNP, the RAD51 135GC, were associated with increased breast cancer risk in BRCA1, BRCA2, or both mutation carriers.[55,56]

Although the FGFR2 locus was associated with breast cancer in all three studies, there was minimal overlap of significantly associated SNPs between the studies. The differences observed may be the result of different population ancestry, sample size, and genotyping platforms.

Limitations and challenges

At present, no genetic testing for clinical practice is possible from the available GWASs. As genetic linkage studies have failed to identify further major genes of breast cancer,[54] the proposed polygenic model widely accepted today is that susceptibility is conferred by a large number of loci, each with a small effect on breast cancer risk.[56] This model is consistent with GWAS findings, which show that many more additional alleles and SNPs will be identified through future GWASs.[20−22] Thus, it will be important to look not only for each one of these gene variants, which separately confers modest relative risk to breast cancer, but also for the multiplicative effects of these alleles, as well as their interactions with environmental risk factors. Existing GWASs lack assessment of these interactive effects, limiting the clinical utility of low-penetrance genes identified by genetic linkage studies such as CHEK2[57] or by GWASs.[21]

Structural genomic variation, beyond SNP variation, also may play an important role in breast tumorigenesis. At present, however, whole-genome analysis to identify and characterize CNVs is expensive and time consuming. For example, the strategy used by J. O. Korbel and colleagues in 2007 currently requires eight months of continuous use of a DNA-sequencing machine, at a cost of 200 thousand US dollars to obtain data on structural genomic variants.[18]

Table 5–3. Incorporating genetics, epigenetics, and personal genomics for a patient-tailored surgery and adjuvant treatment to prevent IBC/CBC in nonmetastatic breast cancer

Population	Cases (n)	SNPs screened (n)	Novel genes and SNPs identified	Future research goals	Ref.
Familial cancer: BRCA-positive					
Antoniou, et al.	8,512 carriers	1: RAD51 135GC	These SNPs (genetic modifiers) moderately increase breast cancer risks	* Identification of additional modifiers (SNPs/CNVs) * nderstanding of interactions between these variants, BRCA1/2 mutations, and environmental factors	55
Antoniou, et al.	10,358 carriers	3: FGFR2 (rs2981482); TNRC9 (rs3803662); MAP3K1 (rs889312)	N/A	* More accurate breast cancer risk estimates and IBC/CBC prediction among individual women and patients with BRCA1/2 mutations	56
BRCA-negative					
Easton, et al.	390 BC	227,876	FGFR2, TNRC9, MAP3K1, LSP1, H19	* Completion of genetic mapping and risk variants (SNPs/CNVs) involved in familial non-BRCA1/2 cancer	20
Gold, et al.	249 BC AJs	150,080	FGFR2; RNF146; ECHDC1 (region of 6q22.33)	* Functional studies for understanding gene-gene and gene-environment interactions	21
Sporadic cancer					
Hunter, et al.	1,145	528,173	FGFR2	* Epigenetics with emphasis on hypermethylation in the CpG islands of genes involved in tumor initiation and metastasis of sporadic cancer * Prospective large-scale studies between patients with and without IBC/CBC, evaluating multiple clinicopathologic, genetic, and genomic risk factors.	22

More recently, specialized companies provide genotypic platforms with one million CNVs at a logical cost.

Another limitation is the large number of low-risk alleles involved in breast cancer initiation. Bert Vogelstein's group sequenced 18,191 genes and found 280 candidates for cancer genes involved in breast cancer and colorectal cancer initiations.[15] Therefore, cancer genes may differ among individual tumors, requiring accurate characterization of the genetic variants in each individual tumor for a subsequent guide on preventive or therapeutic intervention. However, even when the breast cancer gene catalogue will be completed, and the SNPs and CNVs involved in breast cancer characterized, the next hurdle will be to define the precise role of each gene variant in breast carcinogenesis.

Perhaps, one of the most complicated barriers toward a practical personalized cancer approach will be to understand the extreme complexity of the cancer's network biology.[58] Indeed, despite the use of modern technology, including for ribonucleic acid (RNA) interference, genomics, and proteomics, identifying which signaling pathways are deregulated for each individual tumor and defining precisely the intracellular and extracellular interactions of its components (genes and proteins) is uncertain. Further challenges include understanding cancer heterogeneity (including the possible role of cancer stem cells), angiogenesis, tumor microenvironment, dormancy in tumor initiation, progression, and metastasis.[59-65] The elucidation of the functional role of noncoding DNA represents another challenge in achieving personalized oncology.[66]

Over the year 2008, the flood of biomedical discoveries in whole-genome analysis and identification of novel genetic variants has led to the creation of at least three new genomic companies, which for a few thousand dollars, now offer DNA testing — a whole-genome analysis — for the prediction of an individual's risk of developing a complex benign or malignant disease.[67] At present, however, due to its limitations, no genomic testing can be used in clinical practice to determine accurately the breast cancer risk for an individual woman. In a perspective article in the *New England Journal of Medicine*, D. J. Hunter, M. J. Khoury, and J. M. Drazen reported that currently a whole-genome analysis cannot be adopted into medical clinical practice.[68]

Surgical Guidelines

Genetic risk factors usually are not considered for choosing the extent of surgery in routine practice. Since such factors may play an important role in IBC/CBC, beyond the established factors (margin status, multicentricity, and adjuvant treatment), a surgical treatment approach is proposed based on the presence (familial cancer) or absence (sporadic cancer) of family history. All standard clinicopathologic, genetic, and treatment parameters should be considered.

Sporadic and familial BRCA-negative breast cancer

BCS is the standard procedure for stages I-II patients who have no family history (sporadic cancer) or who have a family history and a BRCA-negative test (familial non-BRCA1/2 cancer). However, resection-free margins and absence of multifocal and/or multicentric cancer are important for local control and should be respected by surgeons. In addition, based on current guidelines, adjuvant whole-breast irradiation and systemic treatment — including chemotherapy, targeted hormonal therapy, and trastuzumab[13] — also improve loco-regional tumor control. Although some preliminary data suggest a higher risk of IBC/CBC among specific subsets such as triple-negative cases, particularly for familial non-BRCA1/2 breast cancer cases, evidence is still lacking to support a more aggressive surgery. Perhaps an extensive discussion about the balance of risks and benefits among such individual women might be helpful, but at present, no evidence-based decision for extensive surgery can be made. Future GWASs may lead to patient-tailored surgery.

BRCA1/2-mutation carriers with breast cancer

Patients with BRCA1/2 mutations may benefit from a more aggressive surgery. Recent studies have demonstrated that patients with BRCA1/2 mutations have significantly higher rates of IBC/CBC than have the non-BRCA1/2 carriers, with a 29.5% rate of CBC at ten years after unilateral breast surgery and, perhaps most important, with a highly effective CPM that reduced CBC incidence by up to 97%.[42-44] These clinical data and basic research strongly support BM for patients with BRCA1/2 mutations. However, we note the absence of RCTs, and that in retrospective previous studies the patients had not received trastuzumab and/or AIs, which may have reduced IBC/CBC.

Newer standard targeted agents reduce local failures. However, their efficacy in reducing IBC/CBC in patient subpopulations with BRCA1/2 mutations is unknown, as long-term follow-up data are not yet available. Nevertheless, based on HR/HER2 status of these patients, we may have useful information about the patient's best course of treatment. About 10%–24% of BRCA1-only patients and 65%–70% of BRCA2 patients, having HR-positive tumors,[69,70] may benefit from AIs or tamoxifen treatment regarding IBC/CBC. Given that the vast majority of BRCA1 or BRCA2 patients, at 97%, have HER2-negative tumors,[69] and cannot receive trastuzumab, no local control benefit can be expected. These data reveal that local control benefit provided by targeted therapy is limited to a few patients only, among those with BRCA1/2 mutations. Thus, for most patients with BRCA1/2 mutations, aggressive surgery could be considered.

The timing of genetic testing availability, namely before or after completion of treatment, influences surgical decision. When genetic testing is available before treatment, patients with BRCA1/2 mutations have to choose between BCS or UM of the affected breast and BM. For women with BRCA1 or BRCA2 mutations and early stages I?II breast cancer, HR-negative tumor BM could be considered, whereas for HR-positive disease, particularly for postmenopausal women receiving an AI, BCS could be discussed as an alternative approach.

When BRCA1/2 genetic testing becomes available after treatment completion in disease-free patients, preventive options should include PBSO. Indeed, those patients facing IBC/CBC risk with their BRCA1/2 mutations, and who additionally have a high risk of developing gynecologic cancer (ovarian, fallopian tube or primary peritoneal cancer),[2,45] may benefit from PBSO. Even though PBSO is considered important for preventing breast cancer risk in healthy BRCA1/2 mutation carriers and for reducing IBC/CBC in HR-positive BRCA1/2 patients, its impact on HR-negative patients is uncertain.[71]

Thus, for HR-negative patients with BRCA1/2 mutations, both CPM for patients who had undergone UM in the initial treatment and PBSO should be considered for preventing IBC/CBC and ovarian cancer, respectively. For BRCA1/2 carriers with HR-positive disease, PBSO and intensified screening, including magnetic resonance imaging (MRI), could be discussed as an alternative approach to CPM.

However, it should be emphasized that PBSO reduces breast cancer risk by 50%, but does not eliminate this risk, and that despite intensive screening, including MRI, a substantial proportion of these patients will be diagnosed with node-positive disease or advanced breast cancer stage.[2] Despite advances with genetic testing-based patient-tailored surgery, which accounts for less than 10% of all cases, there currently is no robust marker to guide surgery for the vast majority of women with early breast cancer. Personal genomics and whole-genome analysis hold major promises to achieve this goal of personalized breast cancer surgery.

Future Research Directions

Current whole-genome analysis research has focused precisely and rationally on three distinct subpopulations, with the aim of improving risk stratification. Novel genetic risk variants may further increase the genetic testing-based risk estimation for BRCA1/2 mutation carriers, which is about 70%, and improve risk stratification among women with family history, and BRCA-negative testing with or without family history (sporadic cases).

Table 5–3 lists SNPs associated with increased risk for breast cancer in women, risks that are stratified according to family history, and genetic testing result. New genes and SNPs have been identified in recent GWASs using genotyping platforms with about 150,000 to 500,000 SNPs. With the current availability of genotyping, platforms with one million SNPs and CNVs, it is expected that the number of genetic risk variants will increase dramatically. Given an estimated total number of seven million to fifteen million SNPs in our genome,[19] and the rapid technological advances with next-generation sequencing, it is expected that within a few years, computer chips with several million of genetic variants will become available. Using these new genotyping platforms, which will represent a nearly complete mapping of variants in the human genome, most genetic associations in breast cancer, will be revealed.

Potentially, there are clinical implications arising from such developments. Will genetic tests containing most genetic variants of human genome be available in the clinic as tools for genetic screening and personalized primary prevention of cancers in the population? Could whole-genome scans involving comparison between patients with or without recurrence, and the expected identification of risk variants between these two populations (recurrence, no recurrence), have clinical implications in personalized surgery and loco-regional control?

However, based on current data available,[15,16,20–24,65,72] the answer for the clinic is rather disappointing. There has been an explosion in biomedical research throughout the advent of new technologies. Over 2008 and 2009, GWASs have identified more than 100 new chromosomal regions, at which more than 165 novel DNA variants influence the risk of common human diseases and clinical phenotypes.[72] Nevertheless, despite initial optimism, the clinical implications of these risk variants are being debated.[68]

Assessment of genetic risk variants represents only one part of the puzzle. Given that all of these variants confer, at less than 2%, a small relative risk,[72] there is limited optimism. However, this technological revolution opens new avenues of exploration in other important parts of the puzzle: first, through functional studies, the exact role of each cancer gene and variants and their interactions within the networks of signaling pathways; second, the underlying mechanisms of interactions between all these variants and the environmental and lifestyle factors, in combination with epidemiologic genetic studies; and third, robust classic clinicopathologic factors in the design of future prospective studies.

Epigenetics

Classic genetics alone cannot explain sporadic cancer and cancer development in patients with a weak family history. The concept of epigenetics offers a partial explanation, and may have important clinical implications for these types of cancer. The best-known epigenetic marker is DNA methylation, which occurs in CpG sites (islands), has a critical role in the control of gene activity, and is influenced by modifications in histone structure, which are commonly disrupted in cancer cells.[73]

Hypermethylation of the CpG islands in the promoter regions of tumor-suppressor genes is a major event in the origin of many cancers. It can affect genes involved in the cell cycle, DNA repair, the metabolism of carcinogens, cell-to-cell interaction, apoptosis, and angiogenesis, all of which are involved in the development of cancer.[73] Hypermethylation occurs at different stages in the development of cancer and in different cellular networks, and it interacts with genetic lesions. Such interactions can be seen when hypermethylation inactivates the CpG island of the promoter of the DNA-repair genes hMLH1 (colon and stomach cancers), BRCA1 (breast cancer), and other genes.[74,75] In each case, the silencing of the DNA-repair gene blocks the repair of genetic mistakes, thereby opening the way to neoplastic transformation of the cell. In breast cancer, CpG-island hypermethylation has been identified in BRCA1, E-cadherin (CDH1), target of methylation-mediated silencing (TMS1), and estrogen receptor genes. Hypermethylation of the CpG island has been proposed as a mechanism of inactivation of the tumor-suppressor gene BRCA1.[74,75]

The profiles of hypermethylation of the CpG islands in tumor-suppressor genes are specific to the cancer type.[73] Each tumor type can be assigned a specific, defining DNA 'hypermethylome'. Such patterns of epigenetic inactivation occur not only in sporadic tumors but also in inherited cancer syndromes.[75]

The DNA-methylation and histone-modification patterns associated with the development and progression of cancer have potential clinical use. DNA hypermethylation markers are studied as complementary diagnostic tools, prognostic factors, and predictors of responses to treatment in many cancer types, including breast cancer. DNA methylation techniques permit the sensitive and quantitative detection of hypermethylated tumor-suppressor genes in all types of biologic fluids and biopsy specimens. The establishment of DNA methylation and histone-modification profiles of the primary tumor specimen itself might be a valuable tool in determining the prognosis and in predicting the patient's response to therapies. Prognostic dendrograms similar to those used in gene-expression microarray analyses, combined with hypermethylated markers and CpG-island microarrays, have been developed. These epigenomic profiles are complementary to profiles of gene-expression patterns and can be developed with DNA extracted from archived material.[73]

More recently, the discovery of inactivation of microRNA (miRNA) genes by DNA methylation also may have clinical utility. These miRNAs have short 22-nucleotide noncoding RNAs that regulate gene expression. DNA hypermethylation in the miRNA 5'-regulatory region is a mechanism that can account for the down-regulation of miRNA in tumors.[76,77] The methylation silencing of miR-124a also causes activation of the cyclin D-kinase 6 (CDK6) oncogene, which is a common epigenetic lesion in tumors.[77]

Genetic variants and breast carcinogenesis and local failure

When the catalogue of genetic risk variants is completed and genotyping platforms become available —— a rather 'easy' step —— the next more complicated step will be to look at which combinations of these interactive gene variants with environmental factors lead to treatment resistance and loco-regional events.

Prospective large-scale population-based studies recording tumor characteristics, including HR/HER2-status, host-related and lifestyle factors, family history and BRCA1/2-testing result, and treatment (surgery, radiation, empirical cytotoxic chemotherapy, and targeted therapy), will be required.

Comparing all of these variables between patients with and without recurrence could lead to the development of sophisticated computer-based mathematical models to discriminate between patients at high risk for IBC/CBC from those at low risk. This model could guide patient-tailored surgery for preventing loco-regional recurrence. Personalized surgical decision making might allow aggressive surgery to be tailored only to high-risk patients, while low-risk patients will be treated by BCS. This individualized surgical approach should improve oncological outcomes, surgical morbidity, and overall quality of life. Comprehensive protocols are being developed and proposed for personalized prevention and treatment of solid tumors, based on the latest advances of personal genomics.[6,78] These technological and genomic-based discoveries have yet to be translated into innovative care.

Conclusions

A generalization of aggressive surgery, such as BM, to prevent local events and improve survival, may harm low-risk patients, society and health systems. Instead, a patient-tailored surgery maximizes the benefits, and reduces surgical morbidity and adverse effects on the patient's quality of life.

Currently, BCS is the standard care for women with early-stage familial non-BRCA1/2 or sporadic breast cancer. BM may be considered in high-risk patients with BRCA1/2 mutations. However, there is absence of evidence arising from randomized trials for the superiority of BM versus BCS in patients with BRCA1/2 mutations.

Despite compliance to recent guidelines, the risk of IBC/CBC as isolated events among long-term survivors, after treatment for specific subsets of patients with familial non-BRCA1/2 cancer and sporadic cancer, is alarmingly high. Robust markers are needed urgently to predict these high-risk patients, who may benefit from aggressive surgery.

Latest technological advances, including next-generation DNA sequencing and microarrays, have revolutionized basic sciences. Based on these technologies, research on genetics, epigenetics, gene-expression profiling, and most recently, whole-genome scans has already provided exciting findings, such as the discovery of novel risk alleles. Although at present these discoveries cannot be translated into personalized medicine, current efforts in developing innovative networking and algorithmic approaches to understand, assess, and measure extremely complex gene-gene and gene-environment interactions may lead ultimately to personalized surgery and adjuvant treatment for breast cancer.

Chapter 6

Radiation Therapy

New Strategies of Radiotherapy in Patients with Early Breast Cancer

Rodrigo Arriagada

Summary

Several new radiotherapy strategies for patients with early breast cancer have been developed in the past few years, and importantly have been tested or are being tested in large randomized trials that are better defining treatment indications, so as to increase the disease's local control, decrease treatment sequels, and reduce treatment time, for the major comfort of breast cancer patients.

Introduction: Role of Radiotherapy after Breast-conserving Surgery

Early breast cancer is a common disease in Occidental countries, and its incidence is increasing rapidly in Asia, probably related to changes in lifestyle. Since the 1970s breast-conserving treatment for small tumors has been proposed as an optional strategy, which has been validated in randomized trials.[1] The need for postoperative radiotherapy to the whole breast also has been established, not only to achieve better local control but also with a positive impact on survival.[2,3] We focus this article on the treatment of small tumors, those primarily considered for a breast-conserving surgery. We briefly review some important aspects of radiation effects, such as for local control and survival; we also look at radiation doses, late iatrogenic radiation effects, and loco-regional volumes to be treated; and then we focus on new developments, including their evaluations over recent years.

Table 6–A–1. Radiation dose effect on local control, including boost radiation dose

Study	Radiation dose (conventional fractionation)	RR of local recurrence reduction
Arriagada, et al.[3,4]	35Gy–50Gy	0.26–0.30
EBCTCG[2]	Variable: about 40Gy –50Gy	0.32
Arriagada, et al.[4]	Boost: 15Gy, over 35Gy for regional radiation	0.50
Romenstaing[6]	Boost: 10Gy	0.66
Bartelink[7,8]	Boost: 16Gy	0.51

Treatment Effects on Breast Cancer and Surrounding Tissues and Organs

Radiation dose effect on local control

It has been established that the use of postoperative radiotherapy on the breast or chest wall at a dose of 45 gray (Gy)-50 Gy in conventional fractionation decreases about three-fold the risk of loco-regional recurrences.

A multivariate analysis of a pooled series from the Princess Margaret Hospital in Canada and the Institut Gustave-Roussy in France, including patients with locally advanced breast cancer treated with radiotherapy alone, defined a linear correlation between local control and radiation dose.[4,5] In addition, it was possible to predict that after a total dose of 35 Gy in conventional fractionation, an additional dose of 15 Gy will decrease two-fold the relative risk of local recurrence, including subclinical disease (that is, after breast-conserving surgery). This hypothesis was tested and corroborated by two large randomized trials.[6-8] The data on radiation doses are briefly summarized in Table 6–A–1, and recently published graphically.[9]

Local control and survival effect

For a long time and because of the so-called 'systemic disease' paradigm,[10] it had been considered that local control in breast cancer was only of loco-regional significance, denying any effect on overall patient survival. This hypothesis resulted in an underuse of radiotherapy, mainly after total mastectomy. However, it has been demonstrated clearly by meta-analyses of randomized trials involving worldwide individual patient data that better local control is related to higher survival rates for specific breast cancers and even better overall survival for patients with a high risk of local recurrence.[2] Because of the potential long-term radiation iatrogenic effects, the beneficial effect of better local control on survival is not observed for patients, for whom the absolute risk of local recurrence at ten years is below 10%, for example,

Table 6–A–2. Radiotherapy in breast cancer: Absolute effect at five years on local recurrence reduction and survival effects

Treatment category	Absolute reduction in LRR at 5 years (%)	Breast cancer mortality reduction (%)	Overall mortality reduction (%)
BCS N(−)	16.2	2.9 (10 years)	5.3 (10 years)
BCS N(+)	30.1	8.7 (10 years)	
Post-mastectomy N(−)	4.0	−3.6 (15 years)*	−4.2 (15 years)*
Post-mastectomy N(+)	17.1	5.4 (15 years)	4.4 (15 years)

Note: All reductions or increases are statistically highly significant. *The minus sign denotes a deleterious effect. LRR– Loco-regional recurrence. BCS–Breast-conserving surgery. N(−) – Histologicly negative axillary nodes. N(+) – Histologicly positive axillary nodes.

Table 6–A–3. Excess of contralateral breast cancer, other secondary cancer, cardiac death, and all nonbreast cancer mortality, after breast cancer radiotherapy

Event	Relative risk increase	Absolute increase (%) at 15 years
Contralateral breast cancer	1.18	1.8
Other second cancer	1.20	1.6
Cardiac death	1.27	1.5
Nonbreast cancer mortality	1.12	1.3

Note: All effects are statistically highly significant.

most patients treated with total mastectomy and with histologicly negative axillary nodes (N −). On the contrary, patients treated with breast-conserving surgery have a risk of local recurrence of more than 30% at ten years in the absence of postoperative radiotherapy.[2] A summary of these effects is shown in Table 6–A–2.

Late iatrogenic radiation effects

Analysis of a large randomized series, including more than 30,000 patients with a long follow-up, has measured the extent of late iatrogenic effects relating to the use of adjuvant radiotherapy. These effects include an excess of contralateral breast cancer, other secondary cancers, and cardiac deaths. These three excesses, as shown in Table 6–A–3, are small in absolute figures, but statistically highly significant. Given this analysis, there are two medical requirements of postoperative treatments involving adjuvant radiotherapy: first, a better indication is needed of the adjuvant radiotherapy, including volumes to be treated; and second, radiation techniques need to be improved to significantly decrease the radiation doses to critical organs, such as lung, heart, esophagus, and vertebral bodies.

Table 6–A–4. Effect of the internal mammary chain (IMC) treatment on survival

Study	Type	Number	IMC treatment	Main results
Lacour[12]	Randomized	1,453	Surgery	No difference
Lacour[13]	Randomized	243	Surgery	Advantage on survival for axillary N+ and central/internal tumours in IGR patients
Arriagada[14]	Retrospective	1,195	Surgery or RT	Advantage on survival for axillary N+ and central/internal tumours
Veronesi[15]	Retrospective	68 IMC N+/663	RT in IMC N(+)	95% 5-year survival in IMC N+ patients
Lyon[16]	Randomized	1,334	RT in IMC	Unpublished
EORTC[17]	Randomized	>4,000	RT in IMC	Not available

EORTC–European Organisation for Research and Treatment of Cancer. RT–Radiotherapy. N(+) – Histologicly positive axillary nodes. IGR–Institut Gustave-Roussy.

Volumes to be treated

An indication of volumes to be treated is essential in order to reduce iatrogenic effects. The breast and the tumor bed are indispensable volumes after breast-conserving surgery, as is the chest wall after mastectomy for patients with a high risk of local recurrence (that is, histologicly positive axillary nodes, or N+). The axillary volume should not be treated in cases of N− or N+, where there is a complete (level I and II) axillary dissection. The local recurrence rate in the latter case is very low,[11] and the postoperative irradiation of the axilla clearly increases the risk of the homolateral arm complications. The most controversial volumes are the supraclavicular lymph nodes and the internal mammary chain (IMC). IMC treatment, by surgery or radiotherapy, has been a matter of controversy[12–14] IMC irradiation means an unavoidably high radiation dose to the anterior part of the heart, mainly in left breast-located tumors, and the indication for irradiation should be considered carefully.

We described in a retrospective multivariate analysis[14] that patients with a high risk of IMC involvement (such as those with N+ axillary nodes and central or internal quadrant tumors) may have a beneficial effect in overall survival if an IMC treatment was performed. Umberto Veronesi and colleagues[15] have shown that in patients with histologic-proven IMC involvement a radiation treatment could give optimal results for this high-risk population. The IMC radiation treatment has been tested in the Lyon trial[16] and in a large European Organisation for Research and Treatment of Cancer (EORTC) randomized trial[17], but long-term results of the latter will take some years to be known. These studies are summarized in Table 6–A–4.

New Strategies in Radiotherapy

In the recent years, new questions have been raised on the role of radiotherapy in the formulation of new strategies, covering issues such as:

1. *Irradiated volumes.* The irradiation of the chest wall for intermediate-risk post-mastectomy patients, and the possibility of accelerated partial breast irradiation (APBI).
2. *Radiation dose.* The use of a 'super' boost for patients treated with breast-conserving surgery and who have a high risk of local recurrence; the use of a boost in patients with ductal carcinoma in situ (DCIS), with a high risk of local recurrence; and finally, the use of hypofractionation, allowing for shorter radiation treatments.

Irradiation of the chest wall after mastectomy
The issue on irradiation of the chest wall, summarized in the United Kingdom (UK)-based Selective Use of Postoperative Radiotherapy after Mastectomy (SUPREMO) trial, is addressed in patients with an intermediate risk of local recurrence, which involves factors such as tumor grading and size, intravascular invasion, and low number of involved axillary lymph nodes.

Accelerated partial breast irradiation
For some years, the need to irradiate the whole breast after breast-conserving surgery has been questioned. The main argument is that the truest local recurrences appear in the quadrant in which the primary tumor was located. Indeed, the related figures are quite variable from one series of trials to another, because of different patient selections, but the most accepted rate of local recurrences for patients with a low local recurrence risk is 80% or more. Late local recurrence appearing in other breast quadrant has been interpreted as the appearance of new breast tumors. The main potential advantages of APBI are:

1. A reduced irradiated breast volume, with a decrease in treatment sequels.
2. A lower total radiation time (from one intraoperative fraction to ten fractions).

Three techniques have been used:

1. Interstitial brachytherapy (low- or high-dose rate).
2. Intracavitary therapy, such as orthovoltage photons,[18] intraoperative electrons,[19] or superficial brachytherapy via a balloon inserted in the tumor bed.[20]
3. Three-dimensional external beam radiation therapy.[21–23]

The clear advantage of intraoperative APBI is the easy definition of the

Table 6–A–5. Ongoing randomized trials on accelerated partial breast irradiation (APBI)

Trial	Expected accrual	WBRT dose + boost (Gy)	APBI technique	APBI dose (Gy/fractions/days)
Christie Hospital[24]	708	40	External electrons	40–42.5 / 8 / 10
Yorkshire BCG[25]	174	40	External beams	55 / 20 / 28
NSABP B-39[26]	>4,000	45–50 + 10–16	Interstitial brachytherapy	34 / 10 / 5
RTOG 0413			MammoSite	34 / 10 / 5
			3D conformal external RT	38.5 / 10 / 5
GEC-ESTRO[27]	1,170	50–50.4 + 10	Interstitial brachytherapy:	
			•HDR	32 / 8 /
			•HDR	31.3 / 7 /
			•PDR	50 / /
ELIOT, IEO[28]	824	50 + 10	Intraoperative	21 / 1 /
RAPID, Ontario	2,128	42.5	3D conformal external RT	38.5 / 10 / 5–8
IMPORT-LOW, UK	1,935	40	3D conformal external RT	40 / 15
				36 /
TARGIT[29]	1,600	According to centre	Intraoperative 50 KV	20 / 1 /

WBRT–Whole breast radiotherapy. NSABP–National Surgical Adjuvant Breast and Bowel Project. RTOG–Radiation Oncology Therapy Group. ELIOT–Intraoperative electron beam radiotherapy. TARGIT–Targeted Intraoperative Radiotherapy Trial. RT–Radiotherapy. KV–Kilovolt.

volume to be treated. This can present some difficulties in the postoperative external radiotherapy approach, for which a detailed protocol is required on the position of surgical clips in the tumor bed.

The medical interest in APBI is confirmed by the numerous randomized studies conducted on this subject in Europe and the United States of America. A summary of these trials is presented in Table 6–A–5.[24–29] Some of them, such as the National Surgical Adjuvant Breast and Bowel Project (NSABP) trial,[26] have been very successful in the inclusion of patients. However, the long-term results will only be known in several years. Curiously, two recent reviews[30,31] have been published with some different conclusions, as summarized in Table 6–A–6. Our personal opinion is consistent with the recent St. Gallen[32] consensus that considers this approach as still investigational.

New trials on boost dose

There are two new trials looking at the effect of boosting radiation levels on breast cancer:

1. Invasive breast cancer. It is well known that younger patients treated with breast-conserving treatment present a higher risk of local recurrence compared with those treated with total mastectomy.[8,33] A new trial with a 'super' boost of additional 10 Gy is being tested in a Netherlands-initiated study on patients younger than 50 years of age with T1–T2, and N0–N1 tumors. This study recently has been joined by several teams in France,

Table 6–A–6. Recent reviews and consensus regarding APBI

Review/ consensus	Indication of APBI	Groups if indication	Group characteristics
ASTRO[30]	Suitable for clinical practice	Suitable	•Age 60+yr, T≤2cm, ER+, N(–), and other good prognostic factors
		Cautionary	•Age 50–59yr, T=2.1–3cm, ER–, close surgical margins, and other intermediate prognostic factors
		Unsuitable	•Age<50yr, T>3cm, positive margins, N+, and other high-risk prognostic factors
Danish[31]	•Proper patient selection •Short follow-up of studies •Low comparability among studies •More questions than answers	N/A	N/A
St. Gallen[32]	Experimental	N/A	N/A

N/A–Not applicable.

and should include more than 1,500 patients.

2. DCIS. A trial on boost dose for nonlow-risk DCIS patients was initially proposed by the Trans Tasman Radiation Oncology Group (TROG) and then adopted by the Breast International Group (BIG) 3.07. The trial is proposed as a 2 x 2 factorial phase III design testing of two questions: first, the addition of a boost dose equivalent to 16 Gy; and second, standard versus hypofractionation (42.5 Gy in 16 fractions) on the breast. The following patients are included in the trial — all patients aged less than 50 years and those aged 50 or more — with one of the following factors of symptomatic presentation, palpable tumor, multifocal disease, tumor size 15 mm or more, intermediate to high nuclear grade, central necrosis, comedocarcinoma histology, or radial resection margin less than 10 mm. These trial schedules are summarized in Table 6–A–7.

Hypofractionation

Conventional fractionated radiotherapy is the delivery of 50 Gy in twenty-five fractions over five weeks. Altered fractionations have been used in different tumors: hyperfractionation (accelerated or not) for head and neck or lung cancers[34,35] and hypofractionation for slower growing tumors such as breast and prostate cancer. The background for these altered fractionations is based on the seminal work of J. F. Fowler.[36] The first randomized trial testing the question of equivalence of conventional and hypofractionated schedules was done by T. Whelan and colleagues,[37] comparing a dose of 42.5 Gy in sixteen fractions to the conventional fractionation. The first results showed treatment equivalence,

Table 6–A–7. Ongoing phase III randomized trials evaluating the boost radiation dose

Trial	Expected accrual	Histology	Patients	Treatments
Netherlands Cancer Institute*	>1,500	Invasive BC	BCS: •Age<50yr •T1–T2, N0–N1	Boost 16Gy vs. 26Gy
TROG 07.01,** adopted by BIG 3.07	610	DCIS	•Age<50yr, or •Age>50 yr with at least one risk factor of local recurrence	2x2 factorial design: •Boost 16Gy vs. no boost •Standard vs. shorter fractionation (42.5Gy/16 fractions)

*http://clinicaltrials.gov/ct2/show/NCT00212121-term=young+boost+trial. **http://clinicaltrials.gov/ct2/show/
NCT00470236-term=TROG DCIS&rank=1.

Table 6–A–8. Randomized trials on hypofractionated radiotherapy schedules: Trial designs

Trial	Patients	Hypofractionated schedule (Gy / fractions / weeks)	Median follow-up (years)
Whelan[37, 38]	1,234 N(–)	42.5 / 16 / 3	12
Owen et al[39]	1,410, all N	42.9 / 13 / 5 39.0 / 13 / 5	10
START A[40]	2,236, all N	41.6 / 13 / 5 39.0 / 13 / 5	5
START B[41]	2,215, all N	40.0 / 15 / 3	5
UK FAST[42]	915, N(–)	28.5 / 5 / 5 30.0 / 5 / 5	2.3

but most importantly, the long-term results[38] with a median follow-up of 12.5 years also showed treatment equivalence.

This question also has been explored by large UK randomized trials.[39–42] The characteristics of these trials are shown in Table 6–A–8, and the main reported results are summarized in Table 6–A–9. The START trials still have a relative short follow-up (about five years), and this has been a matter of concern,[43] as evidently long-term follow-up is necessary to evaluate late side effects.[44] The FAST UK study[42] has quite a short follow-up (less than 2.5 years).

Table 6–A–9. Randomized trials on hypofractionated radiotherapy: Main results

Trial	Local recurrence	Breast changes	Survival
Whelan[37,38]	Equivalent	Equivalent	Equivalent
Owen et al[39]	Significantly decreased in the group 42.9Gy	Significantly increased in the group 42.9Gy	Equivalent
START A[40]	Equivalent	Equivalent	Equivalent
START B[41]	Equivalent	Equivalent	Better for the hypofractionated group (40Gy), related to a decreased rate of distant metastases
UK FAST[42]	Equivalent	Equivalent for the group 28.5Gy, and Increased for 30Gy	Too short follow-up

Postmastectomy Radiotherapy in 'Intermediate-risk' Breast Cancer

Ian Kunkler

Summary

There remains significant variation in the use of postmastectomy in 'intermediate-risk' breast cancer, reflecting weaknesses in the current evidence base and differences in its interpretation by investigators. The evidence for recommending postmastectomy radiotherapy (PMRT) to all patients with one to three pathologicly involved nodes is currently insufficient. The Breast International Group (BIG) 2-04/Medical Research Cosuncil (MRC)/EORTC Selective Use of Postoperative Radiotherapy after Mastectomy (SUPREMO) trial will provide valuable information to inform clinical decision making for this group of patients. Clinicians are strongly encouraged to enter patients into the trial to provide a solid base for advising future patients on the risks and benefits of adjuvant irradiation. In the meantime, clinicians will have to weigh the risk factors for recurrence on an individual basis.

Introduction: Defining a Clinical Role for Postmastectomy Radiotherapy

Adjuvant radiotherapy remains one of the cornerstones of loco-regional radiotherapy for early breast cancer. Loco-regional failure after mastectomy and systemic therapy[1] occurs most commonly on the chest wall (12%) and less commonly in the supraclavicular fossa (8%) and axilla (4%). Very rarely does it occur in the internal mammary nodes. Despite a large number of clinical trials,[2-8] there still is uncertainty about the selection of patients for PMRT and appropriate volumes to irradiate.[9] While enthusiasm for PMRT has waxed and waned over the last half century, there has been sustained interest in its clinical role since the publication of the Danish and Canadian trials in 1997 showing a survival advantage from the addition of PMRT to systemic therapy in high-risk premenopausal women[2-3] and a subsequent Danish trial in high-risk postmenopausal women.[4] Added impetus has been given by the results of the 2005 Oxford overview[8] of adjuvant breast radiotherapy trials showing a link between loco-regional control by radiotherapy and breast cancer mortality. That overview estimated that one life is saved for every four breast cancer recurrences prevented by radiotherapy. The mechanism by which loco-regional radiotherapy interacts with systemic therapy to reduce breast cancer mortality is unclear. Systemic therapy is thought to eradicate micrometastases more effectively than loco-regional disease.[10] It is possible that loco-regional radiotherapy may be important in preventing secondary dissemination from residual microscopic disease.[11] Given the impact of PMRT on survival, it is important to identify from the literature which patients are most likely to gain a survival benefit from PMRT in addition to a reduction in local recurrence.

The first overview of trials of adjuvant radiotherapy strongly discouraged the use of PMRT, showing a net increase in mortality in women receiving PMRT.[12] This was attributed to the radiation-induced cardiac mortality in older radiotherapy trials, in which suboptimal field arrangement and irradiation techniques resulted in unwanted irradiation to the heart.[13] However, the inclusion in the overview of trials in which inadequate or excessive doses of irradiation were applied was criticized.[14] Many of the early trials were flawed by inappropriate patient selection (for example, inclusion of node-negative patients), suboptimal radiotherapy technique, and inadequate statistical power to detect clinical significant differences in survival.[15] In contrast, the subsequent overview of more recent radiotherapy trials showed a trend towards survival in the irradiated group, reflecting the inclusion of more recent trials,[16] although the difference was not statistically significant. However, many of these early trials of adjuvant radiotherapy predated the introduction of adjuvant systemic therapy.

This chapter therefore concentrates on PMRT in women with one to three involved axillary nodes at intermediate risk of recurrence (that is, with less than a 20% risk of loco-regional recurrence at ten years),[17] where the role of PMRT remains controversial. It concentrates on clinical study trials in which both PMRT and systemic therapy were given, since only these are relevant to contemporary practice. Previous trials of radiotherapy without systemic therapy are of historical interest only.

International Consensus on Indications for Postmastectomy Radiotherapy

International consensus supports PMRT as a standard of care for patients with four or more pathologicly involved nodes or with a 20% risk of loco-regional recurrence at ten years[17-19]. For patients with a ten-year risk of loco-regional failure of 20%, the absolute benefit in long-term reduction in risk in breast cancer mortality is about 5%.[7,20] For the 'intermediate-risk' group, the National Institutes of Health in its consensus statement felt that there was insufficient evidence to recommend PMRT in intermediate-risk patients with one to three involved nodes.[21] This consensus was supported by the St. Gallen Consensus statement in 2007.[22] In the 2009 St. Gallen consensus statement, the international panel voted by a majority (70%) that PMRT should not be offered to all patients with one to three involved nodes,[23] but should be restricted to young patients and those with other additional poor prognostic features. Practice varies between the Europe and North America, with more radiation oncologists in North America than in Europe recommending PMRT to patients with one to three positive nodes. However, even within Europe, wide variations in practice have been found, with advocates of PMRT varying from 19% in Italy to 74% in Spain and Portugal.[24] These differences in equipoise around PMRT in the 'intermediate risk' group may explain in part the failure of the South Western Oncology Group (SWOG) 9928 trial, addressing the role of PMRT in the one to three node-positive group, to reach its target accrual.

Interpretation of the Danish and Canadian Trials of Postmastectomy Radiotherapy

Much of the current variation in practice of PMRT in the one to three node-positive group of patients is due to different interpretation of the Danish trials and the subsequent subgroup analyses that have been published. The loco-regional recurrence rate in the Danish trials at ten years was more than 30% in the nonirradiated arm. The ten-year loco-regional recurrence rates in the Danish and Canadian trials in the nonirradiated arm for the one to three node-positive group were 30% and 33%, respectively, and for the four or more node-positive group 42% and 46%, respectively.[2-3] This was much higher than in the irradiated arm, possibly reflecting suboptimal surgery of the axilla in the nonirradiated group, in which a median of only seven nodes were removed from the axilla. A minimum of ten nodes would be the current standard for a level III axillary clearance. This is supported by the fact that 40% of the loco-regional recurrences occurred in the axilla. These high loco-regional recurrence rates contrast with the East Cooperative Oncology Group (ECOG) data on 2,016 assessable patients after mastectomy and systemic therapy. These show at a median follow-up of 12.1 years, a cumulative incidence of loco-regional recurrence (including simultaneous distant recurrence) of 13% for the one to three node-positive group, and 29% for those with four or more involved nodes.[1] Thus with good surgery, very low recurrence rates are achievable, and the relative benefit of adjuvant PMRT may be modest. Better attention to surgical technique in the axilla and wider adoption of anthracyclines, taxanes, trastuzumab, and hormonal therapy have reduced local recurrence rates (LRRs).[25] In addition, in the Danish trials, the intensity of the adjuvant systemic therapy with concurrent cyclophosphamide, methotrexate, and 5-fluorouracil (CMF) radiotherapy was considered suboptimal.[17] This challenges the generalizability of these data and subsequent subgroup analyses to contemporary practice. For the 1,885 patients in the Danish Breast Cancer Cooperative Group (DBCG) 82 b&c trials with one to three involved nodes, the overall survival at fourteen years was 10% higher with the addition of PMRT (50% vs. 40%, p = 0.0001). A survival benefit was shown in all subgroups of patients. However, the major benefit accrued to the one to three node-positive group. The survival advantage from adding PMRT to CMF was greater (9%) in small (<21 mm) and intermediate size (21 mm–50 mm) cancers. Findings in the postmenopausal DBCG 82b postmenopausal trial were similar.[4]

A subgroup analysis was published from the Danish 82b and 82c trials on patients with at least eight nodes removed from the axilla.[26] This showed that there was a statistically significant 9% improvement in fifteen-year survival from PMRT in the one to three node-positive group. Some have argued[26,27] that these results justify making PMRT the standard of care for all patients with one to three involved nodes. Others have considered that the loco-regional recurrence rate in the nonirradiated patients was still unusually high at 27% at ten years, again challenging the validity of these data in current practice.[28] In addition, the standard chemotherapy has changed from the combination of CMF in the era of the Danish and Canadian trials to the contemporary standard of anthracycline-based chemotherapy for fit patients with adequate cardiac function. It is noteworthy too that the meta-analysis of adjuvant radiotherapy, in which systemic therapy also was given, shows only a smaller survival gain from PMRT in patients treated by an anthracycline-based regime compared with CMF.[20]

Which Patients Gain Most from Postmastectomy Radiotherapy?

It is possible that loco-regional radiotherapy may confer greater benefit in smaller tumors and in those with few involved nodes,[19] since these tumors are less likely to have metastasized. This hypothesis is supported by both randomized and nonrandomized data. In a subgroup analysis of the DBCG 82 b&c trials,[29] the greatest survival benefit was found in patients with the lower risk of local recurrence. The authors concluded that translation of a reduction in local recurrence to a reduction in breast cancer mortality was heterogeneous. In addition, the European Organisation for Research and Treatment of Cancer (EORTC) adjuvant breast cancer trials[30] demonstrated the largest survival benefit in patients with one to three involved nodes, at a relative risk (RR) of 0.48 and a 99% confidence interval (CI) of 0.31−0.75 ($p \leq 0.001$). Nonetheless, this data should be interpreted with caution, since it is a retrospective analysis. The twenty-year follow-up of the Canadian trial of PMRT[31] shows a 7% gain in overall survival (57% vs. 50%) from the addition of loco-regional radiotherapy to systemic therapy in the one to three node-positive group. However, we remain dependent on subgroup analyses for this subset of patients.

The Importance of Biological Factors in Selecting Patient for Postmastectomy Radiotherapy

Traditionally, patients have been selected for postmastectomy on the basis of clinicopathologic factors, such as the number of pathologicly involved axillary nodes, tumor size, histologic grade, and lymphovascular invasion. However, these do not define the 60%−80% of patients, from whom radiotherapy might be omitted safely.[32] The importance of biological factors, such as estrogen receptor (ER), progesterone receptor (PR), and human epidermal growth factor receptor 2 (HER2), is demonstrated in a subgroup analysis of more than 1,000 patients, in whom these factors were recorded in the DBCG 82 b&c trials.[33] A survival advantage was shown in the ER positive, PR positive, and HER2 negative patients, but not in the ER negative, PR negative, and HER2 positive patients. The reasons for this difference are not clear. The authors speculated that patients with poor prognostic features (for example, hormone receptor negative or HER2 positive) are more likely to have disseminated cancer cells to distant sites at the time of diagnosis, and therefore such patients have little to gain in survival from loco-regional radiotherapy. This hypothesis is supported by a more recent subset analysis of the DBCG 82 b&c trials, which shows that the group with the largest reduction in local recurrence from PMRT does not translate into the largest gain in overall survival.

Interpreting the Oxford Overview in Relation to Postmastectomy Radiotherapy

The Oxford overview provides a valuable assessment of the overall impact of adjuvant radiotherapy after mastectomy in randomized trials. The 2000 Oxford overview of more than 20,000 patients in randomized trials of radiotherapy demonstrated a 5% reduction in breast cancer mortality at fifteen years in axillary node-positive patients treated by mastectomy, axillary clearance, and PMRT.[7] The overview also identified nonbreast cancer events, principally cardiac, as a significant cause of mortality in irradiated patients.

The 2005 overview showed a reduction in local recurrence and survival advantage from PMRT, irrespective of the number of nodes involved. The impact of PMRT on survival is reported to be even stronger in the latest overview (not yet published). Some have argued that the current evidence base is sufficient to apply PMRT routinely in all patients with one to three positive nodes.[34] There are a number of arguments against this interpretation of the latest overview. First, the dataset of the overview is so dominated by the Danish trials that its conclusions mirror those of these trials and the flaws in their quality outlined above. As a result, the overall beneficial effects of radiotherapy are likely to be overestimated. The arguments about the value of PMRT from the overview and the Danish trials are circular, since they reflect the same data.

Second, most of the trials included in the overview employed comprehensive loco-regional radiotherapy encompassing the chest-wall internal mammary and the supraclavicular and axillary nodes. However, the current practice in the United Kingdom (UK) is for most patients to undergo a level III clearance if they are treated by mastectomy, and the axilla is not routinely irradiated. A meta-analysis of adjuvant trials of PMRT by dose, fractionation, and irradiated volume showed a 6.4% benefit in ten-year survival from comprehensive loco-regional radiotherapy compared with chest-wall irradiation alone where adequate dosage was given.[35] Whether the same survival benefit can be conferred by treating the chest wall alone (where most loco-regional relapses occur) for patients with one to three involved nodes or node-negative patients with other risk factors (grade 3 histology and/or lymphovascular invasion) is being investigated in the ongoing BIG 2-04/MRC/EORTC SUPREMO trial.[28]

Table 6–B–1. Recommendations for postmastectomy irradiation[36]

Recommendations: Offer adjuvant chest-wall radiotherapy to patients with early invasive breast cancer who have had a mastectomy and are at a high risk of local recurrence. Patients at a high risk of local recurrence include those with four or more positive axillary lymph nodes or involved resection margins.

Consider entering patients who have had a mastectomy for early invasive breast cancer and who are at an intermediate risk of local recurrence into the current UK trial. This trial, which is called SUPREMO (Selective Use of Postoperative Radiotherapy after Mastectomy), is assessing the value of postoperative radiotherapy. Patients at an intermediate risk of local recurrence include those with one to three lymph nodes involved, lymphovascular invasion, histologic grade-3 tumors, estrogen receptor (ER)-negative tumors, and those aged under forty years of age.

Do not offer radiotherapy following mastectomy to patients with early invasive breast cancer who are at low risk of local recurrence (for example, most patients who are lymph node negative).

Qualifying statement: These recommendations are based on strong evidence from randomized clinical trials (RCTs).

The SUPREMO trial includes a biological substudy TRANS-SUPREMO, in which a tissue microarray is being constructed for the study population to identify biological markers of radiation response/resistance. The recent 2009 guidelines of the National Institute for Health and Clinical Excellence (NICE)[36] endorses entry of patients into the SUPREMO trial (Table 6–B–1). Such markers may help refine the selection of patients with intermediate-risk breast cancer for PMRT.

Third, in most of the trials, adjuvant chemotherapy was given with CMF regimes. The majority of younger intermediate-risk patients with adequate cardiac function are now normally treated with anthracycline-based chemotherapy. Anthracycline-based chemotherapy followed by CMF has been shown to reduce a five-year relapse free survival and increase overall survival by 7% compared with CMF alone[37]. It is likely, but not yet proven, that LRRs after quality-assured surgery and contemporary anthracycline-based chemotherapy will be lower than reported in the Danish trials, and the absolute benefits of radiotherapy on LRRs and overall survival proportionally less.

Which Anatomical Areas Should Be Irradiated?

Identification of the volumes to be irradiated has been reviewed extensively.[38] The Danish and Canadian trials,[2–4] which established the survival advantage of PMRT when added to systemic therapy, employed comprehensive loco-regional irradiation. On this basis, it could be argued that irradiation of the chest wall and all the peripheral lymphatics should be the standard of care for PMRT. However, this perspective simply reflects, as S. M. MacDonald and colleagues pointed out in 2009, that the existing data are for comprehensive nodal irradiation and that few data are available to justify chest-wall irradiation alone. However, many patients in these trials did not undergo a formal level I or II axillary dissection. Currently, a full-level III axillary dissection is carried out for most patients undergoing mastectomy, at least in the UK. It would be considered inappropriate to irradiate an axilla that has been fully dissected because of a substantial increase in the risk of lymphedema (about 30%–40%).[39] The axilla should only be irradiated after a level III clearance if there is evidence of residual disease at surgery. The role of axillary radiotherapy with sentinel node biopsy is currently being investigated in the After Mapping of the Axilla: Radiotherapy or Surgery (AMAROS) trial.[40] For patients with a positive axillary node sample, the risk of axillary recurrence justifies axillary irradiation. A policy of selective nodal irradiation in node-positive patients has been shown to be as effective as axillary clearance.[41] A general consensus is that patients with four or more involved nodes should receive, at the minimum, irradiation of the chest wall and supraclavicular fossa.[42]

As J. Kurtz in 2002 has argued,[43] the clinical benefit from PMRT is presumed to be in direct proportion to the risk of loco-regional failure expected in the absence of radiotherapy. Following modified radical mastectomy, the chest wall is the principal site of recurrence. It seems likely (and is currently being tested in the SUPREMO trial)[28] that the survival benefit from loco-regional control arises from irradiation of the chest wall. There is some nonrandomized data on chest-wall irradiation alone in women with one to three involved nodes. In 2009 MacDonald and colleagues showed in a retrospective series of 238 patients with stage II disease that loco-regional recurrence and disease-free survival were improved by PMRT (5 and 10 years without PMRT at 85% and 75%, respectively, and with PMRT at 93% at 5 and 10 years, p = 0.03).

For patients with less than four positive nodes, the risk of supra/infraclavicular recurrence is low (that is, less than 10%).[1] For such patients, the risk is sufficiently low to omit adjuvant irradiation of the medial supraclavicular fossa following a level III dissection. This does not apply to patients who have had a level I or II dissection.[43]

Although there is a substantial surgical literature that testifies to the microscopic involvement of the internal mammary nodes in patients who are axillary node-positive, clinical recurrence in internal mammary nodes is rare. At present, there is no evidence that internal mammary nodal irradiation increases survival.[44,45] The EORTC trial 22922/10923 has evaluated the role of adjuvant internal mammary irradiation with tight radiotherapy quality assurance.[46] Its results are eagerly awaited.

Toxicity of Postmastectomy Radiotherapy

Older radiotherapy trials were associated with an increase in nonbreast cancer cardiac-related deaths.[7] Particular factors relating to radiation-induced cardiac morbidity and mortality are left-sided tumors and the use of an anterior photon field to treat the internal mammary nodes.[47] Increased cardiac mortality may offset any potential survival advantage. There is a lack of data on lesser degrees of late radiation-induced cardiac damage. Nonetheless, it seems likely that nonfatal ischaemic heart disease is also induced. The excess of cardiac mortality is apparent at about seven years after radiotherapy and increases cumulatively over subsequent years.[48] To minimize cardiac toxicity, three-dimensional (3D) conformal radiotherapy is progressively being introduced while providing adequate coverage of the target volume. A study of successive decades of patients treated by adjuvant radiotherapy in the Surveillance, Epidemiology, and End Results (SEER) program in the United States of America (USA) shows a progressive fall in cardiac deaths.[49] This is likely, but not proven, to be due to the introduction of 3D treatment planning for breast cancer in the USA. The Danish 82 b&c trial of PMRT showed no excess of cardiac deaths arising from the use of an electron field of limited penetration over the medial part of the chest wall.[50] However, this technique has not been adopted widely. Avoiding irradiation of the peripheral lymphatics reduces the risk of late toxicity to lung, brachial plexus, normal lymphatics, vasculature, and bone.[42] Symptomatic pneumonitis after tangential chest-wall irradiation is rare at less than 1%, but rises to at least 4% or more if the regional nodes are irradiated. Higher rates of pneumonitis are reported if radiotherapy is combined with chemotherapy.[51] In addition, radiation-induced brachial plexopathy is a serious, painful, and disabling complication of axillary or supraclavicular nodal irradiation.[52]

Current Pattern of Care in Radiation Therapy in Korea, China, and Japan

Sung Whan Ha, Jiayi Chen, and Michihide Mitsumori

Summary

In this chapter, current practice of radiation therapy (RT) as a component of initial treatment for breast cancer in Eastern Asia is described, along with new trends in RT, such as hypofractionated RT and partial breast irradiation.

Introduction: Radiation Therapy on the Increase in Eastern Asia

The natural history of breast cancer in Eastern Asia is quite different from that of the digestive-tract cancers, which are more common and generally less sensitive to RT. Physicians treating breast cancer in the region therefore have been cautious in adopting the Western concept of minimal local treatment, which involves taking full advantage of RT. Significantly, fear and hate of radiation has been an obstacle to the popularization of RT in medical treatments, especially in Japan. Recently, as clinical evidence regarding the benefits of RT accumulate, more and more physicians and patients in Korea, China, and Japan are opting for RT as a treatment for breast cancer.

Incidence and Treatment of Breast Cancer

Nationwide patient registrations appear scant in Korea and China, and only estimated data exists in Japan, but hospital records in Korea and China, and registry records in Japan, all point to a rapidly increasing incidence of breast cancer, matched by treatments in the region.

The exact extent and causes of the rising number of breast cancer cases in

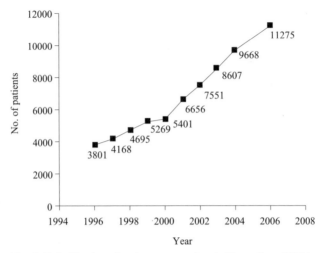

Fig. 6–C–1. Number of patients operated on in Korea from 1996 to
          2006

Eastern Asia is unclear. One possible explanation for the increased incidence
is associated with rising Westernization in the region, namely lifestyle
changes such as diets. The rollout and uptake of screening programs, such as
mammography, in hospitals and populations may also have some impact, but
the magnitnde is still uncertain because, in Japan, only about 20% of eligible
women receive screening mammography, which is one-quarter of that in the
United States of America (USA).

Korea
Breast cancer is one of the most frequent cancers among Korean females. In a
study of 105 hospitals, there were 11,275 breast cancer patients in 2006. That
number had increased by 13% every year between 2000 and 2006 (Figure 6–C–
1). In 2006, 48.8% of patients were given breast-conserving surgery (BCS).[1,2]
According to an RT study analyzing data from eighteen large hospitals with
more than 150 patients a year (Table 6–C–1), the number of breast cancer
patients treated with RT increased by 16% every year from 2002 to 2006.
Consequently, 9% of the patients with breast cancer who were treated in 2006
underwent RT in Korea.[3]

China
Breast cancer is the most common cancer in metropolitan China. In Shanghai,
in 2006, there were 3,835 newly diagnosed breast cancer patients and 942
deaths from breast cancer. Among the most common cancers, it ranks fifth in

Table 6–C–1. List and number of patients in 18 hospitals included in trials

Name of Hospital	No of Patients*	Name of Hospital	No of Patients*
Asan Medical Center	1050	Koshin Medical Center	197
Seoul National Univ Hosp	725	Kyungpook Univ Hosp	188
Samsung Medical Center	667	Chonnam Univ Hosp	187
KIRS & Medical Science	503	St. Mary's Hosp	184
National Cancer Center	473	NHIC Ilsan Hosp	180
Yonsei Univ Hosp	326	Donga Univ Hosp	170
Yeungnam Univ Hosp	271	Keimyung Univ Hosp	156
Pusan Univ Hosp	229	Gachon Univ Hosp	150
Ajou Univ Hosp	210	Chungnam Univ Hosp	147

*Patient numbers are as at 2004. Univ–University. Hosp–Hospital. KIRS–Korean Institute of Radiological Science. NHIC–National Health Insurance Clinic.

mortality, following lung (including trachea and bronchus), stomach, colorectal, and liver cancers.[4] Between 1975 and 2004, incidence rates continuously increased across all age groups. The crude rate had risen from 20.16 to 71.46 per 100,000 women between 1975 and 2004, and overall age-adjusted incidence had risen from 17.19 per 100,000 in 1975 to 40.22 per 100,000 in 2004. The peak age of incidence used to be the 40–44 year-old group in the previous two decades, but this has shifted to the 50–54 year-old group in the most recent decade. Median age at diagnosis has increased from 47.5 years in 1990 to 50 years in 2007.[5]

A review of surgical trends in the Fudan University Cancer Hospital showed that extended radical mastectomy (ERM), radical mastectomy (RM), modified radical mastectomy (MRM), simple mastectomy (SM), and BCS were used in 8%, 27.2%, 55.7%, 1.5%, and 6.3% of patients, respectively, in the 16 years between 1990 and 2005, and 1.3% of patients received immediate reconstruction after mastectomy. Although MRM still ranks first in all of the surgical modalities, the overall trend is towards less extensive surgery. The prevalence of BCS began to increase since the mid-1990s and currently represents about 12% of all surgical types, and the rate of reconstruction also has increased to 5%.[6]

Japan
Breast cancer is the most common cancer in Japanese women, with estimated 45,716 patients in 2003[7] (Figure 6–C–2) and 11,323 deaths in 2007 (Figure 6–C–3), and by mortality, it is the fourth-largest cancer in Japan.[7,8] Data from the Japanese Breast Cancer Society (JBCS) indicates that 59.3% of patients were treated with BCS, and 82.4% of them were treated with postoperative RT in 2006.[9]

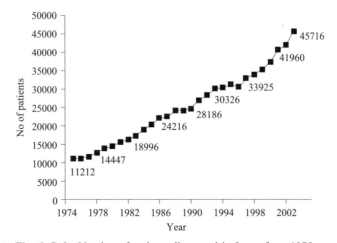

Fig. 6–C–2. Number of patients diagnosed in Japan from 1975 to 2003

Note–Numbers indicate patients every four years from 1976, the last one being for 2003.

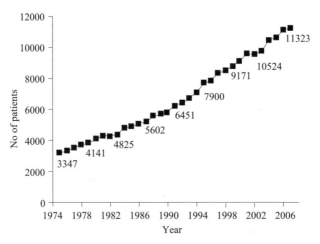

Fig. 6–C–3. Number of patients who died in Japan from 1975 to 2007.

Note–Numbers indicate patients every four years from 1976, the last one being for 2007.

The national breast cancer registry, which is conducted by JBCS, reported that about 12% of MRM patients (792 out of 6,413) underwent postoperative RT in the year 2006. It should be noted that this registry only includes patients from hospitals with a JBCS-approved breast cancer program.[10]

Radiation Therapy After Radical or Modified Radical Mastectomy

It is well known that postmastectomy radiation therapy (PMRT) improves local control and long-term survival. It has been recommended for patients with tumor 3 (T3) or T4, patients with four or more diagnosed positive axillary nodes (pN2), and patients with more advanced lesions

In a meta-analysis of 13,199 patients globally, 7,330 patients were 'treated adequately', and the mortality was different in favor of mastectomy plus RT at five years (difference of 2.9%, p = 0.006) and also at ten years (difference of 6.4%, p < 0.001). Loco-regional recurrence (LRR) also decreased (p < 0.001).[11]

Korea

In sixteen of the eighteen hospitals analyzed for PMRT, a total dose of 50.0 gray (Gy)-50.4 Gy is given to the entire chest wall, when the primary tumor is T3 or more advanced. In two hospitals, a dose of 45 Gy is given ⸺ in one, patients have their whole breast irradiated (left, right, or both), while in the other, such treatment is restricted to left-sided breast cancer patients with the disease.

In one hospital, all patients with T greater than 1.0 cm have their breast cancers irradiated. Boost treatment is not given in twelve of the hospitals, but in six of hospitals, 3.6 Gy-10 Gy of boost is given.

Supraclavicular lymph node (LN) treatment is included in fourteen hospitals if the cancer is N2 or higher; in three hospitals, for N1 or higher cancers; and in one hospital, the treatment is provided to every patient. The internal mammary node (IMN) is treated in four hospitals for patients with medial lesions and N1−N2 or higher cancers; in three hospitals, for every patient, and, if positron emission tomography (PET) scans are positive, in three hospitals. IMN is not treated with irradiation in seven hospitals.

China

PMRT is routinely delivered to patients with T3 and above and to patients with more than four positive axillary nodes (pN2). Previously, the supraclavicular region and IMN was the most common target of RT in 2002 and earlier, according to a questionnaire survey involving 210 responses from 715 hospitals in China. The data showed that PMRT for T3 tumors and four or more positive axillary nodes was noted by 97.1% of the respondents, and 87.6% for stages T1−T2 and one to three positive LNs. There were 63.8% of the respondents who selected PMRT for T1−T2, N0 tumors located in the center or inner quadrant of the breast. Delivering PMRT to T1−T2, N0 patients regardless of the location of the primary tumors was answered in 11.9% of the respondents. The supraclavicular region was the most common radiation target used by the respondents (96.2%), followed by the IMN (85.2%), chest wall (79.0%), and axilla (74.8%).[12] Currently, the major target is the chest-wall and supraclavicular regions. IMN irradiation is still controversial. The Chinese version of the National Comprehensive Cancer Network (NCCN) guidelines for breast cancer recommends irradiation to the IMN for patients whose primary tumor is located in the inner quadrants with positive axillary nodes.[13]

As to the sequence of adjuvant chemotherapy (CT) and RT, in the survey of 2002 the median interval between surgery and PMRT was six weeks. 'Sandwich' sequencing of CT and PMRT was the most common combination, according to 75.5% of the respondents. With the increasing use of anthraycline and taxanes in the adjuvant setting, the sequence of modality has shifted to delivering PMRT after the completion of adjuvant CT.

Generally, compared with the diversity in the indication of PMRT, the techniques used for radiation delivery are relatively consistent. For chest-wall irradiation, a tangential field with a 6 megavolt (MV) photon beam is the most common technique, with a tissue-equivalent bolus applied in one-third of the respondents to increase their surface dose to chest-wall irradiation. A boost dose to the scar was found in less than 10% of the respondents. Supraclavicular and IMN fields are irradiated more frequently by mixed beams of photons and electrons.

Japan

According to the national breast cancer registry conducted by JBCS, 93% of patients (739 out of 792) received radiation to the chest wall, and 63% to regional LNs, after mastectomy

Patterns of care study (PCS) for patients who underwent mastectomy between 1999 and 2001 revealed that the RT target volume included the chest wall in 63% of patients. The RT target volume included the regional LN area, such as the supraclavicular fossa and internal mammary LNs in 79% of patients. The RT target volume included both chest wall and regional LN area in 44% of patients. In the academic facilities, the proportions of patients who received both chest-wall irradiation and regional LN irradiation were 58%. In contrast, the proportion of patients receiving both treatments were 36% in the nonacademic facilities (p<0.001).[14]

Radiation Therapy After Breast-conserving Surgery

Following a BCS, the breast itself is the most common recurrence site. The National Institutes of Health (NIH) recommended postoperative RT after BCS.[15]

The Early Breast Cancer Trialists' Collaborative Group (EBCTCG) reported its meta-analysis result for 42,080 patients from 78 trials.[16] Five-year risk of local recurrence (LR) was 7.3% for BCS plus RT, and 25.9% for BCS only (2p $<$0.00001). The fifteen-year risk of breast cancer mortality was 30.5% and 35.9%, respectively (2p$<$0.0002).

Korea

Post surgery, whole-breast irradiation with a total dose of 50.0 Gy-50.4 Gy over five to six weeks is carried out for right-sided lesions in all of the eighteen hospitals. In two hospitals, 45 Gy or 48.6 Gy is given for left-sided lesions, to reduce dosage to the heart. Boost target volume is determined by surgical defect at seven hospitals, use of surgical clips at five hospitals, pre-radiation therapy computed tomography (CT scan) at five, and preoperative scans using magnetic resonance imaging (MRI) at one. In one hospital, two types of boost doses are used. For patients with a negative resection margin, the boost radiation dose is 9 Gy-10 Gy at sixteen hospitals or 16 Gy for treatments of the left breast at one hospital. In two hospitals, RT boosts are not given at all. At nine hospitals, the boost dose is the same for patients with a positive or close margin as it is for those with a negative margin. In eight hospitals, a higher boost dose of 9 Gy-16 Gy is given, while a 20-Gy dose is given in one hospital.

The supraclavicular LN is treated in seventeen hospitals for N2 or higher. At one hospital, the supraclavicular area is treated for positive cancer nodes, or N(+). At eight hospitals, IMN is not included in the treatment. At five hospitals, IMN is irradiated for medial-side lesions, with or without N(+). At three hospitals, patients who exhibit PET(+) are treated for their IMN medial-side lesions.

China

After BCS for invasive breast cancer, postoperative RT to the whole breast for positive and negative regional LNs are given in China, except for patients more than 70 years of age with favorable histologic subtype or contra-indicated to radiation. A retrospective analysis of 355 patients, staged 0-II, treated at Fudan University Cancer Hospital between October 1995 and September 2005 showed that a tumor-bed boost with a dose of 10 Gy delivered in five fractions (F) in one week (wk), after a whole-breast irradiation of 50 Gy-50.4 Gy/25F−28F over 5 wk–6 wk was given in 96% of the patients. Irradiation of regional LNs was delivered to 81% of the patients (64 out of 79) with positive axillary nodes. The five-year rate of loco-regional and ipsilateral breast control was 94.5% and 95.6%, respectively.[17]

As in the PMRT setting, there has been controversy regarding the sequence of adjuvant CT and RT. Of 248 premenopausal patients with stages I–II invasive cancer who were treated with BCS, adjuvant CT, and whole-breast irradiation, the chemo-radiation sequences included chemo-first (155 patients), concomitant (69 patients), and 'sandwich' (24 patients) treatments. In addition, the chemo-first percentage was 93.5% (144 out of 154) in patients operated on since 2003 compared with 11.7% (11 out of 94) operated on between 1995 and 2002. This shift showed a strong time-trend towards sequential RT after the completion of adjuvant CT.[18]

There has been, and continues to be, an evolution in techniques for whole-breast irradiation. Before 2002, most of the reported treatment techniques were based on two-dimensional (2-D) planning. In Fudan University Cancer Hospital, the percentage of treatments based on three-dimensional (3-D) assessments of patients operated on before 2003 was 8.9% (11 out of 123) compared with 83.2% (193 out of 232) between 2003 and 2005. Intensity-modulated radiation therapy (IMRT) using forward and inverse planning was implemented after initial dosimetrical studies,[19] and currently is applied routinely to patients with BCS and whole-breast irradiation. The boost technique was primarily an en-face electron beam followed by mini-tangents of photons, with only one report of an interstitial implant.[20]

Japan
According to the PCS study of patients who underwent BCT between 1999 and 2001, the most common dose and fractionation for breast conservation was 50 Gy/25 F. Boost RT to the tumor bed was given in 83.5% of patients with microscopically positive margins, 64.1% of patients with close (2 mm or less) margins, and 15.5% of patients with negative margins. Radiation dose for the boost was 10 Gy in 56.8% of patients.

Irradiation to regional LN is rarely given in Japan. In the PCS study, provisional data on patients from 2003 to 2005 revealed that the axillary node is treated in 1.3% (1.2% for N0, 1.6% for N+) of cases, supraclavicular LN in 1.9% (0% for N0, 7.0% for N+), and IMN in 0.6% (0% for N0, 2.3% for N+).[21]

Hypofractionated Radiation Therapy

Canada

In Ontario (Canada), 292 patients were treated with 40 Gy/16 F daily. At five years, LR occurred in 3.5% of cases, while cosmetic result was satisfactory at 96.5%.[22]

In Ontario and Quebec, after lumpectomy 1,234 patients with T1–T2, N0 were treated with 50 Gy/25 F/5 wk or 42.5 Gy/16 F/3 wk. Five-year LR occurred in 3.2% and 2.8% of patients, respectively. Cosmetic result was excellent or good at 77.0% and 76.8%, respectively.[23]

United Kingdom

At Royal Marsden Hospital (RMH) and Gloucestershire Oncology Center (GOC), 1,410 patients were treated. Patients had T1–T3 and N0–N1 lesions, and were less than seventy-five years of age. Afterwards, BCS patients were treated once daily to the whole breast with either 50 Gy/25 F/5 wk, 42.9 Gy/13 F/5 wk, or 39 Gy/13 F/5 wk doses. A boost dose of 14 Gy/7 F was given daily to 1,051 patients. Cosmetic result was excellent or good in 39.1%, 34.2%, and 49.4% of cases, respectively.[24] At ten years, the LR rate was 12.1%, 9.6%, and 14.8%, respectively (p = 0.027 between the last two groups).[25]

In Standardisation of Breast Radiotherapy (START) Trial A, 2,236 patients with T1–T3a and N0–N1 lesions were treated in the United Kingdom (UK). After BCS, postoperative RT with 50 Gy/25 F/5 wk, 41.6 Gy/13 F/5 wk, or 39 Gy/13 F/5 wk was given. LLR rates at five years were 3.6%, 3.5%, and 5.2%, respectively.[26]

In START Trial B, 2,215 patients with T1–T3a and N0–N1 lesions were treated in the UK. After BCS, postoperative RT with 50 Gy/25 F/5 wk or 40 Gy/15 F/3 wk was given. LLR at five years was 3.3% and 2.2%, respectively.[27]

Korea

Hypofractionated RT is performed only at the National Cancer Center, after BCS and without LN metastasis. Whole breast is treated daily with 39 Gy/13 F, and a boost of 9 Gy/3 F. About 250 patients were treated during the past two years.

China

Hypofractionated RT is not routinely performed in China. In a prospective trial at Guiyang, sixty postmastectomy patients with stages II–III disease were randomized into hypofractionated 23 Gy/4 F/17 days (d) (5.0 Gy on d1, d3; 6.5 Gy on d15, d17) and conventional 50 Gy/25 F/5 wk-6 wk groups. Radiation fields included supraclavicular and IMN regions for patients with T1–T2 tumor and less than four positive axillary nodes; additional chest-wall irradiation is given to patients with a tumor of T3 or above, and with at least four positive nodes. The five-year loco-regional failure rate was 10.7% and 7.4% (p>0.05) in the hypofractionated and conventional group, respectively. No statistical difference in overall survival was observed between the two groups.[28] Retrospective data from the Cancer Institute at the Chinese Academy of Medical Sciences in Beijing also reported similar therapeutic results and toxicities for two hypofractionated regimes 23 Gy/4 F/17 d and 45 Gy/15 F/5 wk, compared with the conventional 50 Gy/25 F/5 wk regime, delivered once daily.[29]

Japan

During 1999–2001 of the PCS study, the use of hypofractionated RT in Japan was limited and accounted for less than 2% of the entire cohort. For example, patients living in remote area who did not want hospitalization for RT were offered hypofractionated treatment. Recently, with workloads increasing for radiation oncology departments, some hospitals are starting to use hypofractionation to decrease the waiting time of patients. The Japan Clinical Oncology Group (JCOG) is planning to conduct a multicenter bridging trial to test the feasibility of such a short-course RT for Japanese patients. In this trial, a total of 42.56 Gy/16 F is given once daily to the whole breast over twenty-two days. Patients with close resection margin ($\leq$ 5 mm) and less than four positive axillary LNs are eligible for the trial. Depending on the results of this trial, hypofractionated RT may become mainstream for patients who received BCS.

Accelerated Partial Breast Irradiation for Invasive Breast Cancer

There are a number of accelerated partial breast irradiation (APBI) methods, which variously use intraoperative radiation therapy (IORT) with electron or soft X-ray; external beam radiation therapy (EBRT) using photon (with or without electrons) or proton beams; interstitial implants; or intracavitary brachytherapy using a MammoSite® balloon.

In oriental patients, breast size is smaller and surgery is performed with wider margins (2 cm). Radiation dose to skin can be excessive and external beam planning may not be easy. After BCS, there may not be enough space for insertion of a MammoSite® balloon.

Table 6–C–2. Devices for IORT

Device	Radiation	Dose	Weight (kg)
Intrabeam*	50 kVp X-ray	20 Gy in 25–30 min	1.8
Mobetron**	4–12 MeV electron	20 Gy in 3–5 min	1275
Novac 7***	4–12 MeV electron	20 Gy in 3–5 min	650

IORT–Intraoperative radiotherapy. *Made by Carl Zeiss Inc., Germany. **Intraop Medical Co. USA. ***Hitesys Inc., Italy. kVp–Kilovolt peak. MeV–Mega-electron volt. Gy - Gray.

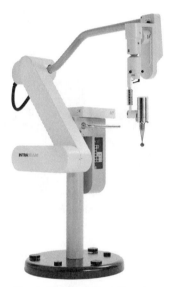

Fig. 6–C–4. Intrabeam® system

Intraoperative radiation therapy

There are two kinds of IORT devices available —— Intrabeam® and Mobetron®. The characteristics of these devices are shown in Table 6–C–2.

Intrabeam® IORT was used at University College London, in England. From 1998, twenty-five patients with tumor size up to 4 cm were treated, and no LLR or major complication was reported at two years.[30]

A randomized trial involving sixteen centers located in the USA, Europe, and Australia compared BCS plus IORT versus BCS plus external beam RT (EBRT). A total of 779 patients with an age profile of forty-five years or more were accrued.[31]

In another study, 301 patients were treated in five hospitals in the UK, Germany, Italy, Australia, and the USA, from 1998 to 2005. A IORT dose of 20 Gy was used as a boost before 45 Gy-50 Gy RT was applied once daily to the whole breast. At five years, LR was only 2.6%.[32]

A mobile linear accelerator (mobile Linac) was used at the European Institute

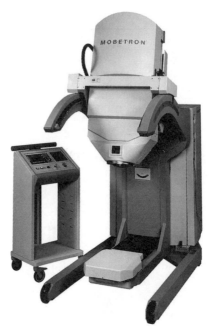

Fig. 6–C–5. Mobetron® system

of Oncology, in Milan. From 1999 to 2003, 590 patients with tumor sizes less than or equal to 2.5 cm were treated — in 574 patients with RT only, and in sixteen patients as a boost. At two years, 0.5% of the patients showed an LR, severe fibrosis appeared in 0.2%, and fat necrosis in 2.5%.[33]

Another study was conducted at Santa Chiara Hospital, in Trento, Italy. There, forty-seven patients at the T1 stage with an age profile of 45 years or more were treated with doses of 20 Gy-24 Gy using an 8 mega-electron volt (MeV)-12 MeV electron beam from the hospital's Linac. There was no LR until the four-year follow-up. Cosmetic result was good or excellent in 92% of patients. Grade-3 complications appeared in 6% of patients.[34]

External beam with photon and/or electron

Three hundred and fifty-three patients were treated by electron beam at Christie Hospital, in the UK. Tumor size was equal to or less than 4 cm, in patients with an age profile of not more than seventy years. An electron beam at 8 MeV-14 MeV was used to deliver 40 Gy-42.5 Gy/8 F over ten days. At eight years, LR was 25%, higher than conventional RT at 13%.[35]

At New York University Hospital, forty-seven postmenopausal patients with T1, N0 who refused the conventional six-week RT were treated with a photon beam of 30 Gy/5 F every second day over two weeks or less, using 2-D planning. At 1.5 years, no patient had LR, and the cosmetic result was excellent or good in 95.7% of cases.[36] Despite its small series and short follow-up, this fractionation treatment is unique given its outcome.

At William Beaumont Hospital, ninety-one patients with an age profile equal to or greater than fifty years and tumor sizes not larger than 3 cm were treated with a photon beam of 34 Gy–38.5 Gy/10 F twice daily (BID; from Latin *bis in die*) using 3-D planning. At two years, there was no LR, and the cosmetic result was excellent or good in 91% of cases.[37]

In Italy, 201 patients were treated with IMRT. In the Modulated Accelerated Radiotherapy in Adjuvant Treatment of Breast Cancer (MARA-1) group, ninety-nine postmenopausal patients with T1–T3 and less than three axillary nodes received a 40 Gy/16 F treatment over three weeks, plus a concomitant boost of 4 Gy/16 F. In the MARA-2 group, 102 pre and postmenopausal patients with T1–T4 and more than two axillary nodes, with a close resection margin, received a 50 Gy/25 F/5 wk treatment plus a concomitant boost of 0.4 Gy in every fraction to the tumor bed. There was no LR at five to forty-four months.[38]

External beam with proton

A new approach on the horizon is partial breast irradiation using a proton beam. Currently not a standard treatment because proton facility availability is limited and operational costs are high, proton therapy will become a realistic option in the future for some patients. Twenty patients with T1, N0 were treated with a proton beam at Massachusetts General Hospital. Patients with resection margins equal to or greater than 2 mm were treated with a cobalt-32 gray equivalent (CGE)/8 F BID/4 d. At one year, the cosmetic result was excellent or good in 100% of the cases, and there was no LR.[39] Despite the small series (fifty is normally considered the minimal number of patients in a trial), the results look promising.

Brachytherapy with a low-dose rate implant

Twenty-four patients with an age profile equal to or more than sixty years at stage T1, N0 were treated at the University of Kansas. Using a low-dose implant of iridium (Ir)-192, 20 Gy-25 Gy was given in one to two days. At four years, the cosmetic result was excellent or good in 100% of the cases, and there was no LR.[40]

Forty-eight patients at stage T1, N0 with ages greater than eighteen years were treated with low-dose rate (LDR) brachytherapy at Massachusetts General Hospital. At 3 cm from the resection margin, a treatment of 50 Gy, 55 Gy, or

60 Gy was given over 100 to 120 hours. At two years, the cosmetic result was excellent or good in 91.8% of cases, and there was no LR.[41]

At William Beaumont Hospital in Michigan in the USA, 120 patients with tumor sizes equal to or less than 3 cm, at stages N0–N1, at ages equal to or more than forty years, were treated with LDR brachytherapy. A dose of 50 Gy was given over four days using iodine (I)-125 seeds. The cosmetic result was excellent or good at 99%. There was infield recurrence in 0.9% of cases.[42,43]

At Guys Hospital in the UK, twenty-seven patients with an age profile of less than seventy years and tumor sizes less than or equal to 4 cm were treated using Ir-192 sources. A total of 55 Gy was given in five to six days. At six years, LR occurred in 37% of cases, and the researchers concluded that their treatment was not good.[44] The other 49 patients, at ages more than seventy years, tumor sizes less than or equal to 4 cm, and stages N0-N1, were given 45 Gy/4 F/4 d using cesium (Cs)-137 source. The cosmetic result was excellent or good in 81% of cases, and there was LR in 18% of the patients (seven of the nine LRs were at a primary site).[45]

Thirty-three patients with tumor size less than or equal to 3 cm, at stages N0–N1, and ages more than thirty years, were treated using the Radiation Therapy Oncology Group (RTOG) 95-17 protocol. Forty-five Gy was given over 3.5 d-5 d, using Ir-192 sources. At five years, 6% had LR, and late complications of grade 3 appeared in 18%.[46,47]

Brachytherapy with high-dose rate or pulsed-dose rate implant

At London Regional Cancer Center (Canada), thirty-nine patients with T1–T2 lesions were each treated with a high-dose rate (HDR) implant. Using Ir-192 sources, 37.2 Gy was given in ten fractions BID. LR was 16.2% at five years (two of the six LRs were found within radiation field).[48]

At National Institute of Oncology (Hungary), forty-five patients with T1, N0–N1mi (single nodal micrometastasis) were treated with Ir-192 doses of 30.3 Gy or 36.4 Gy in seven fractions BID. The cosmetic result was excellent or good in 84.4% of cases, and LR occurred in 9.0%.[49]

At William Beaumont Hospital (USA), seventy-nine patients with tumor sizes equal to or less than 3 cm, diseases at stages N0–N1, and age equal to or more than forty years were treated with HDR brachytherapy. Treatment consisted of 32 Gy/8 F BID/4 d or 34 Gy/10 F BID/5 d. The cosmetic result was excellent or good in 99% of cases. There was no infield recurrence, but there was out-of-field recurrence in 1.5% of cases.[42,43]

At three hospitals in the USA —— Tufts New England Medical Center (Tufts-NEMC), Brown University Hospital, and Virginia Commonwealth University —— seventy-five patients with T1–T2, N0–N1 breast cancers were each treated with 34 Gy/10F BID/5 d, using Ir-192. The cosmetic result was excellent or good in 91%. There was no infield recurrence.[50,51]

At Tufts-NEMC in Boston, thirty-two patients were treated. Patients had T1–T2, N0–N1 diseases, and were given 34 Gy/10 F BID/5 d with Ir-192. The cosmetic result was excellent or good in 88.9% of cases. LR rate at five years was 6.1%, all out-of-field recurrences.[52]

In another study at National Institute of Oncology, 128 patients with T1, N0–N1mi were treated with an electron beam —— eighty-eight patients at 36.4 Gy/7 F BID/4 d and the remaining at 50 Gy/25 F/5 wk once daily. The cosmetic result was excellent or good in 77.6% of cases. LR occurred in 4.7% at five years, including 1.6 % with a true recurrence/marginal miss (TR/MM).[53]

At four hospitals in Germany (University Hospital Erlangen, University Hospital Leipzig) and Austria (University Hospital AKH Wien, Barmherzige Schwestern Hospital), 274 patients, age profile of thirty-five years or older, and tumor sizes equal to or less than 3 cm, were treated using brachytherapy. There were 99 N0 patients treated with HDR brachytherapy, and 175 patients treated with pulsed-dose rate (PDR). For HDR, 32 Gy/8F BID/4 d was given, and for PDR, 49.8 Gy/83 F/5 d was given once daily. The cosmetic result was excellent or good in 94% of patients. LR appeared in 0.4% at three years, and grade-3 complications in 1.8% of cases.[54]

Sixty-six N0–N1 patients with tumor size less than or equal to 3 cm were treated using the RTOG 95-17 protocol, with 34 Gy/10F BID/5 d. At five years, 3% of patients had LR. Late complications of grade 3 appeared in 4% of cases.[47,55]

Seventy patients with T1–T2 lesions were treated with a cobalt (Co)-60 source, with 28 Gy given in a single dose. The cosmetic result was excellent or good in 50% of cases. There were grade-3 or higher complications in 59% of cases. At twelve years, LR occurred in 24% of cases, and 17 % with TR/MM.[56,57]

At Orebro University Hospital in Sweden, fifty patients with T1–T2, N0–N1 lesions were treated with PDR, at 50 Gy/60 F/5 d. The cosmetic result was excellent or good in 56% of cases and late complications (grade 3) appeared in 8% of cases. LR occurred in three cases, including one case with TR/MM.[58]

Brachytherapy with high- or low-dose rate implant
At Ochsner Clinic in Jefferson in Louisiana (USA), fifty patients with tumor sizes equal to or less than 4 cm, N0-N1 were treated with LDR (45 Gy over four days) or HDR (32 Gy in eight fractions BID). Cosmetic result was excellent or good in 75%. LR rate was 2% and regional recurrence rate was 6% at median follow-up of seventy-five months.[59]

Brachytherapy with high-dose rate intracavitary implant (MammoSite®)

MammoSite® (with Ir−192) is the most frequently used intracavitary implant.

At eighty-seven hospitals in the USA, 1,237 patients with stages 0−II were treated with 34 Gy/10 F BID/5 d. The cosmetic result was excellent or good in 92.3% of cases. LR occurred in only one patient (0.1%).[60]

Forty-four patients were treated using this technique at six hospitals in Europe. The age profile was equal to or higher than sixty years, and patients had T1 lesions. For twenty-eight patients, 34 Gy/10 F BID/5 d was given, and for sixteen patients, a boost of 7.5 Gy-15 Gy BID was added to the primary tumor site. The cosmetic result was excellent or good in 85% of patients (with or without boost), and there was no LR.[61]

At William Beaumont Hospital, eighty patients with stages 0−II were treated with 34 Gy/10 F BID/5 days. The cosmetic result was excellent or good in 88.2% of patients, and LR occurred in 2.9% of cases.[62]

At Kaiser Permanente Los Angeles Medical Center in California (USA), fifty-one patients with an age profile of forty-five years or older, T1 patients were treated with same dose schedule. The cosmetic result was excellent or good in 95.6%. There was no LR.[63]

At nine hospitals in the USA, 483 patients with an age profile equal to or higher than forty-five years, and T1, N0−N1 were treated with 34 Gy/10 F BID/5 d. The cosmetic result was excellent or good in 91% of cases, and LR occurred in 1.24% of patients (0.41% infield recurrence).[64]

In the USA, ninety-seven hospitals performed APBI using an Ir-192 MammoSite® balloon. According to the American Society of Breast Surgeons, 1,255 patients were treated by MammoSite® breast brachytherapy between May 4, 2002 and July 30, 2004. Patients with an age profile equal to or more than forty years and with T1 were treated with 34 Gy/10 F BID/5 d. At two years and three years, LR occurred in 1.11% and 2.04%, and axillary failure in 0.44% and 0.70%, of cases, respectively. The cosmetic result was excellent or good in 93% of cases at four years.[65]

Korea

APBI after BCS has been given in two hospitals. At Asan Medical Center, seventy-two patients (May 2005−July 2008) with an age profile equal to or more than forty years, tumor size equal to or less than 1.0 cm, and with N0 were treated with a beam of photons (from two to three ports) plus electrons (from one port). A total dose of 52.5 Gy was given in fifteen fractions. There was no local or distant failure.

At the National Cancer Center, 28 patients with an age profile equal to or more than forty year, tumor size less than 3.0 cm, and with N0 were treated with a proton beam of 30 Gy in total.

Korean Society for Therapeutic Radiology and Oncology (KROG) recently started its APBI treatment protocol with 3-D or IMRT, giving a total dose of 40 Gy in ten fractions, but patient recruitment has been slow.

China

APBI is now an emerging trend for clinical research in China, although most of the reports up to now are limited to technical exploration.[66] External beams with 3-D conformal therapy with or without a subfield technique is the major applied technique. Improved precision with image-guidance or breath-hold techniques have been implemented at certain centers. At Fudan University Cancer Hospital, twenty-two patients with stages 0–I diseases, who underwent BCS with axillary dissection or sentinel nodes biopsy, were treated with APBI of 38.5 Gy/10 F/5 d from June 2008 to August 2009. All of these patients received an online cone-beam CT scan for position verification after initial setup with skin marker and another CT scan at the end of each fraction to analyze the intrafraction error. Yet there is no report regarding brachytherapy or IORT for partial breast irradiation in China.

Japan

Partial breast irradiation is still under clinical/experimental evaluation and in Japan is offered only in a clinical trial setting. Yasuhiro Kosaka and colleagues[67] evaluated 'virtual' 3-D external beam treatment planning using CT scan data of Japanese women with the same dose-constraint employed in the National Surgical Adjuvant Breast and Bowel Project (NSABP) B-39/RTOG 0413 trial. They concluded that, on average, for Japanese women with a tumor located in the inner quadrant, achieving RTOG constraint is difficult because of an excessive dose to the contralateral breast. Recently, initial clinical results of APBI using MammoSite®, Mobetron®, and 3-D conformal RT were reported in the annual meeting of JBCS. The MammoSite® technique is reported to be often impossible because of an excessive dose to the overlying skin. IORT using Movetron® was reported to be feasible, but relatively large ski incision over the tumor may be problematic, as it can deteriorate a patient's cosmesis.

Accelerated Partial Breast Irradiation for Ductal Carcinoma in Situ

One hundred and ninety-four patients were treated with MammoSite® in ninety-seven hospitals in the USA. Patients were treated with 34 Gy in ten fractions BID. The cosmetic result overall was excellent or good, including for invasive cancers, in 93% of patients, and LR occurred in 0.59% and regional recurrence (axilla) in 0.59% of cases.[65]

In twelve hospitals in the USA, 100 patients with an age profile equal to forty-five years or older, tumor size up to 5 cm, N0, and RM equal to or greater than 1 mm were treated with 34 Gy in ten fractions BID. Cosmetic result was excellent or good in 98% of cases. LR occurred in three patients (one TR/MM case).[68]

The Role of Radiation Therapy After Initial Chemotherapy

Eric A Strom and Michihide Mitsumori

Summary

Initial chemotherapy has become a standard treatment option for locally advanced breast cancer (LABC), and useful in the downstaging of a large tumor that can then be amenable to breast-conserving surgery (BCS).

After downstaging a large tumor with initial chemotherapy, breast-conserving therapy (BCT) trials, involving surgery and radiation therapy, yield excellent local control and equivalent survival with early breast cancer patients.

A complete workup —— including proper localization of primary tumor and all possible lymph nodes —— is essential before starting initial chemotherapy to facilitate subsequent radiation therapy.

Introduction: Successful Early Experiences with Initial Chemotherapy

Before the advent of chemotherapy, women with LABC —— whose tumor was inoperable —— were subjected to definite radiation therapy. However, the radiation dose necessary to eradicate breast cancer with a 1-cm size range was about 60 gray (Gy) and for larger tumors in excess of 80 Gy-100 Gy. However, giving such a high dose of radiation imparted severe toxicity to the surrounding normal tissue.

Early experience with initial chemotherapy came from treating patients with LABC. To overcome unsatisfactory local control and severe damage to normal tissue due to an excessive dose of radiation, patients were treated first with chemotherapy in an attempt to provide a curative option for LABC. This attempt resulted in great response rates in the order of 80%, and occasionally a complete response was encountered in a patient. Based on this experience with LABC, the initial chemotherapy was extended to patients with a smaller tumor.

Still, the majority of patients receiving initial chemotherapy have an advanced breast cancer. Consequently, the following clinical advice applies to patients with stage III breast cancer, those with very large tumors or those that involve skin and advanced regional nodal presentations, and some patients with inflammatory breast cancer. The statements probably also apply to patients with loco-regionally recurrent breast cancers after initial mastectomy but without radiation.

The Staging and Initial Assessment of Patients with Advanced Breast Cancer

Initial chemotherapy, while used with increasing frequency in the treatment of operable breast cancer, leads to a number of clinical challenges. The extent of disease and other important pathologic information are no longer available after initial chemotherapy, particularly when there is a pathologic complete response (pCR). Therefore, a thorough workup should be done before starting initial chemotherapy. This includes full delineation of the entire extent of the loco-regional disease, and a clear statement of the tumor, nodes, and metastases, or TNM, stage. A photographic documentation of the initial state, including subtle cutaneous change, is also important.

However, the biggest problem is not breast diagnosis, but assessing the regional nodes. Many of the common diagnostic tools are inadequate for accurately assessing the regional extent of disease. All studies comparing pathologic versus clinical findings demonstrate that about one-third of the time the pathologic assessment is not concordant with the clinical findings.

Therefore, in addition to detailed history taking and physical examination, a comprehensive imaging strategy is necessary. At MD Anderson Cancer Center (MDACC), all patients are staged comprehensively not only with ultrasound (US) to the breast but also with all of the regional-level basins. This ultrasound approach can detect very small metastases, which can be confirmed pathologicly with fine needle aspiration. When assessing the US image, internal architecture rather than size is the important parameter. It is possible that positron emission tomography (PET) scanning and computed tomography (CT) may be able to complement US, although the benefits of adding PET and/ or CT have not yet been fully investigated.

Whether there is involvement of an extra-axillary nodal area is critical information for the radiation oncologist planning to perform radiation therapy after primary chemotherapy. In data presented at the 2008 San Antonio Breast Cancer Symposium, of the 865 locally advanced breast cancer patients treated at MDACC between 1996 and 2000, comprehensive imaging of the regional lymphatics revealed that more than one-third of patients had involvement of the extra-axillary region (that is, in the infraclavicular fossa, supraclavicular fossa, and internal mammary nodes).

Of note, while CT detects small lymph nodes, the technique has a considerable rate of false negatives, because its criteria is based on size only. Therefore, even small lymph nodes should be biopsied, whenever possible.

PET is another tool for detecting extra-axillary involvement, but PET generally requires an even larger lesion than US or CT.

No matter what modalities are used, the important factor is to resolve all diagnostic ambiguities associated with breast imaging before starting the initial chemotherapy. These ambiguities include a second lesion in the ipsilateral breast or a suspicious lesion on the opposite side. Additional biopsies are often needed to evaluate image-detected abnormalities. Since the administration of systemic therapy can further confuse the picture, the time to perform any additional diagnostic procedures is before the initiation of treatment.

Who Might Be Offered Breast Conservation after Initial Chemotherapy

Historically, the advent of initial chemotherapy took place at a time when such BCT trials following chemotherapy yielded equivalent survival rates with mastectomy. These successes raised the question on whether a good response to initial chemotherapy for advanced breast cancers might be achievable with intermediate stage tumors, which were not good candidates for breast conservation.

In the seminal analysis by Eva Singletary and colleagues published in *Cancer* in 1992, a major response was observed in the majority of 143 patients mostly with large stage II tumors and stage III tumors. All underwent a planned extended simple mastectomy, and the entire specimen was carefully reviewed pathologicly.[1]

Nearly one-quarter of these patients could have been offered breast conservation based on the pathologic evaluation of the breast. The clinical factors that predicted the ability to offer patients breast conservation included resolution of any focal skin edema at presentation and significant shrinkage of the tumor. The tumor must be unicentric on examination and by imaging studies, and show absence of lymphovascular space invasion. As lymphovascular space invasion is a very high predictor of multifocality and multicentricity in the breast, patients with lymphovascular invasion generally are not thought to be good candidates for breast conservation. A core biopsy of the breast is strongly advised, preferably several of them, before beginning the initial chemotherapy.

It is well established that the patients with LABC who are offered BCS after initial chemotherapy should receive postoperative radiation therapy even if the tumor showed a pCR, although the magnitude of the benefit of radiation therapy has not been confirmed in randomized clinical trials. In such a situation, it is crucial to clearly identify the extent of the disease before initial chemotherapy to facilitate later treatment planning by radiation therapy.

H. M. Kuerer and colleagues evaluated 372 patients treated with neoadjuvant chemotherapy for LABC, about one-third of these patients received BCS as a result of their good response to chemotherapy. The biggest concern for patients who underwent BCT after initial chemotherapy is whether such a strategy might compromise their survival by offering them anything short of a mastectomy. Surprisingly, patients treated with breast conservation had an improved five-year survival compared with mastectomy patients. Breast conservation was surrogate for a favorable response, and offering breast conservation to responding patients did not appear to have compromised survival.[2]

In a 2005 review, A. M. Chen concluded that patients with stage III and large stage II breast cancers, who were treated with initial chemotherapy, lumpectomy, axillary dissection, and radiation therapy to the breast and to the comprehensive regional nodal basins, had less than a 10% local failure rate at the six-year follow-up.[3]

Patients Who Ought Not To Receive Breast Conservation after Initial Chemotherapy

There also are some patients who will never become candidates for breast conservation — those with multiple primary tumors, malignant microcalcifications throughout the breast, and inflammatory carcinoma.

In addition, there are a few subgroups of patients for whom application of breast preservation is controversial. If a central segmentectomy is recommended as the method of operation, the patient needs to decide whether that option is acceptable from a cosmetic standpoint. Patients with a multifocal tumor — meaning a tumor that is within about a 4-cm sphere, but comprising several subunits — also might not be a good candidate for breast conservation. If a large tumor shrinks from a single mass into a cluster of smaller tumors, the net amount of downstaging might not be large enough to offer BCS.

Chapter 7

Preoperative Therapy

How To Optimize Neoadjuvant Chemotherapy in Breast Cancer Patients —— Experience of the German Breast Group

Mattea Linder and Gunter von Minckwitz

Summary

In this paper, we discuss promising key results of two German-based breast group trials, arising from the integrated meta-analysis of breast cancer patients treated with neoadjuvant anthracycline- and taxane- (plus trastuzumab) containing chemotherapy.

Introduction: Benefits of Neoadjuvant Systemic Chemotherapy

The German Breast Group (GBG) is a leading study group covering the complete field of clinical breast cancer research in Europe. A network of more than 650 national and international centres participates in our GBG trials. In 2008 more than 4,250 patients were enrolled in GBG studies, which is about 8.5% of all new diagnosed breast cancer patients in Germany. Overall, about 11% all primary breast cancer patients receive their adjuvant and neoadjuvant therapies within a clinical trial.

This approach, first to apply systemic therapy and then to operate it, has been widely accepted in Germany. The reason neoadjuvant studies in breast cancer are particularly popular and successful in Germany probably lies in the way breast cancer is treated. Diagnostic, systemic, as well as surgical treatment generally is in the hand of the gynaecologist, who cooperates in a multidisciplinary team. Therefore, there is a single point of contact for patients, which reduces time and enhances treatment.

Given GBG's expertise over the past decade, this chapter gives an overview of its clinical and therapeutic experiences to help further improve the world's knowledge about breast cancer and of its treatment.

Alongside other therapy modalities, neoadjuvant systemic chemotherapy

(NACT) presents an effective therapy option involving loco-regional and postoperative treatment for patients with operable breast cancer. Previously, NACT was thought to be a treatment modality to gain operability for patients with initially inoperable or inflammatory breast cancer. However, meta-analysis of these cohorts demonstrated an equal long-term effect to patients treated with adjuvant chemotherapy regimes, and therefore NACT gained popularity also for patients with primary operable breast cancer. Even though NACT could not be shown to improve overall survival (OS), the advantages became obvious:

1. It is an 'in vivo' testing of the chemosensitivity, and therefore predictive of the patients' prognosis. Patients with a pathologic complete response (pCR), or remission, after NACT have a better long-term prognosis than those without pCR.
2. It increases the rate of operability and breast-conserving therapy (BCT). Initially inoperable tumor masses can be reduced to operable tumors, and 60%–80% of the tumors can be treated by BCT.
3. By gaining more information about the tumor's biology, NACT offers patients with the option of individualized therapy over the near term. For patients without pCR, there especially is a great need to develop further treatment strategies post-NACT to significantly improve patient prognosis.

Integrated Meta-analysis of Early Breast Cancer Patients in Trials

Extensive knowledge about NACT in Germany has been gained from this meta-analysis of 6,634 patients with early breast cancer.[1] This study is the largest integrated meta-analysis of breast cancer patients treated with neoadjuvant anthracyclines and taxanes worldwide, and includes German data between 1998 and 2006. In a more recent study, human epidermal growth factor receptor 2 (HER2)-positive patients received trastuzumab. In this meta-analysis, data from eight trials run by GBG and the Arbeitsgemeinschaft Gynäkologische Onkologie (AGO Breast Study Group) were evaluated. These were the five German Preoperative Adriamycin and Docetaxel (GerparDo) trials of GeparDo, GeparDuo, GeparTrio (pilot phase[2] and main phase[3]), and GeparQuattro,[4,5] and the three trials of AGO-1, Taxol-Epirubicin-Cyclophosphamid-Herceptin Neoadjuvant (TECHNO), and Preoperative Epirubicin Paclitaxel Aranesp® (PREPARE). For reliable results of this analysis, high-quality data was essential. This was achieved by using individual patient data, homogenous eligibility criteria, and homogenous definitions of pCR within all eight clinical trials. For evaluation of pathologic response, the following two definitions were used in GBG's neoadjuvant studies:

Table 7–A–1. Tumor characteristics of the meta-analysis

	1998–2002 n = 2,108 (%)	2003–2006 n = 4,526 (%)
Age < 40 years	15.2	17.0
cT4	7.0	13.5
cN +	45.6	51.2
Lobular type	14.7	12.5
Grade 3	38.0	37.5
ER and PR negative	27.2	35.5
HER2 positive	3.6	29.4
Treated with trastuzumab	0.0	44.0

1. Pathologic complete response of breast and lymph nodes (pCR breast and nodes). No microscopic evidence of residual viable tumor cells (invasive or noninvasive) in any resected specimens of the breast and axillary nodes.
2. Pathologic complete response of invasive tumor and nodes (pCR invasive and nodes). No microscopic evidence of residual invasive tumor cells in all resected specimens of the breast and no microscopic evidence of residual viable tumor cells in axillary nodes.

The goal of this analysis was to assess the pCR invasive and nodes rate according to different treatment groups (trastuzumab, dose density, treatment duration, and administration of concomitant or sequential chemotherapy), and to define predictive factors for pCR so as to better predict each patient's prognosis and individualize therapy options. Table 7–A–1 summarizes the baseline data of the cohort in the meta-analysis

Prognostic Factors

Choosing the appropriate patient for a neoadjuvant chemotherapy is profound for successful treatment. NACT is the treatment of choice for patients with inflammatory and inoperable disease and also for patients with large tumors, for whom the first approach would be a mastectomy, but who wish a breast-conserving approach. In general, NACT is indicated in all patients needing chemotherapy postoperatively due to their tumor constellation.

The following prognostic factors for a complete pathologic response are revealed from the analysis:
1. *Tumor grading.* The most important prognostic factor to achieve a pCR turned out to be tumor grading. As our data show, G3 tumors (high grade) have a significant higher chance for a complete response than G1 and G2

tumors (27.8%, 4.7%, and 12.9%, respectively; p>0.001). So, patients with low-differentiated or badly differentiated tumors especially benefit from neoadjuvant chemotherapy.

2. *Hormone receptor status.* In hormone receptor negative tumors (estrogen and progesterone receptor negative), the chance for a pCR is about 30.8%, which is significantly higher than that for other hormone receptor constellations (estrogen and/or progesterone receptor positive; p>0.001).

3. *Histologic type.* The histologic type of the tumor cannot be considered as an independent prognostic factor, as it is highly correlated with tumor grading, hormone receptor status, and HER2 status. The pCR in lobular carcinomas is worse than in ductal carcinomas. However, this is due to the higher probability being hormone receptor positive, low grade, and HER2 negative. Therefore, the prognosis is better for patients with lobular carcinomas and a low pCR than for patients with ductal carcinomas and a low pCR. Within the lobular carcinomas, patients with the G1 tumor have the least chance for a pCR, but still have a good prognosis. In ductal carcinomas and other histological types, the meta-analysis showed a pCR of more than 20%.

4. *Age.* The patient's age is important as an independent prognostic factor. The younger the patient is, the higher the chance for a pCR. In the meta-analysis, patients under thirty-five years of age had a pCR rate of 30.2% (n = 424), which steadily decreased to only 16.2% in the patients' group older than sixty years of age (n = 1,365; p<0.001).

5. *Tumor size.* The clinical-measured tumor size at diagnosis also needs to be considered for the prediction of a pCR (p<0.001). In patients with a tumor size of less than 2 cm (cT1), a pCR was detected in nearly one-quarter of the patients (24.8%). For the T2 tumor, the pCR decreased to 21.3%. It further decreased to 14% in the patients' group with T3 tumors, and then to only 13.5% in the T4a-c group. It slightly increased to 15.7% in patients with inflammatory diseases.

6. *Nodal status.* Looking only at the patients' nodal status, there is again a relationship between the clinical assessment N0 and N+ (p<0.001). Patients with cN0 have a pCR rate of 21.5%, which decreases to 9.8% in patients with cN3 (cN1: 18.3%; cN2: 14.8%).

But most important, the constellation of age, tumor size, and nodal status should be considered. The younger the patient is (<35 years of age), the smaller the tumor diameter is (cT1 and cT2); and the less lymph node invasion before therapy is detected, the higher the chance for a pCR. Figure 7–A–1 shows results from the multivariable analysis regarding prognostic factors for a pCR.

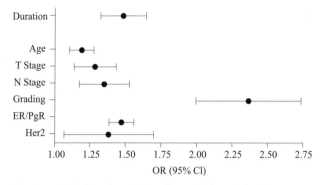

Fig. 7–A–1. Multivariate backward stepwise* analysis of prognostic treatment and baseline factors**

Note–Analysis excludes patients with missing values or trastuzumab treatment, n = 5,172. *Dose density, concomitant and sequential, histologic type, triple (ER/PR/HER) receptor status were removed because of p > 0.05. **Factors grouped as in a histogram.

As a biological marker to assess the aggressiveness of the tumor, the HER2 status should be determined. The result of the meta-analysis revealed it to be an independent, but less relevant prognostic factor for reaching pCR, if an anthracycline-taxane-based regimen is used. In HER2-negative patients, only 18.3% reached a pCR, whereas in HER2-positive patients, 22.7% had a pCR detected, regardless of other prognostic factors. Nevertheless, the most important determinant of HER2 status today remains the indication whether the patient should receive anti-HER2 therapy.

In conclusion, this data underlines the need for chemotherapy in patients with biological aggressive tumors. Though the pCR rate is significant lower in less aggressive tumors with a low proliferation rate as in G1 tumors, this does not imply a bad prognosis for their treatment. It only raises the question of the need versus the harm of chemotherapy in this population, and underscores the need for further targeted options to individualize breast cancer therapy.

HER2 Positive Disease: Characteristics in Neoadjuvant Setting

Since the introduction of trastuzumab in the treatment of HER2-positive breast cancer in 1998, the response and survival rates have improved dramatically. The therapy for HER2-positive patients, who formerly had a poor prognosis due to their aggressive disease, has become better in the setting of an anti-HER2 therapy. In HER2-positive breast cancer patients, the addition of trastuzumab to neoadjuvant chemotherapy almost doubles the rate of pCR.

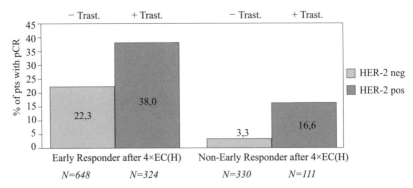

Fig. 7–A–2. Early versus late response effects of trastuzumab in chemotherapy regimen: Results of GeparQuattro trial

Note–Trastuzumab given after four lots, or cycles, of epirubicin and cyclophosphamide (EC).

This has been demonstrated in a small single institutional study by the MD Anderson Cancer Center (MDACC), in the USA, which was discontinued early on the advice of the Independent Data Monitoring Committee (IDMC) because of highly significant differences in the pCR rates in favor of the trastuzumab plus chemotherapy arm.[6] This result has been confirmed in other studies. In the German meta-analysis, the pCR rate increased from 22.7% to 41.1% when trastuzumab was added concomitantly to chemotherapy (p<0.001) in HER2-positive patients. Results of the GeparQuattro study reveal that the largest benefit can be achieved for patients without an early response to the first couple of chemotherapy cycles. This group generally achieves a pCR rate of 3%–5% irrespective of the chemotherapy regimen used. When trastuzumab is added to chemotherapy, the pCR rate could be increased five times, whereas in the group of patients with early response, the addition of trastuzumab only doubles the pCR rate (Figure 7–A–2).

Up to now, there are no large data sets regarding the addition of lapatinib to neoadjuvant chemotherapy regimes. The NeoAdjuvant Lapatinib and/or Trastuzumab Treatment Optimisation (Neo ALTTO) study and the GeparQuinto trial hopefully will determine whether lapatinib is as effective as trastuzumab, by comparing whether the combination of lapatinib and trastuzumab is better than trastuzumab alone.

Recommended Duration of Neoadjuvant Chemotherapy Regimes

Especially in the treatment of patients with a rather aggressive tumor constellation, the question of the appropriate lengths of chemotherapy arises regularly. Could a longer application regime improve the response of patients to the treatment? As a result of the German meta-analysis, the recommended treatment duration for patients receiving taxane- or antracyclines-containing chemotherapy is eighteen weeks reaching a pCR of about 19%, compared with only 9.5% with shorter durations of between eight to seventeen weeks. According to the data, a longer treatment duration of twenty-four to thirty-six weeks does not significantly improve the pCR (19.3%). The successful use of dose-dense regimes in the neoadjuvant setting is also bound to the duration of the chemotherapy. Applying two comparable neoadjuvant chemotherapy regimes, one in a dose-dense schedule and the other in the common application schedule, the pCR rate reached in the dose-dense arm was lower than that of the conventional arm (9.2%–16.9% depending on the regime vs. 18.1%, respectively). Based on these observations, dose-dense regimes in the neoadjuvant setting should only be used when a duration of at least eighteen weeks is maintained.

Cardiac Events Arising from Trastuzumab-Anthracyclines Combination

Anthracyclines are one of the most effective cytotoxic drugs and are widely prescribed for the treatment of breast cancer. However, the utility of anthracyclines are limited due to the cardiotoxic side effects, which are bound to the cumulative dose and generally unrecoverable. It can lead to progressive myocardial damage and to congestive heart failure. Anthracyclines act as a primary cardiotoxin that promotes production of free radicals, resulting in mitochondrial damage to myocytes and in myocardial cell death.[7]

Trastuzumab also has cardiotoxic side effects. It is a humanized monoclonal antibody that selectively inhibits the growth and proliferation of breast cancer cells overexpressing the type-1 tyrosine kinase membrane receptor and the HER2/neu site[8]. The HER2 site has also been detected on myocardial cells, which probably leads to cardiotoxic side-effects, with congestive heart failure and a decrease in the left ventricular ejection fraction (LVEF). The risk of cardiotoxicity with trastuzumab has been reported to be 4% with monotherapy and 27% when administered in combination with an anthracycline and cyclophosphamide[9] in a population with unknown preexisting cardiac morbidities and no monitoring of LVEF.

As anthracyclines are commonly used drugs for the treatment of primary breast cancer, the combination of both agents in patients with HER2-positive breast cancer is desirable. Based on recent results, cardiac-healthy younger patients with a left ventricular function above the upper normal limit of 55% before the start of treatment can receive a combination of both drugs without risk, if LVEF is monitored three times a month during the treatment. In the GeparQuattro trial, trastuzumab was given in combination with epirubicin and cyclophosphamide (EC), where these precautions were taken. The incidence of chronic heart failure (CHF) was only 0.2 % in this population. The trial included a total of 1,495 patients, of which 453 were HER2 positive and received trastuzumab. Six cardiac events were reported in the HER2-positive group. In four cases, a transient asymptomatic decrease in LVEF to less than 45% occurred; and in three of these patients, cardiac function had recovered before surgery. CHF and cardiac ischemia occurred in only one case each. In comparison, in 1,042 patients with HER2-negative tumors, CHF and cardiac ischemia (probably related to capecitabine) was reported in two cases each. As there was no routine monitoring of LVEF in HER2-negative patients, no data was available regarding the asymptomatic LVEF decrease in this cohort. Other clinical trials also were focusing on the question of whether it was safe to combine two agents, without potential cardiatoxic effects.

The Neoadjuvant Herceptin (NOAH) study investigated the neoadjuvant use of trastuzumab concomitant to chemotherapy with a regime containing doxorubicin (60 mg/m^2) versus cyclophosphamide, methotrexate, and 5-fluorouracil (CMF) in 327 patients with locally advanced breast cancer.[10] The HERCULES[11] study investigated cardiac safety in two cohorts of anthracycline-naive patients with metastatic breast cancer. They received trastuzumab plus either epirubicin 90 mg/m^2 or 60 mg/m^2 and cyclophosphamide as the first-line therapy. The Herceptin study at MDACC evaluated the addition of trastuzumab to standard chemotherapy — trastuzumab plus taxol, followed by FE$_{75}$C, was the experimental arm — in a neoadjuvant setting for operable breast cancer. All three studies reported cardiac toxicities at similar low frequencies.

A steady state of trastuzumab is reached only after at least twelve weeks of treatment. If trastuzumab is added to the taxane part of a sequential anthracycline-taxane regimen, this might not lead to a sufficiently long treatment duration. Results from the TECHNO study, in which the standard chemotherapy of EC was followed by a twelve week-only treatment of paclitaxel and trastuzumab, revealed a pCR rate of 32%, which appears to be lower than the pCR rate of 40% observed in the GeparQuattro trial (EC-trastuzumab followed by docetaxel-trastuzumab), where trastuzumab was given during all chemotherapy cycles over a period of twenty-four weeks.

The results from the GeparQuattro study, as well as the data from other clinical trials, support the concomitant use of trastuzumab and anthracyclines to achieve the best response and increase the overall survival of breast cancer patients. A careful selection of the patients and close monitoring of the LVEF are prerequisites when considering a combination of trastuzumab and anthracycline.

Individualized Neoadjuvant Treatment

Patients receiving neoadjuvant chemotherapy should be monitored closely regarding their tumor response, so early interventions can be done in case of progressive disease. Breast ultrasound is the preferred examination to evaluate the patient's response to NACT; however, if sonography appears not to provide valid results or if it is not performed, other imaging tests will be considered, in the following priority: magnetic resonance imaging (MRI), mammography, and positron emission tomography (PET).

Given the chance of higher pCR rates with therapy durations of about eighteen weeks, patients with a partial response should continue with the same treatment regime until their planned operation. In patients with an early complete response the probability of a pCR is about 60%, subject to further investigations if these patients require less chemotherapy. If the tumor does not show a reduction of more than 50% after the first two-to-four cycles, chemotherapy should also be finished as planned. If possible, switching to a noncross-resistant regime might be worthwhile (if a sequential treatment was not planned upfront), with the aim of achieving a better response with this individualized approach.

In cases of progressive disease, chemotherapy should be stopped and the initially planned operation should be performed immediately. In case of inoperability, radiotherapy offers a further treatment possibility. Such patients are considered chemotherapy resistant and have a biological aggressive tumor, with a higher risk of lymph node involvement, distant metastases, and worse prognosis. Figure 7–A–3 summarizes the course of neoadjuvant chemotherapy that was used in the GeparQuinto trial.

Surgical Approach

Operating on patients after neoadjuvant treatment is a bigger challenge for the surgeon than primary operation on a breast cancer patient. The precise documentation of the tumor's location before, during, and after chemotherapy is essential to estimate sufficient tumor margins. This is even more important in cases of a complete response or a partial response with unclear palpation

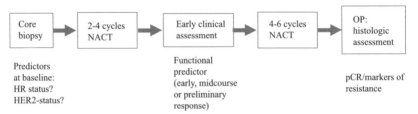

Fig. 7–A–3. Course of neoadjuvant chemotherapy used in GeparQuinto trial

findings. For detailed documentation along the course of therapy, regular photographs of the skin-marked tumor area are helpful to estimate the extent of tumor tissue and therefore the extent of the operation.

The precise excision of the tumor within the new margins is nowadays justifiable, especially for those patients with a complete clinical remission. The rate of secondary resection after NACT is higher (15%–25%). Nevertheless, the standard guidelines for BCT or mastectomy (minimum are microscopically clear margins) has to be followed for patients after NACT, as well as for primary breast operations, and no compromises should be made in surgical margins to obtain better cosmetic results. German guidelines recommend setting the operation date after the leukocyte count reaches a nadir, which is about two to four weeks after the last cycles of chemotherapy.[12,13]

One aim of the neoadjuvant approach is to improve the chance for breast conservation. Despite more effective treatments and increasing pCR rates, the BCT rate has not changed. To further increase the rate of BCT-specific contra-indications for example, T4 or multicentric tumors have to be reassessed, especially in case of a complete response. Our data show that patients treated by mastectomy have a pCR rate as high as 20%, signaling a high degree of surgical overtreatment.

In the AGO-1 study and the GeparTrio trial, the rate of BCT was 33% in locally advanced tumors and 13% in inflammatory carcinomas. Up to now, there was no long-term follow-up and no information about the recurrence rate, so the safety of this procedure cannot yet be assessed.

Evaluating the sentinel node after preoperative therapy remains a challenge, and there are no clear guidelines on how to handle this issue. Is the axillary dissection really necessary in initially clinical node-positive patients with a clinical complete response in the breast, as well as in the axilla? So far, studies evaluating the sentinel node biopsy after NACT are inconsistent on feasibility and efficacy, and therefore it cannot be recommended outside clinical trials. The SENTINA trial, also implemented as a subprotocol in the GeparQuinto trial, is looking for clear answers on this topic.[14] The SENTINA protocol was implemented as a prospective, multicenter, observational substudy to assess the feasibility, efficacy, and safety of sentinel node biopsy in patients after neoadjuvant chemotherapy, where treatment follows a specific algorithm. Patients with clinically negative axilla receive a sentinel node biopsy before neoadjuvant chemotherapy. Regardless of the results, patients start with their therapy. Afterwards, in case of a positive sentinel node, they receive a second sentinel node biopsy, immediately followed by an axillary clearance and their planned breast surgery. In case of a negative sentinel, no further interventions in the axilla is recommended. Initially node-positive patients receive their chemotherapy straight away. After completion, a reassessment of the nodal status follows. The node-negative patients receive a sentinel node biopsy, in addition to the axillary clearance. The patients with persisting node-positive status receive an axillary clearance without a sentinel node biopsy. It is expected that with this algorithm about 65% of complete axillary dissections will be avoided.

Post Neoadjuvant Systemic Treatment Options

The extent of responses to primary systemic chemotherapy has been demonstrated to be a reliable prognostic factor in breast cancer for a complete response than for patients with partial response or no change as the best result to preoperative chemotherapy.[15] The best disease-free survival was demonstrated for patients with a pathologicly confirmed complete remission of the tumor. This fact was further investigated using MDACC's data base. Prognosis of patients appeared to depend on the extent of remaining tumor tissue in the breast and in the axilla. In the presence of remaining tumor in the breast and in the axilla, the disease-free survival was poor, whereas it was very favorable if a pathologic complete remission was confirmed in the breast and nodes (Figure 7–A–4).[16] These data strongly support the hypothesis that pathologic response is a valid surrogate marker for long-term outcome. Similar results were presented by C. Liedtke[17] in 2008 (Figure 7–A–5). Their results showed that outcomes for patients were significantly correlated with the residual disease in combination with the hormone receptor status and the HER2 status. Patients with triple negative breast cancer (TNBC) and residual disease had an extremely poor prognosis. The residual tumor after NACT is the most important factor regarding overall survival (p<0.001). Patients with TNBC and residual disease had a 68% chance to be alive after three years, whereas it was 94% after three years in patients with TNBC but who had pCR.

This underscores the great need for further treatment options in patients with

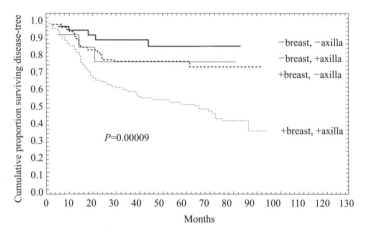

Fig. 7–A–4. Remaining tumor in the breast and/or axilla has a negative impact on disease-free survival[16]

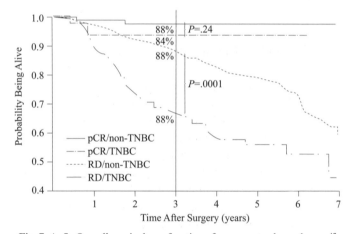

Fig. 7–A–5. Overall survival as a function of response to chemotherapy[17]

residual disease after neoadjuvant chemotherapy. For HER2 positive patients,
trastuzumab is recommended for the duration of one year, and for hormone
receptor positive patients, there are a great range of anti-hormonal therapy
options, like tamoxifen or aromatase inhibitors, for the duration of five to ten
years. But what can be done for patients with TNBC, which does not allow
for these options, and who have residual tumor tissue after the neoadjuvant
treatment?

Until now, no new effective strategy has been developed on how the poor
prognosis for TNBC patients can be improved by further postoperative
treatment. Postoperative chemotherapy does not represent a valuable option,

as resistance to chemotherapy has to be postulated after extensive preoperative treatment, and it is expected that many patients will not tolerate further toxic treatments. In addition, data of a retrospective analysis from M. Knauer[18] did not show a significant benefit in the disease-free survival of patients treated with neoadjuvant chemotherapy, followed by adjuvant chemotherapy combinations after the completed operation. Therefore, nontoxic approaches, with mechanism of action different to cytotoxic agents, have to be investigated.

One approach is the use of zoledronic acid. There is increasing evidence from a range of cell-line experiments that zoledronic acid can inhibit tumor cell adhesion and invasion.[19] There also is evidence from two adjuvant zoledronic acid studies — Austrian Breast and Colorectal Cancer Study Group trial — 12 (ABCSG-12) and Zo-Fast trial[20] — showing a lower recurrence rate after two to five years of treatment. This approach is under investigation in several clinical trials like the GAIN study conducted by the GBG, or the AZURE study (Adjuvant Zoledronic Acid to Reduce Recurrence) by the Clinical Trials Research Unit (CTRU) at the University of Leeds, in the United Kingdom.

In the NaTaN study, a prospective, randomized, open, multinational phase III study, patients with residual tumor after neoadjuvant chemotherapy were randomized to receive either ibandronate (oral) for two years as postneoadjuvant systemic therapy or were only observed over the same period. The study, which has been closed for recruitment in June 2009, has an overall 693 German patients, and the study's first safety evaluation demonstrated a feasible approach. The final efficacy analysis is awaited.

Further development of new therapeutic strategies for postoperative approaches requires an understanding of basic breast cancer biology. Extensive laboratory data and substantial evidence from preclinical and clinical studies show that angiogenesis plays an essential role in tumor growth, invasiveness, and metastasis. Studies have shown an inverse correlation between vascular endothelial growth factor (VEGF) expression and overall survival in both node-positive and node-negative patients.[21,22,23,24] Incorporation of antiangiogenic therapies in the treatment of breast cancer has shown significant improvements in outcomes.[25] Therefore, inhibition of the VEGF pathway with an anti-VEGF is currently an important strategy being actively investigated for the development of new drugs used in breast cancer treatment. Other therapy options for patients with residual tumor after neoadjuvant chemotherapy include anti-HER2 agents, such as lapatinib, pertuzumab, and T-DM1, and or other multi-tyrosin kinase inhibitors, such as sorafenib.

Conclusion

More than 6,600 patients have participated in the GBG and AGO trials, which are the largest, integrated meta-analysis of breast cancer patients treated with neoadjuvant anthracycline- and taxane- (plus trastuzumab) containing chemotherapy.

Key results of the GBG and other trials are as follows:

1. Increase of pCR rates over time is achieved by longer duration (≥18 weeks) of treatments and the additional use of trastuzumab in HER2-positive patients.
2. Characteristics of patients signaling a high chance for pCR are:
    · Young age (<35 years)
    · Small tumor size (T1 and T2)
    · Undifferentiated tumor pattern (Grade III)
    · Node-negative disease
    · Negative hormone-receptor status
    · Positive HER2 status.
3. Conventional contra-indications for breast conservation have to be reassessed in patients with clinical complete remissions.
4. Residual disease after effective neoadjuvant treatment should be considered as a new treatment indication.
5. New treatment options for those patients are of urgent need. Bisphos-phonates and anti-VEGF agents may play a role.

Acknowledgments

We want to thank the members of the Neoadjuvant Subboard of the GBG for their advisory role and all centers and patients participating in the GBG and AGO Breast studies. Without their engagement and support, the results of this clinical research would not have been possible.

Local Management After Preoperative Chemotherapy: A Surgical Perspective

Raimund Jakesz and Karl Thomanek

Summary

Preoperative chemotherapy (PCT) provides an excellent setting to determine the most efficient treatment approach for individual patients. Among various benefits, PCT assesses in vivo the tumor response to different regimens without requiring long-term follow-up, and also serves as a predictive marker of outcome. Ongoing clinical investigations should help to identify the subset of patients most likely to benefit from the use of PCT, and to establish the most effective PCT regimen and determine optimal multidisciplinary approaches in the management of breast cancer.

Introduction: Cancer Downstaging by Preoperative Chemotherapy

PCT —— also known as neoadjuvant or primary systemic treatment —— has become a frequently used and standard option for primary operable breast cancer in patients who are candidates for adjuvant systemic therapy. In particular, PCT is an established part of the management of large and locally advanced breast cancers. PCT for operable breast cancer has several potential advantages. Although not serving to improve overall survival (OS) or disease-free survival (DFS), PCT enhances the amount of breast-conserving interventions by facilitating downstaging. Furthermore, this tool allows clinicians to obtain in vivo sensitivity, along with prognostic, information.

To date, the evidence supports the hypothesis that the optimal regimens for adjuvant therapy are likely to be the optimal agents for PCT as well. The clinical trial emphasis preferably should be on whether subsets of patients can be identified needing a particular regimen, based on the molecular features of the cancer and the development of novel approaches to patient management, regardless of whether the therapy is adjuvant or PCT.

Preoperative administration of cytotoxic agents is the treatment of choice whenever breast-conserving surgery (BCS) is unfeasible or likely to have inadequate cosmesis. This strategy also is considered in patients whose tumors express markers of good response to chemotherapy, for example, low or absent hormone receptor (HR) status, high-grade non-lobular invasive histology, high counts of the the proliferation antigen Ki67, or luminal B tumors. PCT is commonly completed before surgery, except in rare cases where the disease's progression during treatment presents a hazard to surgery. PCT is given for at least six cycles over an interval of four to six months. However, it is accepted today that more PCT does not necessarily translate to a further increase in BCS.

Re-excision Factors

Various factors indicate increased re-excision rates after attempted BCS.

The German GeparDuo trial randomly assigned 607 patients to the two preoperative treatments of doxorubicin plus docetaxel, versus doxorubicin plus cyclophosphamide followed by docetaxel.[1] One hundred and four patients (21%) underwent breast-conserving re-excision or subsequent mastectomy as final pathologic analysis presented either involved or close surgical margins. The re-excision rate after attempted BCS was significantly higher in patients with invasive lobular cancer (ILC) than in patients with invasive ductal cancer (IDC) or other histologic diagnoses (32.4% vs. 14.6%, p<0.0001). Re-excision was more frequent after lumpectomy than after segmentectomy or quadrantectomy (24.1% vs 19.3%, p = Not significant) and significantly less frequent (13.3% vs. 27.0%, p<0.0001) when intraoperative frozen-section analysis was performed for margin evaluation.

In conclusion, improved breast-imaging modalities are necessary for an improved detection of residual disease after PCT, especially in the presence of ILC histology. Margin assessment by intraoperative frozen-section analysis is useful in avoiding the need for re-excision.

Ipsilateral Breast Tumor Recurrence

Loco-regional failure subsequent to BCS is associated with increased risk of distant disease and death. Ipsilateral breast tumor recurrence (IBTR) following BCS and radiation for early-stage invasive cancer occurs in about 15% of all patients at 10 years and is reduced with surgically achieved negative margins.

Table 7–B–1. Adverse prognostic factors for IBTR after PCT and BCS

Author/citation	Prognostic factors
Huang, 2006[2]	Score out of: clinical N2 and N3, lymphovascular invasion, tumor size at surgery>2cm, and multifocality
Loibl, 2006[1]	No pCR, pathologicly positive nodes, lymphovascular invasion, and multifocality
Oh, 2006[3]	Age<35 years, but no multicentric or multifocal disease
Rouzier, 2001[4]	Age<40 years, margin<2mm, and tumor size at surgery>2cm

IBTR–Ipsilateral breast tumor recurrence. PCT–Preoperative chemotherapy. BCS–Breast-conserving surgery. pCR–pathologic complete response.

It appears that early IBTR is a significant predictor of distant metastasis. Table 7–B–1 lists adverse prognostic factors in connection with IBTR.

The objective of an investigation by R. Rouzier and co-workers was to determine the incidence and prognostic value of IBTR in 257 patients treated with PCT and BCS.[4] These authors found that early recurrence is associated with a higher risk of distant metastases, but a later IBTR is also an independent predictor of distant disease.

Concludingly, IBTR is shown to be a strong predictor of distant metastases. There are implications for BCS after tumor downstaging and therapy at the time of IBTR. Whether early breast cancer relapse is a marker for, or cause of, distant metastasis remains a controversial and unresolved issue.

Challenges to Surgery

It is well known that BCS is associated with a higher loco-regional recurrence rate than mastectomy, without however affecting long-term OS.[5] The main problem with surgery and PCT is the lack of prospectively conceived surgical questions and evaluation of surgical aspects within randomized clinical trials. Most commonly, surgical data are only derived from retrospective analyses and are not powered to address and resolve aspects of surgery. The reason for this is that surgeons are less intensively involved in preparing clinical protocols for PCT. Moreover, histopathologic examination is very time consuming in preoperative diagnosis and the surgical specimen. Overall, due to a variety of confounding factors, including subjective bias and consideration toward patients' preferences, it has proven difficult to standardize the surgical criteria for primary tumor operability among patients receiving PCT.

Including techniques such as lumpectomy, wide excision, and quadrantectomy,[6] breast surgery after PCT should be performed according to the guidelines for adjuvant breast surgery.[7] BCS is the treatment of choice in all patients with lesions smaller than 3 cm in diameter, irrespective of age of patient, localization of the disease, or whether the disease is in situ, invasive, or multifocal, as long as free margins are feasible.

Dermoglandular flaps can be used to manage the excision site in midsize and larger organs.[8.] Clips should be applied to the initial tumor location if intramammary glandular flaps or reduction mammoplasty techniques are used, thus allowing clinicians to plan subsequent radiotherapy of the breast.[1] Postoperative radiotherapy is indicated in most cases of mastectomy, and breast reconstruction should be postponed until six to twelve months after completion of irradiation.

Diagnostic Biopsy

In diagnostic biopsy, core biopsy is recommendable with multiple cores, at various locations, and with needles of at least gauge size 14. An accurate determination of histology would consider invasive versus in situ disease, extensive intraductal component (EIC), and lymphovascular invasion (LVI). Preoperative risk evaluation draws on factors such as age, tumor stage, grading, receptor status, HER2 status, and status of tumor suppressor p53 (protein 53 kilodaltons). The insertion of a clip in the biopsy site is mandatory.

BCS after PCT depends on the ability to completely resect residual disease and maintain an acceptable esthetic outcome, as well as complete resolution of skin edema. Regardless of response, patients not qualifying for BCS after PCT typically present with inadequate tumor response, LVI, skin-chest wall fixation, collagen vascular disease, diffuse microcalcification, or multicentric disease. It is not clear that such patients would benefit from PCT outside of clinical trials, unless they present with locally advanced or inoperable breast cancer.

Younger women ($<$40 years) who undergo BCS that would not have been possible without PCT may have a higher local recurrence rate than other patients, but this does not necessarily compromise patient survival, and may reflect biological factors. As younger women often request BCS, age should not constrain the use of PCT to achieve this goal.

There are various factors that may influence the success of BCS, such as tumor size, LVI, or nodal status. The aim of a study by S. Sadetzky and co-workers was to create a quantitative tool to preoperatively evaluate the successful outcome of BCS in patients with locally advanced tumors.[9] One hundred consecutive patients designated for lumpectomy or mastectomy received PCT. Three factors were found to be the main predictors for successful BCS: absence of diffuse microcalcification as seen in the pretreatment mammogram, a postchemotherapy tumor size of less than 25 mm, and the existence of a circumscribed lesion on mammography. These authors concluded that the use of such criteria as a basis for deciding on the type of surgery may lower the number of avoidable procedures.

Similarly, the purpose of a trial by A. M. Chen and co-workers was to develop a prognostic index to help refine selection criteria and to serve as a general framework for clinical decision making.[10] The investigators previously determined four statistically significant predictors of IBTR and loco-regional recurrence: clinical N2 or N3 disease, residual pathologic tumor size larger than 2 cm, multifocal pattern of residual disease, and LVI in the specimen.

Planning and performing surgery subsequent to PCT needs to consider the size of the original tumor and the patient's response to PCT. The indication for, and planning of, postoperative radiotherapy relies on accurate documentation of tumor location, thus enabling the surgeon to assess the initial tumor size in case of tumor shrinkage.[7]

Sentinel Node Biopsy

Axillary metastases can be identified with either sentinel node biopsy (SNB) or ultrasound-guided fine-needle aspiration (FNA) before PCT. The standard surgical procedure for staging the axilla has been axillary node dissection (AND), aiming at removing at least ten axillary lymph nodes. In early-stage disease, SNB instead of AND is a widely accepted method of staging the axilla before chemotherapy. In this setting, SNB yields an identification rate of 86%–93% and a false-negative rate of 7%–13%.[11]

An important question relates to the timing of axillary staging, before or after PCT. A single-institution study by J. L. Jones and co-workers showed that sentinel node identification rates were significantly better when mapping was performed before rather than after PCT (100% vs. 80.6%, respectively).[12] Failure to map after chemotherapy was correlated with clinically positive nodal disease at presentation and residual disease at AND.

Intraoperative frozen sections of the sentinel node are advisable. In subsequent paraffin histology, step sections, as well as immunohistochemical staining for epithelial markers such as cytokeratins, should be performed. Standard AND is not required, and the axilla can be considered free of tumor cells, if the frozen section and the definitive histology show no tumor cells in the sentinel node. Conversely, if sentinel node mapping fails or if that node is positive for metastasis (>0.2 mm), AND should be carried out.[13]

The accuracy of SNB for determining lymph node status before primary surgery has been confirmed in a meta-analysis with pooled data from sixty-nine trials and more than 8,000 patients, with 30% of T1 tumor patients having involved lymph nodes.[14] Although performing an SNB with or without an AND before PCT will necessitate two different surgical procedures, many surgeons argue that axillary staging should be done before initiating systemic therapy to avoid confounding.

Axillary staging before PCT would probably not alter plans for systemic therapy, but might impact regional lymph node management. SNB before PCT does not offer particular clinical advantages, and reduces the number of patients who could benefit from the downstaging effects of PCT in the axillary nodes.

SNB after PCT is an acceptable approach in patients with clinically tumor-free axillary lymph nodes after PCT.[15] The procedure may be performed in such patients with an accuracy comparable to that of primary surgery patients.[16]

The large-scale National Surgical Adjuvant Breast and Bowel Project (NSABP) B-27 trial randomized 2,344 patients to receive preoperative doxorubicin and cyclophosphamide (AC), preoperative AC followed by docetaxel (T), or AC followed by surgery and then T.[17] The results demonstrated that the addition of T to AC did not significantly impact DFS or OS, but preoperative T added to AC significantly increased the proportion of patients having pCR compared with preoperative AC alone (26% vs. 13%, p <0.0001). Results showed that the frequency of successful BCS was similar among women who received preoperative AC only and those who received both preoperative AC and preoperative T (61.6% vs. 63.7%, p $= 0.33$). Pathologic primary breast tumor response was a significant predictor of pathologic nodal status (p <0.001).

Investigators opposing SNB after PCT mainly argue that SNB is not as efficient as before PCT, and also that important information on further patient management is lost. A suggested disadvantage of PCT is alteration of the lymphatic network, hampering the accuracy of SNB.[18] However, a recently published meta-analysis has demontrated equivalent accuracy of SNB after PCT and primary surgery.[19]

The apparent safety of this procedure after chemotherapy could decrease the need for AND, thereby reducing morbidity.[20] Whether this will affect prognosis, particularly in the situation of a clinically suspect axilla, remains unclear.

The identification rate and false-negative rate for SNB reported in that meta-analysis were similar for patients with and without PCT.[19] The SNB procedure and histologic examination should be performed according to consensus recommendations.[21,22] A relevant question remains whether patients are at higher risk for local recurrence or distant relapse (Table 7-B-2).

Table 7–B–2. Comparison of false-negative rates between multicenter studies after PCT

Author/citation	FNR (%)	SN − /SN +
Julian, 2004[23]	10	75/766
Krag, 1998[24]	11	13/114
McMasters, 2000[25]	7	24/333
Mamounas, 2005[26]	11	15/140
Tafra, 2001[27]	13	25/193
Veronesi, 2003[28]	9	8/91
Xing, 2005[19]	12	65/540

In summary, optimal candidates for SNB after PCT should have a low risk for a positive nonsentinel node. The SNB inaccuracy rate is a function of the false-negative rate and the rate of axillary node positivity. SNB after PCT is feasible and accurate with similar performance characteristics to those of SNB before systemic therapy.[29] By performing SNB after PCT, up to 40% of patients who present with involved axillary nodes may be spared axillary dissection.

Conclusion: Preoperative Chemotherapy To Individualize Treatment

Today's surgical approaches, including a focus on the role of SNB after PCT, are evolving strongly. Despite a multitude of clinical trials using PCT in breast cancer patients, we still are faced with certain fundamental questions (Table 7–B–3).

Overall, PCT offers an excellent setting in which to determine the most efficient treatment approach for an individual patient. Probably, the main benefit of PCT is assessing in vivo the tumor response to different regimens without requiring long-term follow-up, and also serving as a predictive marker of outcome. Also, PCT might identify nonresponders early in the course of therapy and allow for a change in treatment with potentially improved response and less toxicity. Early identification of better responders could then permit administration of a shorter course of PCT, thus minimizing toxicity.

Finally, PCT has advantages for future clinical trials evaluating novel drugs and combinations of agents in the systemic treatment of breast cancer patients. Ongoing clinical investigations will help to identify the subset of patients who would most benefit from the use of PCT, establish the most effective PCT regimen, and determine optimal multidisciplinary approaches in the management of breast cancer.

Table 7–B–3. PCT and BCS-Topics to be addressed in the future

---

* Development of radiological criteria to better define the extent of remission

---

* Optimal management of patients with residual disease in the breast or axilla, subsequent to maximum PCT
* Optimal management of patients who do not respond to initial PCT
* Better definition of who needs PCT and who is not at an increased risk for IBTR after BCS
* Implementation of more accurate predictive markers for pCR and IBTR (gene profiling)
* Role of combination chemotherapy plus endocrine treatment for patients with ER + /PR + tumors
* Role of biologicals, such as trastuzumab, bevacizumab, and lapatinib

Local Management After Preoperative Chemotherapy: An Imaging Modality Perspective

Hiroyasu Yamashiro, Masahiro Takada, and Masakazu Toi

Summary

Local management after neoadjuvant chemotherapy (NAC) for primary breast cancer (PBC) is affected by predictability of treatment response according to tumor phenotypes. Although evaluation of residual tumor burden after NAC by imaging has improved, controversy still remains. This article focuses on the prediction of pathologic response and the imaging of clinical response from the point of local management following NAC in the patients with PBC.

Introduction: Can Neoadjuvant Chemotherapy (NAC) Strategies Further Improve Patient Care?

NAC for PBC was indicated for advanced breast cancer when the technique was introduced into clinical practice in the 1970s. However, based on many clinical trials on NAC performed thereafter, the indication of NAC became similar to that of postoperative adjuvant therapy, and now NAC is considered one of the standard selections for operable breast cancer. This remarkable change in the strategy of systemic therapy has affected the subsequent local management of breast cancer.

NAC's Role in Optimal Systemic Therapy

One aspect of NAC for PBC is the in vivo drug sensitivity test. Its combination with translational research has made a marked contribution to elucidating cancer biology, including host reactions. Such attempts may continue in the future, but at present, the clinical benefits of NAC may be summarized as follows:

1. Downstaging increases the opportunity for breast-conserving surgery (BCS).

2. Pathologic response of the primary lesion can be used as a surrogate marker of long-term outcome, because outcomes —— such as disease-free survival (DFS) and overall survival (OS) —— are improved when a pathologic complete response (pCR) is achieved.

3. Residual tumor burden after NAC contains therapy-resistant phenotype, which helps to tailor the postoperative systemic and local treatment.

Estrogen receptor (ER), human epidermal growth factor receptor 2 (HER2), and tumor grade have been reported as predictive factors in the response of patients to NAC.[1] The Japan Breast Cancer Research Group-01 (JBCRG01)[2] study, which evaluated the efficacy and safety of a four course of 5-fluorouracil/epirubicin/cyclophosphamide (FEC) followed by a four course of docetaxel as NAC treatment for early breast cancers, showed a pathologic response rate (pCR) that was different according to tumor phenotype. The quasi-pathologic complete response (QpCR) rate of ER positive/HER2 negative tumors was 13%, while that of ER negative/HER2 positive tumors was 67%. Furthermore, HER2 was an independent predictor of pCR. R. Rouzier and co-workers showed that basal-like and HER2 type breast cancer were more sensitivity to NAC compared with other types.[3] In estimating the residual tumor burden after NAC, we should take into account the relationship between tumor phenotype and treatment response to NAC.

In clinical trials of NAC, such as National Surgical Adjuvant Breast and Bowel Project (NSABP) B-27[4] and Aberdeen[5] studies, the additional administration of chemotherapeutic drugs without cross resistance increased the response rate. An interesting point regarding the results of the NSABP B-27 and JBCRG01 studies was that the effect of additional taxane varied, depending on the response to the preceding anthracycline-based regimen. The NSABP B-27 trial showed that partial responders to four courses of AC (doxorubicine/cyclophosphamide) benefited from the addition of preoperative docetaxel treatment (hazard ratio for disease-free survival = 0.71; 95% CI, 0.55–0.91, p = 0.007), whereas non-responders to AC did not. In the JBCRG01 trial, clinical response to FEC was an independent predictive factor of pCR. It might be possible to hypothesize that pan-chemotherapy sensitivity is involved in these clinical phenomena. Therefore, the therapeutic effect should be monitored at an early phase of therapy, and its modality and timing are important (Figure 7–C–1).

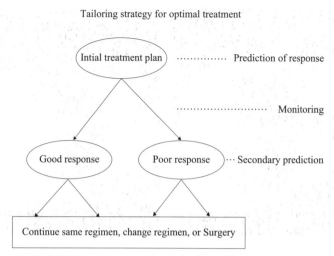

Tailoring strategy for optimal treatment

Fig. 7–C–1. Tailoring strategy for optimal neoadjuvant chemotherapy

Imaging Study for Monitoring Response to NAC

Ultrasonography (US) and mammography (MMG) are relatively simple modalities, but not very accurate in the prediction of pCR.[6] Although magnetic resonance imaging (MRI) previously was considered very sensitive but inferior in specificity,[7] it is now playing an important role in assessing the therapeutic effect after NAC and in deciding the area to be resected. Dynamic contrast-enhanced MRI using gadolinium contrast medium reflects angiogenesis around tumors, increased vascular permeability, and blood flow, and such images show high tissue resolution.

Even if tumor volume changes can be assessed accurately by MRI, they may manifest after changes in the underlying tumor function, such as vascular density or permeability. Therefore, vascular or metabolic parameters might provide a more sensitive indicator of early tumor response. It has been reported that responses to NAC could be predicted by performing MRI after the first one to two cycles of NAC.[8,9] In these reports, in addition to the maximum diameter of the tumor in the late phase of contrast imaging, the functions and characteristics of tumors and surrounding tissue, such as the area under the curve of dynamic contrast-enhanced study and the relative signal intensity of tumors immediately after the contrast medium injection, were given as response-predictive factors.

Magnetic resonance spectroscopy (MRS) is a method to investigate the types and components of molecules in the body, based on the level of slight

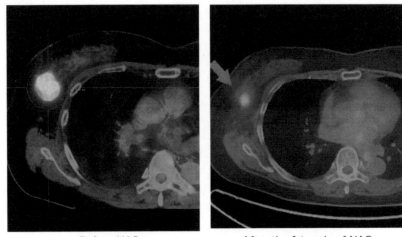

Before NAC   After the 1ˢᵗ cycle of NAC

Fig. 7–C–2. Response to NAC (FDG-PET evaluation)

differences in the resonance frequency (chemical shifts) produced, due to the influence of a magnetic field generated by an adjacent atomic nucleus on the magnetic field of a molecule. It has been reported that malignant tumors contain a high level of metabolites, including choline, compared with normal tissue, and the residual tumor mass may be estimated from the metabolite level, which is useful for the prediction of responses in the early phase of NAC.[10]

18F-fluorodeoxyglucose-positron emission tomography (FDG-PET) may also be useful as another imaging method to predict the effect of chemotherapy, which may be due to changes in the metabolic function of tumor cells preceding tumor size reduction. A high response rate following reduction in the standardized uptake value (SUV) of FDG during therapy and after one to two cycles of NAC has been reported[11,12] (Figure 7–C–2). In addition, studies on changes in the expression levels of gene biomarkers after the first one to two cycles, such as HER2, Ki-67, p-53, and bcl-2,[13] and measurement of cytokeratin 18 and circulating tumor cells, have been progressing,[14] and these may simultaneously serve as effect-predictive factors during NAC. Molecular markers associated with responses to treatment will be identified by a combination of NAC and translational research. The development of the method for NAC response prediction may provide important information for the evaluation of residual tumor burden after NAC, designing the cut margin of the tumor, and tailoring the NAC system to the individual patient.

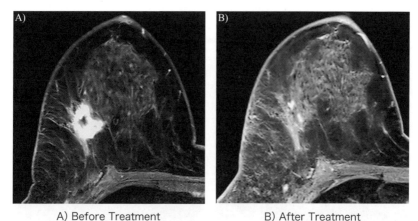

A) Before Treatment   B) After Treatment

Fig. 7–C–3a. Dendritic shrinkage pattern during neoadjuvant chemotherapy
MRI imaging of a patient.

Evaluation of the Residual Tumor Burden and Surgery

Meta-analysis of NAC[15] pointed out an elevation in the local recurrence rate, and accurate evaluation of the resection area is an issue concerning surgery after NAC. Studies have consistently suggested a closer agreement between MRI and the extent of residual disease than that detected with physical examination or conventional imaging study, such as US or MMG.[16] It has been reported that whether the tumor reduction shows a concentric or dendritic shrinkage pattern can be identified by performing MRI before and after NAC, which facilitates the identification of patients appropriate for BCS.[17] In the dendritic pattern, an expansion similar to that of before NAC was noted through MRI along the mammary duct despite a reduction in absolute cancer volume, and its detection by MMG and US is difficult (Figure 7–C–3).

The pre-conference questionnaire results of the Kyoto Breast Cancer Consensus Conference in 2009 clarified that many experts utilize MRI for decision making regarding BCS. To the question of the cut margin after NAC, about two-thirds of the experts answered that they set a new margin —— adjusted for the tumor's extent after NAC —— in cases showing a concentric shrinkage pattern, while one-third maintain the previous margin. In contrast with cases showing a dendritic shrinkage pattern, about one-quarter set a new margin, while most experts kept the previous margin. Regarding clinical complete response (cCR) cases, only a small percentage of the experts surveyed performed needle biopsy to confirm pCR, but about one-half performed only exploratory or limited excision, accounting for a higher rate of respondents than

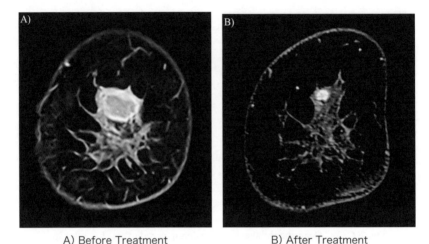

A) Before Treatment   B) After Treatment

Fig. 7–C–3b. Concentric shrinkage pattern during neoadjuvant chemotherapy
MRI imaging of a patient.

those who maintained the previous margin. This suggested that the resection area could be reduced in cases of a concentric shrinkage pattern and cCR (Figure 7–C–4).

We mentioned that the probability of achieving pCR can be predicted by phenotype classification based on the expression of hormone receptors and HER2[2,18] and clinical response to NAC. It is also possible that tumor shrinkage pattern differs among hormone receptor-positive, HER2-positive, and triple negative breast cancers. These differences in the tumor phenotype may determine the reliability of the expansion, shrinkage pattern, and cCR evaluation by imaging such as MRI. Hormone receptor positivity implies a dendritic pattern, but no predictor has been identified definitively.

Residual Tumor Burden as a Prognostic Marker

Under the current consensus that identifiable residual lesions should be resected, there are no differences in the local recurrence or survival rates between cases in which all invasive cancer and ductal carcinoma in situ (DCIS) were eradicated with NAC and cases in which only residual DCIS remains.[19] Although DCIS is usually difficult to be detected by MMG and US, it was probably controlled by postoperative radiotherapy and adjuvant therapy. However, MRI detects DCIS due to its relative high sensitivity, which may lead to oversurgery,[20] because the local recurrence rate following radiotherapy-combined BCS was not reduced

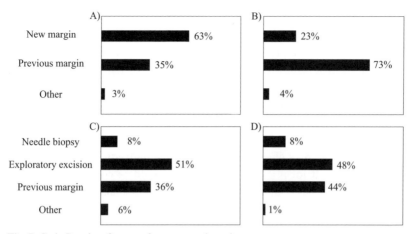

Fig. 7–C–4. Results of pre-conference questionnaire
Breast-conserving surgery for (A) patients with concentric shrinkage pattern and (B) patients with
dendritic shrinkage pattern. Surgery for complete clinical response cases (C) with HER2-negative
breast cancer and (D) with HER2-positive breast cancer.

when the tumor was evaluated by MRI.[21] Whether all of the lesions identified
by MRI after NAC should be completely resected or not should be re-discussed
between the doctors and patients. Together, they should also address problems
on whether local recurrence will influence survival and whether postoperative
adjuvant therapy should be performed in patients who do not achieve pCR to
NAC.

It also has been reported that the outcomes of NAC can be predicted by a
scoring system using the clinical stage before therapy, the pathologic stage
after NAC, the presence or absence of ER, and nuclear grade.[21] A nomogram
that predicts probability of pCR and distant metastasis-free survival using
some clinicopathologic parameters has been developed. The American Joint
Committee on Cancer (AJCC) system of pathologic stages for resected tissue
also may be a prognostic factor after NAC.[22] Studies on the prediction of
outcomes after NAC are progressing, but these discussions are based on the
appropriate resection. Therefore, mapping techniques that accurately reflect
the extent of tumor before NAC and residual cancer burden after NAC are
important.

Residual Tumor Phenotype After NAC

After NAC, it is known that the phenotype of a residual tumor is changed by
the treatment. For example, the phenotype of hormone receptors and HER2

is occasionally changed by the systemic therapy. It is difficult to predict these changes by the treatment before starting. There is controversy whether clinicians should use post-treatment status or pre-treatment status for the selection of treatment, for instance, for hormonal therapy. It also has been shown that nuclear factor kappa B (NF-κB) expression in the residual tumor is a marker of poor prognosis. Therefore, it might be important to measure these markers before and after treatment, because the knowledge will help to develop novel therapeutic concept and tools. Furthermore, recent study results in cancer stem cell biology may give us some ideas on the property of residual tumors and the treatment for it.[23] That information would be crucial, not only for systemic therapy but also for local therapy. Multidisciplinary approaches also are indispensable for the control of residual tumor burden.

Conclusion

The accurate prediction and monitoring of effects and eventual assessment of residual disease are essential to perform optimal local therapy. At present, MRI is the most sensitive modality, which facilitates the identification of the shrinkage pattern and may lead to a reduction in the resection volume for patients with pCR or a dendritic shrinkage pattern. A clinical trial is needed to assess whether MRI is the most appropriate modality.

Local and Systemic Management After Preoperative Anti-HER2 Therapy

Nobuko Sakita, Takayuki Ueno and Masakazu Toi

Summary

Preoperative anti-HER2 therapy, in combination with chemotherapy, achieves very good pCR rates in breast cancer patients with overexpressing HER2, but there are too many unanswered questions for preoperative anti-HER2 therapy to be regarded as a standard treatment of care.

Introduction

Overexpression of the human epidermal growth factor receptor 2 (HER2) occurs in 20%–30% of invasive breast carcinomas. Although patients with overexpression of HER2 have poor prognosis, introduction of anti-HER2 therapy (trastuzumab) in both metastatic and postoperative settings has improved the prognosis of breast cancer patients. Trastuzumab, in combination with chemotherapy, in preoperative settings is the next promising strategy. The reported pathologic complete response (pCR) rate looks higher in patients with trastuzumab than in those without trastuzumab. Since pCR rate is a reliable predictor of prolonged survival, it is reasonable to assume that trastuzumab, in combination with chemotherapy, will become a standard therapy in preoperative settings. In this chapter, we discuss the local management of breast cancer after preoperative anti-HER2 therapy.

Anti-HER2 Drugs

Human epidermal growth factor receptor 2 (HER2)
The HER family consists of four closely related transmembrane tyrosine kinase

receptors:
1. HER1, also known as epidermal growth factor receptor, or EGFR;
2. HER2, also known as HER2/neu (neuro/glioblastoma derived oncogene homolog (avian)), or erbB-2 (v-erb-b2 erythroblastic leukemia viral oncogene homolog 2);
3. HER3; and
4. HER4.

Each of these receptors consists of an extracellular domain, a transmembrane lipophilic segment, and a functional intracellular tyrosine kinase domain (except for HER3). The tyrosine kinase domains are activated by homodimerization and heterodimerization, which are induced by ligand binding (a ligand for HER2 is unknown). HER2 signaling promotes cell proliferation through the RAS-MAPK pathway and inhibits cell death through the PI3K-AKT-mTOR pathway[1] (Figure 7−D−1).

It is reported that HER2 signaling has cross-talks with estrogen receptor (ER)-related signaling and other growth factor signaling, such as insulin-like growth factor 1 receptor (IGFR-1).[2,3] In intrinsic subtypes, HER2 overexpression is observed in the HER2 type and in some part of the luminal B type[4] (Figure 7−D−2).

Trastuzumab

Trastuzumab is the first and successful agent among HER2 targeting agents, and many other agents are being developed.

Mechanisms of action of trastuzumab. Trastuzumab is a recombinant humanized monoclonal antibody targeting the extracellular domain of the HER2 protein on the tumor cells. The mechanism of action of trastuzumab is not sufficiently understood, and there are several hypotheses (Table 7−D−1).

The mechanisms of action are being investigated. Among many hypotheses, antibody-dependent cellular cytotoxicity (ADCC) is one of the mechanisms of trastuzumab action. The Fc domain of trastuzumab binds to the Fcγ receptor of natural killer (NK) cells, then activates them. Activated NK cells put tumor cells into lysis. ADCC has been demonstrated in many cancer cell lines. In clinical data, R. Gennari and colleagues reported that clinical responses have significant correlation with ADCC-mediated killing by patients' peripheral blood monocular cells in preoperative use of trastuzumab plus chemotherapy.[7]

Trastuzumab also induces inhibition of HER2 signaling by binding to the HER2 extrracellular domain (ECD), or by blocking dimerization. As shown in Figure 7−D−3, inhibition of HER2 signaling leads to a reduction in cell proliferation, cell survival, and angiogenesis. p95, one of the causes of resistance to trastuzumab, is a truncated and activated form of receptor that is

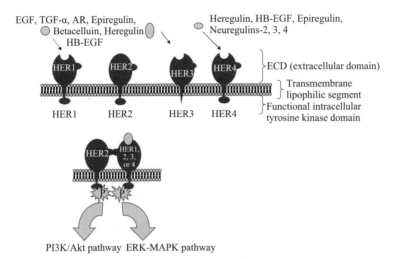

Fig. 7-D-1. HER family members, their structure, and ligands
Dimerization and phosphorylation induce HER2 signaling.

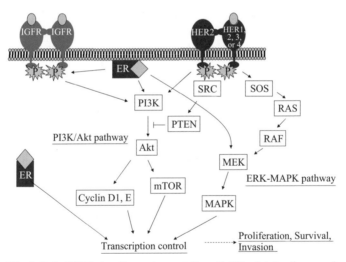

Fig. 7-D-2. HER2 signaling and cross-talks with ER-related pathway and other growth factor signaling

cleaved by the protease (Figure 7-D-4). Trastuzumab is reported to prevent production of p95 by interfering with the protease.

Mechanism of resistance of the HER2-expressing breast cancer cells to trastuzumab. In particular, the mechanisms of resistance to trastuzumab are not proven *sufficiently*, and for which there are several possible explanations (Table 7-D-2). Increased cell signaling in PI3K-Akt pathway and other pathways

Table 7–D–1. Mechanisms of the cancer antibody trastuzumab

Proposed main mechanism	Process of action
ADCC	• Tumor cell lysis
Inhibition of HER2 signaling/ Blocking dimerization	• Inhibition of the pI3-K pathway (G1 arrest and reduction of survival and angiogenesis*)
	• Attenuation of cell signaling
Inhibition of HER2 (ECD) shedding	• Prevention of p95 expression
Endocytosis of HER2	• Degradation (controversial)

*Reduction of angiogenesis may lead to normalization of tumor vessels, resulting in better delivery of chemoagents.[5,6]

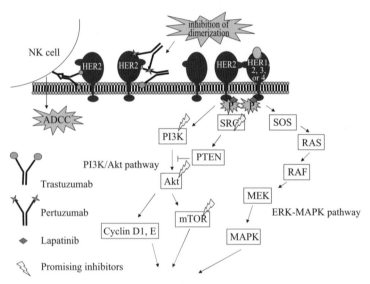

Fig. 7–D–3. Mechanism of action of anti-HER2 therapy

is likely to be one of the mechanisms. In patients with expression of p95, trastuzumab is reported less effective than in those without expression of p95. As the effectiveness of ADCC varies among patients, ADCC activity may also affect trastuzumab efficacy.

Pertuzumab

Pertuzumab is a monoclonal antibody targeting the extracelluar domain of the HER2 protein on the tumor cells, sterically blocking dimerization of HER2 with HER2 or another receptor, including HER3 and HER1 (Figure 7–D–2). The targeting site is different from that of trastuzumab.[9] The mechanism of action is inhibition of intracellular signaling by blocking dimerization. It has not been proven that pertuzumab induces ADCC. In vitro, the combination of trastuzumab and pertuzumab caused more apoptosis and cell growth arrest

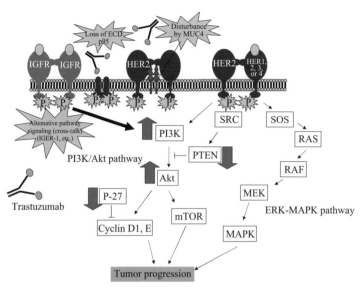

Fig. 7–D–4. Mechanism of resistance of the HER2-expressing breast cancer cells
to trastuzumab

Table 7–D–2. Proposed mechanisms of resistance to trastuzumab

Main mechanisms	Explanation
Unable to bind to ECD	Steric hindrance of receptor by cell surface proteins (MUC4)
	Truncated form of receptor (p95)
Alternative pathway signaling	IGF1R overexpression
	VEGF overexpression
Alternative HER signaling	HER1/HER3 (or HER1) heterodimers
	Increased level of ligands (such as heregulin, EGF, and TGF-α)
	Increased level of TGF-β
Constitutive activation of downstream effectors	Reduced level of PTEN
	Reduced p27^{kip1}
	Increased Akt activity

Source: Modified from ref.8.

than trastuzumab alone.[10] A phase I study showed efficacy of pertuzumab to
a part of solid tumors and tolerance of pertuzumab.[8] The results of the phase
II clinical trial with trastuzumab plus pertuzumab in patients with metastasis,
showed an overall remission rate (ORR) of 14%.[11]

Lapatinib
Lapatinib is a small molecule, dual tyrosin kinase inhibitor, which inhibits
HER1 (EGFR) and HER2. In vitro, lapatinib is effective, not only in HER2-

Table 7–D–3. Anti-HER2 agents under development

Group	Agents
Anti-HER2	Ertumaxomab, trastuzumab-MCC-DM1
Inhibitors of several HER, and TKIs	Canertinib, neratinib, JNJ-28871063
mTOR inhibitor	Everolimus (RAD001), CCI779 (temsirolimus)
PI3K inhibitor	TCN-P (triciribine)
SRC inhibitor	Dasatinib, bosutinib

overexpressing cells, but also in trastuzumab-resistant cell lines (especially p95 expressing cells). In clinical trials, lapatinib (± chemotherapy) was also effective in patients who had received a treatment containing trastuzumab. The advantages of lapatinib are, first, that it is an oral drug; second, that it causes less frequent cardiac events than trastuzumab; and third, it shows possibilities in preventing brain metastasis. Since lapatinib can be effective in trastuzumab-resistant breast cancers, lapatinib seems to be an effective drug in anti-HER2 therapy if biomarkers of trastuzumab resistance (such as p95) are established.

Others

There are many anti-HER2 agents under development. Targeting the downstream signaling pathway from HER2 could be effective, when it is added to current therapies (anti-HER2 agents and chemotherapy) (Table 7–D–3).

A combination of EGFR family inhibitors, anti-angiogenesis agents, and current therapies including anti-HER2 agents is also a possible strategy to overcome resistance.

Clinical Efficacy of Preoperative Anti-HER2 Therapy

Background: Postoperative anti-HER2 therapy improves prognosis in breast cancer patients with overexpressing HER2

The efficacy of postoperative anti-HER2 therapy has been proven in several phase III clinical trials (Table 7–D–4). Postoperative anti-HER2 therapy prolongs both disease-free survival (DFS) and overall survival (OS).[12-14] For example, in the Herceptin Adjvant (HERA) Trial, the hazard ratio (HR) of DFS and OS is 0.64 (p<0.0001) and 0.66 (p<0.0001) at a median follow-up of two years, respectively, and 0.76 (p<0.0001) and 0.85 (p=0.108) at a median follow-up of four years. The trastuzumab-related cardiac dysfunction is one of the adverse effects of great concern in adjuvant setting. In HERA trial at 3.6-year median follow-up, the incidence of cardiac events was higher in the trastuzumab

Table 7-D-4. Summary of clinical trials of postoperative anti-HER2 therapy

study	number of patients	Therapy	DFS (%)	HR for DFS	p value	OS (%)	HR for OS	p value	Median follow-up (m)
NSABP B-31 /NCCTG N-9831	1679	AC x 4→paclitaxel (q3w x 4) or (qw x 12)	2y: 67 4y: 73.1	2y: 0.48 (0.39-0.59) 4y: 0.49 (0.41-0.58)	<0.001 <0.0001	2y: 87 4y: 89.4	2y: 0.67 (0.48-0.93) 4y: 0.63 (0.49-0.81)	0.02 0.000	24 35
(ref. 12, 17)	1672	AC x 4→paclitaxel (q3w x 4) or (qw x 12) + T(qw) x 52	2y: 85 4y: 85.9			2y: 91 4y: 92.6			
HERA	1698	standard adjuvant/neoadjuvant chemotherapy	2y: 74 4y: 72.2	2y: 0.64 (0.54-0.76) 4y: 0.76 (0.66-0.87)	<0.001 0.0001	2y: 90 4y: 87.7	2y: 0.66 (0.47-0.91) 4y: 0.85 (0.70-1.04)	0.011 0.109	23.5 48.4
(ref. 13, 18)	1703	standard chemotherapy→T(q3w) x 18	2y: 81 4y: 78.6			2y: 92 4y: 89.3			
BCIRG 006	1073	AC x 4→DOC (q3w) x 4	3y: 77			3y: 86			
(ref. 19)	1074	AC x 4→DOC (q3w) x 4+T x 1year	3y: 83	3y: 0.61 (0.48-0.76) (vs. T(-) group)	<0.0001	3y: 92	3y: 0.59 (0.42-0.85)	0.004	36
	1075	{DOC + carboplatin} (q3w) x 6+T x 1year	3y: 82	3y: 0.67 (0.54-0.83) (vs. T(-) group)	0.0003	3y: 91	3y: 0.66 (0.47-0.93)	0.017	36
FinHer	116	{vinorelbine (qw) x 8} OR {DOC (q3w) x 3}→CEF x 3	3y: 77.6 5y: 73.3 (DDFS)	3y: 0.42 (0.21-0.83) 5y: 0.65 (0.38-1.12)	0.01 0.12	3y: 89.7 5y: 81.9	3y: 0.66 (0.16-1.08) 5y: 0.55 (0.17-1.83)	0.15 0.094	35-37 62
(ref. 14, 20)	116	{{vinorelbine (qw) x 8} OR {DOC (q3w) x 3}} + T(qw) x 9→CEF x 3	3y: 89.3 5y: 81.9 (DDFS)			3y: 96.5 5y: 89.6			

Source: Modified from ref. 12-14, 17-20.

group than in chemotherapy alone group, with severe chronic heart failure (CHF) at 0.77% vs 0.00%, and confirmed drop in significant left ventricular ejection fraction (LVEF) by 3.57% vs 0.64%.[15] The 80.8% of patients with cardiac adverse effects recovered from LVEF by more than 50% at 6.4-month median follow-up. They also reported that the incidence of cardiac events appears not to increase, but to remain constant after planned one-year treatment of trastuzumab was completed. It appears that one-year treatment of trastuzumab in adjuvant setting has tolerability. The standard strategy in a postoperative setting for HER2 overexpression breast cancers is the combination of anti-HER2 agent and chemotherapy according to National Comprehensive Cancer Network (NCCN) guidelines and the report of St. Gallen consensus meeting in 2009.[16]

However, clinical questions still remain in postoperative anti-HER2 therapy. The questions include:

1. What is the best treatment regimen in combination with trastuzumab?
2. Which is better, using trastuzumab and chemotherapy sequentially or simultaneously?

Table 7–D–5. Summary of clinical trials of preoperative anti-HER2 therapy

	Reference	Number of patients	Therapy	pCR rate	ORR	DFS (%)	Median follow-up (m)
Phase II	Bines, J.	34	T(qw) x 14 + DOC (qw) x 12	14	72	NA	NA
	Coudert, B.P.	33	T(qw) x 18 + DOC (q3w) x 6	47	96	NA	26
	van Pelt, A.E.	22*	T(qw) x 12 + DOC (q3w) x 4	NA	77	NA	15.5: (2-38)
	Lybaert, W.	25	{T + DOC + capecitabine (day 1-14)} (q3w) x 6	45	100	NA	NA
	Tripathy, D.	23 (21 evaluable)	T (qw) x 12 + {DOC + capecitabine (day 1-14)} (q3w) x 4	52	90	NA	NA
	Limentani, S.A.	31	T (qw) x 12 + {DOC + vinorelbine} (q2w) x 6	39	94	83.90%	25
	Coudert, B.P.	70	T (qw) x 18 + {DOC + carboplatin} (q3w) x 6	39	95	NA	25: (16-43)
	Han, H.S.	32 (25 evaluable)	T (qw) x 10 + {DOC + carboplatin} (q2w) x 4	40	NR	NA	NA
	Hurley, J.	48	T (qw) x 12 + {DOC + cisplatin} (q3w) x 4	23	NR	NA	NA
	Burstein, H.J.	40	T (qw) x 12 + paclitaxel (q3w) x 4	18	75	2y: 83.3	25: (9-37)
	Kelly, H.	37	AC (q3w) x 4 → T (qw) + paclitaxel (qw) x 12	19	86	NA	NA
	Anton, A.	26	{liposomal doxorubicin + DOC} (q3w) x 6 → T (qw) x 17	31	96	NA	NA
	Harris, L.N.	42	T (qw) x 12+ vinorelbine (qw) x 12	20	88	NA	2.6: (0.9-3.8)
Phase III	Buzdar, A.U.	23	T (qw) x 12 + paclitaxel (q3w) x 4 → T (qw) x 12 + FEC (q3w) x 4	65	96	3y: 100	36.1: (12.3-54.8)
		19	paclitaxel (q3w) x 4 → FEC (q3w) x 4	26	95	3y: 85.3	NA
	Gianni, L.	115	T + A + paclitaxel (q3w) x 3 → T + paclitaxel (q3w) x 4 → T (q3w) x 4 + CMF (q4w) x 3	43	81	NA	NA
		113	A + paclitaxel (q3w) x 3 → paclitaxel(q3w) x 4 → CMF (q4w) x 3	23	73	NA	NA
Lapatinib	Cristofanilli, M.	30**	lapatinib (q2w) + paclitaxel (qw) x 12	17	77	NA	NA

Note: Only studies with ≥ 20 evaluable patients are included. *Six of stage IV patients are included. **Clinical trials for inflammatory breast cancer.
Source: Modified from ref. 8, 23−37.

3. How long should trastuzumab be used after surgery?
4. Should patients with small tumor (≤1 cm) receive trastuzumab?
5. How should the new anti-HER2 agents (lapatinib, pertuzumab, and so on) be used?

Despite only moderate evidence, preoperative anti-HER2 therapy seems to give great benefits. Since chemotherapy in preoperative settings and postoperative settings brings the same benefits,[21,22] preoperative anti-HER2 therapy seems promising, especially for patients with local advanced cancer. Clinical trials of preoperative anti-HER2 therapy have been, and are being, conducted to test its benefits within a preoperative chemotherapy setting.

Preoperative anti-HER2 therapy improves pCR rate in combination with chemotherapy

The main strategy of preoperative anti-HER2 therapy is the combination of anti-HER2 agent and chemotherapy. There are not enough clinical trials to indicate whether the combination of anti-HER2 agent and chemotherapy prolongs OS.

pCR rate is a reliable predictor of prolonged survival. In most clinical trials, the primary endpoint is pCR rate. The pCR rate of preoperative anti-HER2 therapy varies with regimens (Table 7−D−5). Two randomized phase III trials that compare preoperative therapy with and without trastuzumab are reported.

Both trials show significantly higher pCR rates in the trastuzumab groups (65% and 43%) than in the chemotherapy alone groups (26% and 23%).[23,24]

Since the pCR rate is greatly improved by this strategy, starting further more trials that compare preoperative chemotherapy with and without trastuzumab is not allowed ethically. Recent clinical trials in preoperative anti-HER2 therapy use the combination therapy (anti-HER2 therapy and chemotherapy) as a control arm. In the near future, preoperative anti-HER2 therapy will become a standard therapy. In practice, further investigations will be needed.

Long-term outcome of preoperative anti-HER2 therapy

There are few reports that show long-term outcome of patients in preoperative anti-HER2 therapy. Since most of their primary endpoint is pCR, the sample size is not large enough to ensure reliability of long-term outcome. S. A. Limentani and colleagues reported that the OS in patients with preoperative anti-HER2 therapy was 96.8% (median follow-up: 25 months).[30] A. U. Buzdar and colleagues reported DFS at three years was 100% in the chemotherapy and trasutuzmab group, while 85.3% in the chemotherapy alone group.[23] The combination of chemotherapy and trasutuzmab seems to improve DFS, but it is still unknown whether the preoperative anti-HER2 therapy brings better OS than the postoperative anti-HER2 therapy. Moreover, the breast conservation rate of the two groups was not significantly different. However, this therapy undoubtedly will contribute to the treatment of local advanced cancer, which is inoperable before treatment.

Recurrence pattern after preoperative anti-HER2 therapy

There are few reports that show patterns of recurrence after preoperative anti-HER2 therapy. There is one retrospective analysis of HER2-positive breast cancer patients, who were treated by preoperative chemotherapy (anthracycline plus taxane) with and without trastuzumab (n = 54, 71, respectively). The data show the HR for DFS in the pCR patients over non-pCR patients was 0.09 (95% confidence interval, or CI, 0.01−0.70) in the chemotherapy plus trastuzumab group and 0.62 (95% CI, 0.21−1.83) in the chemotherapy alone group (p = 0.10, according to an interaction test). Also, it is reported that the rate of CNS metastasis within two years of the treatment was higher in patients with chemotherapy plus trastuzumab than in patients with chemotherapy alone.[38] Another report showed that in a retrospective cohort study of patients receiving preoperative trastuzumab plus chemotherapy (n = 40), pCR rate was 55% (or 22 patients). In this report, four of five recurrence patients had not achieved pCR in primary therapy. Brain metastasis was the first recurrence in four patients.[39]

Despite insufficient evidence, it seems that pCR is a good surrogate marker of good prognosis, even in preoperative anti-HER2 therapy. It seems that prevention of brain metastasis will be important in HER2-positive patients after preoperative anti-HER2 therapy.

Questions To Be Solved Before Standardization of Preoperative Anti-HER2 Therapy

Which agents are the best in combination with anti-HER2 therapy in preoperative settings? Which agents are the best among anti-HER2 agents?

Several clinical trials of preoperative anti-HER2 therapy have been reported. The most commonly used treatment is an anthracycline-containing regimen (FEC or AC x 4) followed by taxane (Doc q3w or PTX qw) plus trastuzumab (FEC: cyclophosphamide + epirubicin + fluorouracil; AC: doxorubicin + cyclophosphamide; DOC: docetaxel; and PTX: paclitaxel). However, the best regimen has not been determined yet. Questions include which combinations are better: trastuzumab qw or 3qw, trastuzumab with anthracycline, or anthracycline.

The other important question relates to which anti-HER2 agent should be used in the treatment. Trastuzumab is one of the most successful molecular targeting agents, for which there is much evidence. The problems with trastuzmab are, first, cardiac side effect; second, difficulty in transition to cerebrospinal fluid (CSF); and third, existence of resistant cancers. To overcome these problems, lapatinib is an attractive anti-HER2 agent. There are ongoing three Phase III randomized clinical trials with lapatinib: neo-ALTTO, CALGB40601, and NSABP B-41.

There are other new agents (pertuzumab, ertumaxomab, trustuzumab-MCC-DM1, and so on). Although further investigations and new biomarkers are needed, these anti-HER2 agents will play an important role in individualized therapy.

What kind of patients are an indication for preoperative anti-HER2 therapy?

Patients in past clinical trials ranged from stages II-IIIA to stage IV, including inflammatory breast cancers. Their HER2 overexpression was evaluated in fluorescence in situ hybridization (FISH) and/or immunohistochemistry (IHC) (3+)(2+).

In stage IV cases, it is possible but still controversial that an operation after preoperative anti-HER2 therapy can provide patients with a better chance of a cure. Local advanced cancer will be a good indication for preoperative anti-HER2 therapy, as the NCCN guidelines show.

Patients with Stage I (≥ 1 cm) HER2 overexpressing cancer are also recommended to receive trastuzumab as per the St. Gallen consensus meeting[16] and other guidelines. Whether anti-HER2 therapy is more beneficial in preoperative or postoperative settings will need to be studied in stage I, especially small tumor cases. In preoperative and postoperative anti-HER2 therapy of tumor (≤ 1 cm), further investigation is needed.

What is the best surgical management for shrunk tumor?

Buzdar and colleagues reported that breast conservation rate was not significantly different between chemotherapy alone group and chemotherapy plus trastuzumab group. In cases where the tumor becomes small enough, breast conservation therapy can be done in combination with postoperative radiation. In Buzdar's study, patients with clinically node-negative disease (after primary therapy) underwent sentinel lymph node biopsy (SLNB). There are still many discussions about SLNB in clinically N0 patients receiving preoperative systemic therapy, and it is under investigation. Some surgeons insist (as per NCCN guidelines) that SLNB should be done before primary systemic therapy for the purpose of staging. Others argue that SLNB could be done after primary therapy, and then there are those who insist that SLNB for patients who have received preoperative systemic therapy is early in general practice in the viewpoint of safety. Some researchers believe that tumor status after preoperative therapy is more important than tumor status before starting therapy. They developed the recurrence risk score calculated by the patient's tumor status after preoperative therapy.[40]

What should we do for non-pCR patients after preoperative anti-HER2 therapy?

Non-pCR patients after preoperative anti-HER2 therapy seem to have poor prognosis in past reports. There is no evidence that shows benefit of additional therapy for non-pCR patients after primary systemic therapy. Ongoing clinical trials of additional chemotherapy after primary systemic therapy will provide answers to this question, whereas from the point of mechanism of resistance, chemotherapy plus another anti-HER2 agent or HER2 downstream signaling inhibitor (such as mTOR, or mammalian target of rapamycin, inhibitor) may be more effective than continuing with the same therapy.

Are postoperative therapies necessary for pCR patients?

There is no evidence that shows pCR patients can skip postoperative therapies (radiation, anti-HER2 therapy, or hormonal therapy). If postoperative therapies could be skipped in some patients, this would be great progress toward individualized therapy. In order to identify such patients, new biomarkers will be necessary. Currently, clinical practice is not allowed to skip postoperative therapies for pCR patients.

In Search of a New Perspective

Although there are many unanswered questions, preoperative anti-HER2 therapy is promising. Anti-HER2 and other molecular targeting therapies are different from conventional chemotherapy, in that the former is designed on the molecular biology of the tumor. It has been reported that HER2 regulates cancer stem cells,[41] and that preoperative lapatinib therapy reduces cancer stem cell-like population while conventional chemotherapy increases that population.[42] Considering that ADCC is induced by trastuzumab, the relationship between tumor and immune system is notable. The evidences from clinical trials are important, but considering the tumor biology of each patient's cancer will also be helpful in deciding treatment on an individual basis.

In order to individualize the therapy, it is important not only to investigate the new agents but also to seek useful biomarkers for decision making in the indication or monitoring of treatment.

Individualized therapy will eventuate using the strategy where HER2-overexpressing breast cancer patients can choose anti-HER2 agents, chemotherapy, and/or other molecular targeting drugs, depending on the characteristics of the tumor and the host.

Conclusion

Preoperative anti-HER2 therapy, in combination with chemotherapy, achieves very good pCR rates in breast cancer patients with overexpressing HER2.

Preoperative anti-HER2 therapy is a promising therapy for breast cancer patients with overexpressing HER2, although there are many unanswered questions. These include:

1. Unknown long-term outcome;
2. Establishment of the best regimen of chemotherapy and anti-HER2 agents;
3. Effectiveness of anti-HER2 agents on prevention against brain metastasis;
4. Indication of preoperative anti-HER2 therapy;
5. Appropriate operation;

6. Additional therapy for non-pCR patients;
7. Appropriate postoperative therapy for pCR patients; and
8. Finding new biomarkers for individualized therapy.

Hormone Responsiveness in Neoadjuvant Endocrine Therapy in Breast Carcinoma: Estrogen Receptor Evaluation in Core Needle Biopsy Specimens

Hironobu Sasano

Summary

Immunohistochemical analysis of the estrogen receptor (ER) in core needle biopsy specimens could help to determine the endocrine responsiveness of neoadjuvant endocrine therapy, if handled, processed, and evaluated appropriately. However, it is also important to recognize potential drawbacks or limitations when interpreting results of such analysis.

Introduction: Establishing Estrogen Receptor (ER) Presence, Key to Clinical Response

In breast cancer therapy, an increasing number of patients receive neoadjuvant treatment because it allows for breast-conserving surgery. The treatment offers opportunities to examine the resultant in vivo sensitivity of patients, and therefore its utility as a predictor of the long-term outcome of patients.[1] Neoadjuvant therapy for breast carcinoma patients usually had been synonymous with neoadjuvant chemotherapy.[1] However, the recent advent of endocrine therapy, including an introduction of effective and well-tolerated new generations of aromatase inhibitor therapy into clinical practice,[2-5] and an evaluation of predictive factors for endocrine therapy at routine diagnostic levels, has led to its use as an alternative to chemotherapy in the algorithm of neoadjuvant therapy in breast carcinoma patients.

As expected, at least the presence of estrogen receptor (ER) is a prerequisite for clinical responses in any settings of hormonal therapy in breast carcinoma patients; that is, treatment benefits are not expected in true ER negative cases. It is valid that the presence of ER alone by no means can represent a patient's successful response to endocrine treatment, including new generations of aromatase inhibitors,[1] but ER status in breast carcinoma cells is a very powerful predictive factor for responses to neoadjuvant treatment.[6,7] In addition, in the past, surgical open biopsy was the gold standard of preoperative biopsy, but recently with the advent of radiological techniques ⸺ such as stereotactic radiosurgery ⸺ core needle biopsy has been used widely for preoperative histologic diagnosis. Therefore, it is very important to assess the status of ER as accurately as possible in core needle biopsy specimens before neoadjuvant endocrine treatment in breast carcinoma patients.

In this mini-review, I cover the following two aspects: first, the advantages and potential pitfalls of immunohistochemical evaluation of ER levels (the most effective and widely used method of determination in core needle biopsy specimens); and second, whether the findings obtained in core needle biopsy specimens represent the status of ER in the whole carcinoma tissue, to which neoadjuvant endocrine treatment will be administrated.

Immunohistochemical Evaluation of ER in Core Needle Biopsy

Analysis of ER in clinical materials

At present, evaluation of steroid receptors is done in almost all of the patients diagnosed with breast carcinoma. Historically, biochemical evaluation, including detran-coated charcoal (DCC) assay and enzyme immunoassay (EIA), were used following the discovery of ER. Immunohistochemical evaluation of ER was available only in freshly frozen tissue preparation and at best considered as a research or investigative tool. However, an improvement in the technical aspects of immunohistochemistry, including newly developed monoclonal antibodies and antigen retrieval methodology, made it possible to perform immunostaining of ER and progesterone receptor (PR) in 10% formalin-fixed and paraffin-embedded tissue specimens. Therefore, at present, the evaluation of ER using immunohistochemistry is being performed on archival diagnostic materials at most of the hospitals. Immunohistochemical analysis of ER provides important information as to the status of endocrine responsiveness or prediction of subsequent anti-estrogen therapy.[8] The technique can be performed relatively easily at routine diagnostic laboratories, and accurately localizes the presence of steroid receptor in contrast to biochemical analyses. However, the technique is associated with limitations or drawbacks, which may influence greatly the results of ER positivity. Potential problems associated with the immunohistochemistry of ER in core needle biopsy specimens can be categorized as follows, first, preparation of the specimens; second, techniques of immunostaining; and third, interpretation of the results.

Influence of tissue preparations on the results

The most important factor that influences the results of ER immuno-histochemistry in the process of tissue preparation is related to the fixation of specimens.[9] It has been demonstrated that at least six to eight hours of formalin fixation time is required to obtain reliable or reproducible results of ER in immunohistochemistry.[10] Overfixation has been proposed as detrimental to the results of immunohistochemistry using archival materials.[11,12] However, T. Oyama and colleagues recently demonstrated that overfixation did not influence the results of ER immunohistochemistry, with an exception of specimens fixed for more than three weeks, possibly due to the effects of antigen retrieval.[9] Therefore, when performing ER immunohistochemistry in core needle biopsy specimens, 'one day pathology' examinations using underfixation specimen should be of concern.

The other problems in tissue preparation for the immunohistochemistry of core needle biopsy specimens are delayed fixation or degeneration before fixation, and edge effects. Indeed, a delay in the onset of fixation has affected adversely the results of immunohistochemistry in ER.[13,14] However, unless the specimen is attached to the wall of tubes or containers filled with formalin, delayed fixation is practically rare in cases of core needle biopsy. Rather, interpretation of ER immunohistochemistry may be compromised by edge or crushed effects in such biopsy specimens (Figure 7−E−1). Crushed tumor cells (Figure 7−E−2) can demonstrate false-negativity for ER, and these cells should not be used for diagnosis.

Influence of immunostaining methodology

The appropriate selection of immunostaining methods, including the choice of primary antibodies, is cardinal in obtaining the correct results of immunohistochemistry regardless of the antigens. For the primary antibodies against ER, three antibodies, 1D5,[15] 6F11,[16] and SP1,[17] have been clinically validated; that is, the results of immunohistochemical evaluations of ER using these antibodies were correlated with clinical outcomes and found to be superior to biochemical assays, such as DCC or EIA. These three antibodies have been used for the ER immunohistochemistry of human breast cancer cases in the great majority of diagnostic laboratories around the world.

The next important practical factor for successful and standardized immunohistochemistry is the methodology of staining, especially the selection of manual or automatic staining. K. Arihiro and colleagues compared evaluations for ER and PR in breast carcinoma using two manual and three automated immunohistochemical assays.[18] They demonstrated the differences

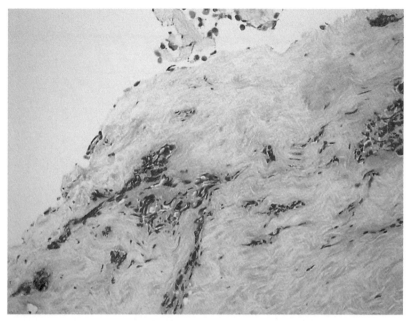

Fig. 7–E–1. Light microscopic features of core needle biopsy specimens associated with edge or crushed artifacts

The nests of carcinoma cells designated by arrows are associated with smashed nuclei. DNA representation in nuclei is by hematoxylin and eosin staining.

among these methodologies, but could not conclude which methodologies provided more inert results.[18] However, P. Regitnig and colleagues[19] demonstrated that the automated immunohistochemical techniques yielded significant advantages over manual techniques regarding interlaboratory variability of ER immunohistochemistry results in ring studies of thirty-two surgical pathology laboratories in Australia. Therefore, considering the recent advent of automatic staining instruments, including possible minimum interlaboratory differences in the technical aspects of staining procedures by these instruments compared with manual staining instruments, immunostaining by an automatic staining instrument should provide more reliable and reproducible results.

It is now possible, when performing immunohistochemistry of ER in core needle biopsy specimens of breast carcinoma, to standardize results with the combination of reliable primary antibodies and an automatic immunostaining instrument. Therefore, the next important step for interpreting ER immunohistochemistry is evaluation of the findings, especially the establishment of a threshold for positivity.

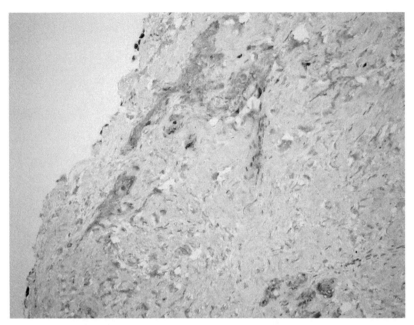

Fig. 7–E–2. Immunohistochemistry of estrogen receptor (ER) sites
Immunohistochemistry of ER sites are for the locations shown in Figure 7–E–1. The areas associated with edge or crushed artifacts were totally negative for ER immunoreactivity.

Evaluation of ER immunoreactivity

Both positive and negative controls of immunostaining are quite important in the interpretation of immunohistochemistry, and ideally the internal controls of immunostaining are much better than external ones for consistency of results. For negative control of immunohistochemistry in ER, stromal cells or peritumoral fibroblasts are usually negative for ER alpha, although sometimes positive for ER beta, antigens. The primary antibodies recognize ER alpha but not ER beta, and the absence of immunoreactivity can serve as a good negative control for immunostaining. In addition, when using the three antibodies 1D5, 6F11, and SP1, positive immunoreactivity is almost exclusively located in the nuclei, and positive staining in the cell membrane or cytoplasm is usually nonspecific background. If these patterns of immunoreactivity are predominant in the specimen, the staining must be repeated and by no means should be interpreted as positive for ER.

For positive control in immunostaining, the non-neoplastic ductal epithelial cells, although their frequency of immunopositivity is far less than that of carcinoma cells, could serve as a good candidate. However, these non-neoplastic ductal cells are usually present in surgically resected specimens, but not necessarily so in the core needle biopsy specimens. When one confirms both positive and negative controls, the next important step is to evaluate immunoreactivity in carcinoma cells.

Two important points on the evaluation of ER immunoreactivity in core needle biopsy specimens are, first, how to present the findings, especially whether relative immunointensity should be considered, and second, how to define ER positive in the cases to be examined.

In the early days of incorporation of ER immunohistochemistry into routine diagnostic practice, many laboratories defined ER positivity as those test biopsy tissues with more than 5% or 10% positive carcinoma cells. The cutoff percentage was quite arbitrary, based on each pathologist's experience rather than on any scientific concept or data; that is, there were no reports regarding the response of patients to endocrine or anti-estrogen therapy. Therefore, the cases of nonabundant ER expression in carcinoma cells were determined positive in one diagnostic laboratory but negative in the other laboratories, even though the same tissue specimens were immunostained in the same manner. This situation was further complicated by the intratumoral heterogeneity in distribution of not only positive carcinoma cells but also ER nuclear immunointensity. Figure 7–E–3 and 7–E–4 demonstrates examples of ER immunohistochemistry, at lower and higher magnification, respectively. It is not necessarily evident at lower magnification, but at higher magnification, one appreciates marked intratumoral or even intratumoral nest heterogeneity of nuclear immunoreactivity of ER. In figure 7–E–3b, the carcinoma cells designated by arrows may be interpreted as positive by almost all qualified and well-trained surgical pathologists, but those designated by arrow heads may be interpreted as positive or negative by the same group of pathologists. Therefore, it is reasonable to postulate that not only the percentage or number of positive cells but also the immunointensity of the cells should be incorporated into the evaluation criteria, if one can provide more standardized or reproducible criteria to the clinicians.

The first attempt at scoring immunoreactivity incorporating immunointensity is the H score proposed by K. S. McCarty and colleagues.[20] The H score is obtained by multiplying the percentage of positive cells by a factor representing the relative immunointensity of nuclear immunoreactivity (1 for weak, 2 for moderate, and 3 for strong), which eventually results in a maximum score of 300. This H score is employed in some institutions, and scores with less than 10 are currently considered negative for ER. This scoring system is comprehensive and provides relatively good correlation with well-controlled biochemical data. We have used this scoring system for more than ten years in evaluating various nuclear antigens in immunohistochemistry, but the scoring takes time and reproducible interpretation requires considerable training with

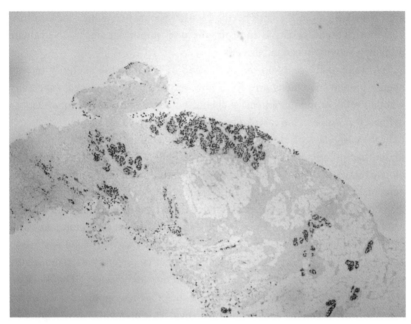

Fig. 7–E–3. The immunohistochemistry of estrogen receptor (ER) sites in core needle biopsy at low-power field microscopy

ER immunoreactivity was detected in many carcinoma cells in this area.

multiheaded light microscopy, which may explain why this rather accurate scoring system has not been widely incorporated into routine diagnostic practice.

J. M. Harvey and colleagues[16] performed the semi-quantitative analysis of ER immunoreactivity by adding two factors, one reflecting the percentage of nuclear positive tumor cells (0: none, 1: less than 1%, 2: 1%–10%, 3: 11%–33%, 4: 34%–66%, and 5: more than 67%), and the other factor representing the relative immunointensity (1: weak, 2: moderate, and 3: strong), which together yielded the maximum score of 8. Applying this Allred scoring system to about 2,000 cases of breast carcinoma, they obtained results that were significantly correlated with the improvement of disease-free survival (DFS) in patients receiving adjuvant endocrine therapy.[16] The cutoff, or threshold, of the Allred score for immunopositivity is for greater than 2, because multivariate analyses demonstrated that the largest number of the patients categorized accordingly could benefit from adjuvant endocrine therapy.[8,16] However, it is also important to note that cases with Allred scores of 3 may include those containing as few as 1% of weakly positive carcinoma cells, which may be missed easily by core needle biopsy.

This Allred score is well designed and relatively easy to be incorporated

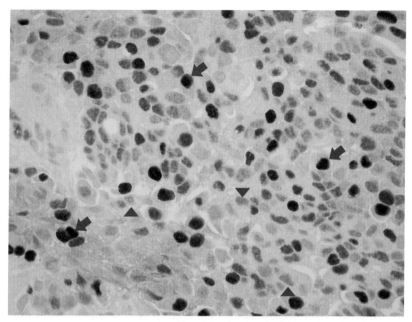

Fig. 7–E–4. The immunohistochemistry of estrogen receptor (ER) sites in core needle biopsy with high-power field microscopy

The immunohistochemistry of ER sites of core needle biopsy is taken from the area shown in Figure 7–E–3, using high-power field. Heterogeneity of immunoreactivity is easily appreciated at this magnification, from relatively strong (designated by arrows) to relatively weak (designated by arrowheads) nuclear immunoreactivity.

into daily clinical practice, but there are several justified criticisms: first, clinical significance or validity of evaluating immunointensity; second, clinical significance or validity of quantification of ER; and third, lack of absolute quantification of the findings.

For the problems of immunointensity, it is well known that the intensity of immunopositive cells are influenced markedly by various factors, including conditions of fixation, methodologies of immunostaining, and especially duration of colorimetric reaction. Therefore, standardization of immunohistochemical procedures is a 'must' for evaluation of immunointensity. However, even under standardized conditions, R. Horii and colleagues[21] reported the usefulness of incorporating immunointensity in both clinical outcome and response of Japanese patients to endocrine therapy. They also demonstrated that intensity and proportion of positive cells were significantly correlated, and that clinical outcome could be predicted based solely on the proportion of ER positive carcinoma cells.[21] Therefore, the J-score, which evaluated only the percentage of positive carcinoma cell (without considering the immunointensity of cells), was proposed by M. Kurosumi.[22]

Whether it is worthwhile to quantitate ER immunoreactivity has been disputed recently.[23,24] Bimodal distribution of ER has been reported using the well-characterized monoclonal antibody 1D5 in cases of breast carcinoma, which suggests that ER is almost always completely either positive or negative.[8,23,24] However, this concept has been challenged,[25] and it requires further investigation for clarification.

Immunohistochemistry is based principally on morphologic evaluation, and reproducibility or absolute quantification always has been in dispute. Therefore, even if the preparation of specimens, the procedures of immunostaining, and the other technical aspects are standardized, interobserver differences, which may be influenced by the experience or training of the pathologist, always could be problematic.[26,27] Recently, several investigators have attempted to employ a novel automated or semi-automated imaging analysis in evaluating ER immun ohistochemistry.[28,29] These approaches may be able to count the positive cells in all carcinoma cells, especially in the cases of core needle biopsy specimens. However, it is still pathologists who determined the locations in tissue for evaluation of carcinoma cells and the nominated threshold of immunointensity. The latter examination still could be subjective if performed by inexperienced observers.

Recently, ER messenger ribonucleic acid (mRNA) levels demonstrated a much wider dynamic range than results of ER immunohistochemical evaluation, by both reverse transcription-polymerase chain reaction (RT-PCR) and genomic microarray methods.[30,31] The possible advantage of these genomic microarray or multiplex RT-PCR assays is that they could detect the expression of multiple relevant genes, and especially downstream pathways of estrogen signals in carcinoma cells, which may be closely correlated with the response to endocrine therapy in patients with ER positive carcinoma.[30,32] However, from the viewpoint of the stability of RNA in formalin-fixed and paraffin-embedded tissue specimens, and the lack of in situ analysis unless time-consuming laser capture microscopy is employed, the introduction of a panel of reliable antibodies against the components of downstream signals molecules of ER pathway is considered a more plausible and practical diagnostic approach.

Does ER evaluation in biopsy represent the whole tumor?

With the widespread application of core needle biopsy, it is important to know whether such specimens provide better information than the histologic diagnosis of the lesions, especially regarding the status of expression of predictive factors in the whole breast carcinoma. S. Usami and colleagues studied 111 cases of breast cancer in patients who underwent core needle biopsy and subsequent surgical excision, and reported the almost perfect concordance of ER values between the specimens obtained by core needle biopsy and surgical resection.[33] Z. Hodi and colleagues[34] also reported nearly 100% concordance of results in ER immunohistochemistry between core needle biopsy and subsequent resection specimens, if both of them were processed adequately. Therefore, the information regarding ER status obtained from core needle biopsy specimens reflect its status in the whole carcinoma tissues, if core needle biopsy specimens are taken by experienced breast surgeons under appropriate modes of image evaluation and are appropriately processed in a well-controlled manner and evaluated by experienced pathologists.

Bibliography

Chapter 1

Section A

1. Izuo, M. (2004), 'Medical history: Seishu Hanaoka and his success in breast cancer surgery under general anesthesia two hundred years ago', *Breast Cancer*, 11 (4): 319–24.
2. Bigelow, H. J. (1846), 'Insensibility during surgical operations produced by inhalation', *Boston Med Surg J*, 35: 309–17.
3. Hinkley, R. C. (1882), 'First operation under ether', Painting, Boston Medical Library.
4. Semmelweis, I. P. (1858), 'A gyermekágyi láz kóroktana [The etiology of childbed fever]', *Orvosi Hetilap*, 2, in Wikipedia <http://en.wikipedia.org/wiki/Ignaz_Semmelweis>.
5. Fisher, R. A. (1925), *Statistical Methods for Research Workers* (ISBN 0-05-002170-2).
6. Early Breast Cancer Trialists' Collaborative Group (1998), 'Effects of adjuvant tamoxifen and of cytotoxic therapy on mortality in early breast cancer: An overview of 61 randomized trials among 28,896 women', *N Eng J Med*, 319: 1681–92.
7. Early Breast Cancer Trialists' Collaborative Group (2005), 'Effects of chemotherapy and hormonal therapy for early breast cancer on recurrence and 15-year survival: An overview of the randomized trials', *Lancet*, 365 (9472): 1687–717.
8. Forbes, J. F. and Cuzick J. (2005), 'Systemic adjuvant therapies for early breast cancer: 15-year results for recurrence and survival', *Med J Aust* (Editorial), 183 (9): 447–8.
9. Gralow, J. R., Zujewski, J. A. and Winer, E. (2008), 'Preoperative therapy in invasive breast cancer: Reviewing the state of the science and exploring new research directions', *J Clin Oncol*, 26 (5): 696–7.
10. Gralow, J. R., Burstein, H. J., Wood, W., et al. (2008), 'Preoperative therapy in invasive breast cancer: pathologic assessment and systemic

therapy issues in operable disease', *J Clin Oncol*, 26 (5): 814–19.

11. Wolff, A. C., Berry, D., Carey, L. A., et al. (2008), 'Research issues affecting preoperative systemic therapy for operable breast cancer', *J Clin Oncol*, 26 (5): 806–13.

12. Vaidya, J. S. (2007), 'Partial breast irradiation using targeted intraoperative radiotherapy (Targit)', *Nat Clin Pract Oncol*, 4 (7): 384–5.

13. TARGIT Trial: <http://www.dundee.ac.uk/surgery/targit/targitpapers.htm>.

14. Cuzick, J., Forbes, J. F., Sestak, I., Cawthorn, S., et al., for the International Breast Cancer Intervention Study (IBIS) I investigators (2007), 'Long-term results of tamoxifen prophylaxis for breast cancer – 96-month follow-up of the randomized IBIS-I trial', *J Natl Cancer Inst*, 99 (4): 272–82.

15. Visvanathan, K, Chlebowski, R. T., Hurley, P., et al. (2009), 'American Society of Clinical Oncology Clinical Practice Guideline Update on the Use of Pharmacologic Interventions Including Tamoxifen, Raloxifene, and Aromatase Inhibition for Breast Cancer Risk Reduction', *J Clin Oncol*, 27 (19): 3235–58.

16. Forbes, J. F., Cuzick, J., Buzdar, A., et al. for the Arimidex, Tamoxifen, Alone or in Combination (ATAC) Trialists' Group (2008), 'Effect of anastrozole and tamoxifen as adjuvant treatment for early-stage breast cancer: 100-month analysis of the ATAC trial', *Lancet Oncol*, 9 (1): 45–53.

17. Cuzick, J. (2005), 'Aromatase inhibitors for breast cancer prevention', *J Clin Oncol*, 23 (8): 1636–43.

18. IBIS II: <http://www.ibis-trials.org> (Home Page).

19. LATER: <http://anzbctg.org/contentaspx?page=laterpart>.

20. Fong, P. C., Boss, D. S., Yap, T. A., et al. (2009), 'Inhibition of poly(ADP-ribose) polymerase in tumors from BRCA mutation carriers', *N Eng J Med*, 361 (2): 123–34.

21. Iglehart, J. D. and Silver, D. (2009), 'Synthetic lethality – A new direction in cancer-drug development', *N Eng J Med*, 361 (2): 189–91.

22. Jemal, A., Siegel, R., Ward, E., et al. (2007), 'Cancer statistics, 2007', *CA Cancer J Clin*, 57 (1): 43–66.

Chapter 2

Section A

1. Fisher, B., Ravidin, R. G., Ausman, R. K., et al. (1968), 'Surgical adjuvant chemotherapy in cancer of the breast: Results of a decade of cooperative investigation', *Ann Surg*, 168: 337–56.

2. Fisher, B., Slack, N., Katrych, D., et al. (1975), 'Ten year follow-up results

of patients with carcinoma of the breast in a co-operative clinical trial evaluating surgical adjuvant chemotherapy', *Surg Gynecol Obstet*, 140: 528–34.

3. National Institutes of Health Consensus Development Conference Statement (2001), 'Adjuvant therapy for breast cancer', *J Natl Cancer Inst Monogr*, 30: 5–15.

4. Giuliano, A. E., Kirgan, D. M., Guenther, J. M. and Morton, D. L. (1994), 'Lymphatic mapping and sentinel/lymphadenectomy for breast cancer', *Ann Surg*, 220: 391–401.

5. Zavagno, G., De Salvo, G. L., Scalco, G., et al. (2008), 'A randomized clinical trial on sentinel lymph node biopsy versus axillary lymph node dissection in breast cancer results of the Sentinella/GIVOM Trial', *Ann Surg*, 247 (2): 207–13.

6. Veronesi, U., Luini, A., Galimberti, V., et al. (1990), 'Extent of metastatic axillary involvement in 1446 cases of breast cancer', *Eur J Surg Oncol*, 16: 127–33.

7. Rosen, P. P., Lesser, M. L., Kinne, D. W. and Beattie, E. J. (1983), 'Discontinuous or "skip" metastases in breast carcinoma: Analysis of 1228 axillary dissections', *Ann Surg*, 197: 276–83.

8. Van Lancker, M., Goor, C., Sacre, R., et al. (1995), 'Patterns of axillary lymph node metastasis in breast cancer', Am J Clin Oncol, 18: 267–72.

9. Krag, D., Weaver, D., Ashikaga, T., et al. (1998), 'The sentinel node in breast cancer - A multicenter validation study', *N Engl J Med*, 339: 941–95.

10. Theodore, K., Giuliano, A. E. and Lyman, G. H. (2006), 'Lymphatic mapping and sentinel lymph node biopsy in early-stage breast carcinoma: A metaanalysis', *Cancer*, 106: 4–16.

11. Krag, D. N., Anderson, S. J., Julian, T. B., et al., for the National Surgical Adjuvant Breast and Bowel Project (NSABP) (2007), 'Technical outcomes of sentinel-lymph-node resection and conventional axillary-lymph-node dissection in patients with clinically node-negative breast cancer: Results from the NSABP B–32 randomised phase III trial', *Lancet Oncol*, 7 (10): 881–8.

12. Veronesi, U., Paganelli, G., Viale, G., et al. (2006), 'Sentinel-lymph-node biopsy as a staging procedure in breast cancer: Update of a randomised controlled study', *Lancet Oncol*, 7 (12): 983–90.

13. Canavese, G., Catturich1, A., Vecchio, C., et al. (2009), 'Sentinel node biopsy compared with complete axillary dissection for staging early breast cancer with clinically negative lymph nodes: Results of randomized trial', *Ann Oncol*, 20: 1001–7.

14. Naik, A. M., Fey, J., Gemignani, M., et al. (2004), 'The risk of axillary relapse after sentinel lymph node biopsy for breast cancer is comparable with that of axillary lymph node dissection: A follow-up study of 4008 procedures', *Ann Surg*, 240: 462–71.

15. Bergkvist, L., de Boniface, J., Jönsson, P. -E., et al., on behalf of the Swedish Breast Cancer Group and the Swedish Society of Breast Surgeons (2008), 'Axillary recurrence rate after negative sentinel node biopsy in breast cancer: Three-year follow-up of the Swedish Multicenter Cohort Study', *Ann Surg*, 247: 150–6.

16. Lyman, G. H., Giuliano, A. E., Somerfield, M. R., et al. (2005), 'American Society of Clinical Oncology guideline recommendations for sentinel lymph node biopsy in early-stage breast cancer', *J Clin Oncol*, 23: 7703–20.

17. Silverstein, M. J., Skinner, K. A. and Lomis, T. J. (2001), 'Predicting axillary nodal positivity in 2282 patients with breast carcinoma', *World J Surg*, 25: 767–72.

18. Intra, M., Rotmensz, N., Mattar, D., et al. (2007), 'Unnecessary axillary node dissections in the sentinel lymph node era', *Eur J Surg*, 43: 2664–8.

19. Bedrosian, I., Reynolds, C., Mick, R., et al. (2000), 'Accuracy of sentinel lymph node biopsy in patients with large primary breast tumors', *Cancer*, 88 (11): 2540–5.

20. Chung, M. H., Ye, W. and Giuliano, A. E. (2001), 'Role for sentinel lymph node dissection in the management of large (= 5 cm) invasive breast cancer', *Ann Surg Oncol*, 8 (9): 688–92.

21. Lelievre, L., Houvenaeghel, G., Buttarelli, M., et al., (2007), 'Value of the sentinel lymph node procedure in patients with large size breast cancer', *Ann Surg Oncol* 14 (2): 621–26.

22. Wong, S. L., Chao, C., Edwards, M. J., et al. (2001), 'Accuracy of sentinel lymph node biopsy for patients with T2 and T3 breast cancers', *Am Surgeon*, 67: 522–8.

23. Meretoja, T. J., Leidenius, M. H., Heikkilä, P. S. and Joensuu, H. (2009), 'Sentinel node biopsy in breast cancer patients with large or multifocal tumors', *Ann Surg Oncol*, 16: 1148–55.

24. Damera, A., Evans, A. J., Cornford, E. J., et al. (2003), 'Diagnosis of axillary nodal metastases by ultrasound-guided core biopsy in primary operable breast cancer', *British Journal of Cancer*, 89: 1310–13.

25. Abe, H., Schmidt, R. A., Kulkarni, K., et al (2009), 'Axillary lymph nodes suspicious for breast cancer metastasis: Sampling with US-guided 14-gauge core-needle biopsy—Clinical experience in 100 patients', *Radiology*, 25: 41–49.

26. Bonnema, J., van Geel, A. N., van Ooijen, B., et al. (1997), 'Ultrasound-guided aspiration biopsy for detection of nonpalpable axillary node metastases in breast cancer patients: New diagnostic method', *World J Surg*, 21: 270–4.

27. de Kanter, A. Y., van Eijck, C. H. J., van Geel, A. N., et al. (1999). 'Multicentre study of ultrasonographically guided axillary node biopsy in patients with breast cancer', *Br J Surg*, 86: 1459–62.

28. Kuenen-Boumeester, V., Menke-Pluymers, M., de Kanter, A. Y., et al. (2003), 'Ultrasound-guided fine needle aspiration cytology of axillary lymph nodes in breast cancer patients. A preoperative staging procedure', *Eur J Surg*, 39: 170–4.

29. Bedrosian, I., Bedi, D., Kuerer, H. M., et al. (2003), 'Impact of clinicopathological factors on sensitivity of axillary ultrasonography in the detection of axillary nodal metastases in patients with breast cancer', *Ann Surg Oncol*, 10 (9): 1025–30.

30. Deurloo, E. E., Tanis, P. J., Gilhuijs, K. G. A., et al. (2003), 'Reduction in the number of sentinel lymph node procedures by preoperative ultrasonography of the axilla in breast cancer', *Eur J Surg*, 39: 1068–73.

31. van Rijk, M. C., Deurloo, E. E., Nieweg, O. E., et al. (2006), 'Ultrasonography and fine-needle aspiration cytology can spare breast cancer patients unnecessary sentinel lymph node biopsy', *Ann Surg Oncol*, 13 (1): 31–35.

32. Hinson, J. L., McGrath, P., Moore, A., et al. (2008), 'The critical role of axillary ultrasound and aspiration biopsy in the management of breast cancer patients with clinically negative axilla', *Ann Surg Oncol*, 15 (1): 250–5.

33. Koelliker, S. L., Chung, M. A., Mainiero, M. B., et al. (2008), 'Axillary lymph nodes: US-guided fine-needle aspiration for initial staging of breast cancer—Correlation with primary tumor size', *Radiology*, 246 (1): 81–9.

34. Gilissen, F., Oostenbroek, R., Storm, R., et al. (2008), 'Prevention of futile sentinel node procedures in breast cancer: Ultrasonography of the axilla and fine-needle aspiration cytology are obligatory', *Eur J Surg Oncol*, 34: 497–500.

35. Swinson, C., Ravichandran, D., Nayagam, M. and Allen, S. (2009), 'Ultrasound and fine needle aspiration cytology of the axilla in the pre-operative identification of axillary nodal involvement in breast cancer', *Eur J Surg Oncol*, 35 (11): 1152–1157.

36. Dauway, E. L., Giuliano, R., Haddad, F., Pendas, S., Costello, D., Cox, C. E., et al. (1999), 'Lymphatic mapping in breast cancer', *Hematol Oncol Clin North Am*, 13 (2): 349–71.

37. Sato, K., Tamaki, K., Tsuda, H., et al. (2004), 'Utility of axillary ultrasound examination to select breast cancer patients suited for optimal sentinel node biopsy', *Am J Surg*, 187: 679–83.

38. Somasundar, P., Gass, J., Steinhoff, M., et al. (2006), 'Role of ultrasound-guided axillary fine-needle aspiration in the management of invasive breast cancer', *Am J Surg*, 192: 458–61.

39. Krishnamurthy, S., Sneige, N., Bedi, D. G., et al. (2002), 'Role of ultrasound-guided fine–needle aspiration of indeterminate and suspicious axillary lymph nodes in the initial staging of breast carcinoma', *Cancer*, 95 (5): 982–8.

40. Mamounas, E. P., Brown, A., Anderson, S., et al. (2005), 'Sentinel node biopsy after neoadjuvant chemotherapy in breast cancer: Results from National Surgical Adjuvant Breast and Bowel Project Protocol B–27', *J Clin Oncol*, 23: 2694–702.

41. Classe, J. -M., Bordes, V., Campion, L., et al. (2009), 'Sentinel lymph node biopsy after neoadjuvant chemotherapy for advanced breast cancer: Results of Ganglion Sentinelle et Chimiothérapie Neoadjuvante, a French prospective multicentric study', *J Clin Oncol*, 27 (5): 726–32.

42. Kelly, A. M., Dwamena, B., Cronin, P. and Carlos, R. C. (2009), 'Breast cancer sentinel node identification and classification after neoadjuvant chemotherapy – Systematic review and meta analysis', *Academic Radiology*, 16 (5): 551–63.

43. van Deurzen, C., Vriens, B., Tjan-Heijnen, V., et al. (2009), 'Accuracy of sentinel node biopsy after neoadjuvant chemotherapy in breast cancer patients: A systematic review', *Eur J Cancer*, 45: 3124–30.

44. Gimbergues, P., Abrial, C., Durando, S., et al. (2008), 'Sentinel lymph node biopsy after neoadjuvant chemotherapy is accurate in breast cancer patients with a clinically negative axillary nodal status at presentation', *Ann Surg Oncol*, 15 (5): 1316–21.

45. Khan, A., Sabel, M. S., Nees, A., et al. (2005), 'Comprehensive axillary evaluation in neoadjuvant chemotherapy patients with ultrasonography and sentinel lymph node biopsy', *Ann Surg Oncol*, 12 (9): 697–704.

46. Newman, E. A., Sabel, M., Nees, A. V., et al. (2007), 'Sentinel lymph node biopsy performed after neoadjuvant chemotherapy is accurate in patients with documented node-positive breast cancer at presentation', *Ann Surg Oncol*, 14 (20): 2946–52.

47. Lee, S., Kim, E. Y., Kang, S. H., et al. (2007), 'Sentinel node identification rate, but not accuracy, is significantly decreased after pre-operative chemotherapy in axillary node-positive breast cancer patients', *Breast Cancer Res Treat*, 102 (3): 283–288.

48. Shen, J., Gilcrease, M. Z., Babiera, G. V., et al. (2007), 'Feasibility and accuracy of sentinel lymph node biopsy after preoperative chemotherapy in breast cancer patients with documented axillary metastases', *Cancer*, 109 (7): 1255–63.

49. Yu, J. -C., Hsu, G. -C., Hsieh, C. -B., et al. (2006), 'Role of sentinel lymphadenectomy combined with intraoperative ultrasound in the assessment of locally advanced breast cancer after neoadjuvant chemotherapy', *Ann Surg Oncol*, 14 (1): 174–80.

Section B

1. Veronesi, U., Paganelli, G., Viale, G., et al. (2003), 'A randomized comparison of sentinel-node biopsy with routine axillary dissection in breast cancer', *N Eng J Med*, 349 (6): 546–53.

2. Krag, D. N., Anderson, S. J., Julian, T. B., et al. (2007), 'Technical outcome of sentinel-lymph-node resection and conventional axillary-lymph-node dissection in patients with clinically node-negative breast cancer: Results from the NSABP B–32 randomised phase III trial', *Lancet Oncol*, 8: 881–8.

3. Mansel, R. E., Fallowfield, J., Kissin, M., et al. (2006), 'Randomized multicenter trial of sentinel node biopsy versus standard axillary treatment in operable breast cancer: The ALMANAC Trial', *J Natl Cancer Inst*, 98 (9): 599–609.

4. Zavagno, G., De Salvo, G. L., Scalco, G., et al. (2008), 'A randomized clinical trial on sentinel lymph node biopsy versus axillary lymph node dissection in breast cancer: Results of the Sentinella/GIVOM trial', *Ann Surg*, 247 (2): 207–13.

5. Krag, D. N., Weaver, O. J., Alex, J. C., et al. (1993), 'Surgical resection and radiolocalization of the sentinel lymph node in breast cancer using a gamma probe', *Surg Oncol*, 2: 335–40.

6. Giuliano, A. E., Kirgan, D. M., Guenther, J. M., et al. (1994), 'Lymphatic mapping and sentinel lymphadecectomy for breast cancer', *Ann Surg*, 220: 391–401.

7. Kitai, T., Inomoto, T., Shikayama T., et al. (2005), 'Fluorescence navigation with indocyanine green for detecting sentinel lymph nodes in breast cancer', *Breast Cancer*, 12 (3): 211–15.

8. Tagaya, N., Yamazaki, R., Nakakawa, A., et al. (2008), 'Intraoperative identification of sentinel lymph nodes by near infrared fluorescence imaging in patients with breast cancer', *Am J Surg*, 195: 850–3.

9. Giuliano, A. E, Jones, R. C, Brennan, M., et al. (1997), 'Sentinel lymphadenectomy in breast cancer', *J Clin Oncol*, 15: 2345–50.

10. Motomura, K., Inaji, H., Komoike, Y., et al. (1999), 'Sentinel node biopsy

guided by indocyanin green dye in breast cancer patients', *Jpn J Clin Oncol*, 29: 604–7.

11. Benson, R. C. and Kues, H. A. (1978), 'Fluorescence properties of indocyanine green as related to angiography', *Phys Med Biol*, 23 (1): 159–63.

12. Yoshiya, I., Shimada, Y., Tanaka, K., et al. (1980), 'Spectrophotometric monitoring of arterial oxygen saturation in the finger tip', *Med Biol Exp Comp*, 18: 27–32.

13. Kitai, T., Miwa, M., Liu, H., et al. (1999), 'Application of near-infrared time-resolved spectroscopy to rat liver – A preliminary report for surgical application', *Phys Med Biol*, 44: 2049–61.

14. Wilson, B. C. (1991) 'Optical properties of tissues', in *Encyclopedia of Human Biology*, Academic Press, St. Louis, vol. 5: 587–97.

15. Sevick, E. M., Chance, B., Leigh, J., et al. (1991), 'Quantitation of time- and frequency-resolved optical spectra for the determination of tissue oxygenation', *Anal Biochem*, 195 (2): 330–51.

16. Kitai, T., Beauvoit, B. and Chance B. (1996), 'Optical determination of fatty change of the graft liver with near-infrared time-resolved spectroscopy', *Transplantation*, 62: 642–7.

17. Beauvoit, B. and Chance, B. (1998), 'Time-resolved spectroscopy of mitochondria, cells and tissues under normal and pathological condition', *Mol Cell Biochem*, 184 (1–2): 445–55.

18. Borgstein, P. J., Meijer, S., Pijpers, R. J., et al. (2000), 'Functional lymphatic anatomy for sentinel node biopsy in breast cancer. Echoes from the past and the periareolar blue method', *Ann Surg*, 232: 81–9.

Section C

1. Buchholz, T. A., Lehman, C. D., Harris, J. R., et al. (2008), *J Clin Oncol*, 26: 791–7.

2. Veronesi, U., De Cicco, C., Galimberti, V. E., et al. (2007), *Ann Oncol*, 18: 473–8.

3. Menard, J. P., Extra, J. M., Jacquemier, J., et al. (2009), *Eur J Surg Oncol*, 35: 916–20.

4. Kilbride, K. E., Lee, M. C., Nees, A. V., et al. (2008), *Ann Surg Oncol*, 15: 3252–8.

5. Papa, M. Z., Zippel, D., Kaufman, B., et al. (2008), *J Surg Oncol*, 98: 403–6.

6. Abe, H., Schmidt, R. A., Kulkarni, K., et al. (2009), *Radiology*, 250: 41–9.

7. Kelly, A. M., Dwamena, B., Cronin, P. and Carlos, R. C. (2009), *Acad Radiol*, 16: 551–63.

8. Arkenau, H. T., Chong, G., Cunningham, D., et al. (2007), *Ann Oncol*, 18:

541–5.
9. Lee, S., Kim, E. Y., Kang, S. H., et al. (2007), *Breast Cancer Res Treat*, 102: 283–8.
10. Kang, S. H., Kim, S. K., Kwon, Y., et al. (2004), *World J Surg*, 28: 1019–24.
11. van Rijk, M. C., Nieweg, O. E., Rutgers, E. J., et al. (2006), *Ann Surg Oncol*, 13: 475–9.
12. East, J. M., Valentine, C. S., Kanchev, E. and Blake, G. O. (2009), *BMC Surg*, 9: 2.
13. Jones, J. L., Zabicki, K., Christian, R. L., et al. (2005), *Ann Surg Oncol*, 190: 517–20.
14. Schrenk, P., Tausch, C., Wölfl, S., et al. (2008), *Am J Surg*, 196: 176–83.
15. Lehman, C. D., DeMartini, W, Anderson, B. O. and Edge, S. B. (2009), *J Natl Compr Canc Netw*, 7: 193–201.
16. Liu, Y., Bellomi, M., Gatti, G. and Ping, X. (2007), *Breast Cancer Res*, 9: R40, 1–7.
17. Ogasawara, Y., Doihara, H., Shiraiwa, M. and Ishihara, S. (2008), *Surg Today*, 38: 104–8.
18. Hsiang, D. J., Yamamoto, M., Mehta, R. S., et al. (2007), *Arch Surg*, 142: 855–61.

Section D

1. Luini, A., Gatti, G., Ballardini, B., et al. (2005), 'Development of axillary surgery in breast cancer,' *Ann Oncol*, 16 (2): 259–62.
2. Fisher, B., Jeong, J. H., Anderson, S., et al. (2002), 'Twenty-five year follow-up of a randomized trial comparing radical mastectomy, total mastectomy, and total mastectomy followed by irradiation', *N Engl J Med*, 347 (16): 567–75.
3. Krag, D. N., Weaver, D. L, Alex, J. C. and Fairbank, J. T. (1993), 'Surgical resection and radiolocalization of the sentinel lymph node in breast cancer using a gamma probe', *Surg Oncol*, 2 (6): 335–9.
4. Giuliano, A. I., Kirgan, D. M., Guenther, J. M. and Morton, D. L. (1994), 'Lymphatic mapping and sentinel lymphadenectomy for breast cancer', *Ann Surg*, 220 (3): 391–8.
5. Kim, T., Giuliano, A. E. and Lyman, G. H. (2006), 'Lymphatic mapping and sentinel lymph node biopsy in early-stage breast carcinoma', *Cancer*, 106 (1): 4–16.
6. Krag, D., Weaver, D., Ashikaga, T., et al. (1998), 'The sentinel node in breast cancer. A multicenter validation study', *N Engl J Med*, 339 (14): 941–6.

7. Edge, S. B., Niland, J. C., Bookman, M. A., et al. (2003), 'Emergence of sentinel node biopsy in breast cancer as standard-of-care in academic comprehensive cancer centers', *J Natl Cancer Inst*, 95 (20): 1514–21.
8. Chen, A. Y., Halpern, M. T., Schrag, N. M., et al. (2008), 'Disparities and trends in sentinel node biopsy among early-stage breast cancer patients (1998–2005)', *J Natl Cancer Inst*, 100 (7): 462–74.
9. Krag, D. N. and Julian, T. B. (2003), 'Practice patterns of sentinel node biopsy at five comprehensive cancer centers', *J Natl Cancer Inst*, 95 (20): 1498–9.
10. Lyman, G. H., Guiliano, A. E., Somerfield, M. R., et al. (2005), 'American Society of Clinical Oncology guideline recommendations for sentinel lymph node biopsy in early stage breast cancer', *J Clin Oncol*, 23 (30): 7703–20.
11. Early Breast Cancer Trialists' Collaborative Group (2005), 'Effects of radiotherapy and of differences in the extent of surgery for early breast cancer on local recurrence and 15-year survival: An overview of the randomized trials', *Lancet*, 366 (9503): 2087–106.
12. Truong, P. T., Bernstein, V., Wai, E., et al. (2002), 'Age-related variations in the use of axillary dissection: A survival analysis of 9038 women with T1–T2 breast cancer', *Int J Radiat Oncol Biol Phys*, 54 (3): 637–9.
13. Hewitt, M. and Simone, J. V. (eds) (1999), *Ensuring Quality Cancer Care*, Washington, DC: National Cancer Policy Board, National Academy Press.
14. Edge, S. B. (2008), 'Early adoption and disturbing disparities in sentinel node biopsy in breast cancer', *J Natl Cancer Inst*, 100 (7): 449–50.
15. van Deurzen, C., Vriens, B., Tjan-Heijnen, V. et al. (2009), 'Accuracy of sentinel node biopsy after neoadjuvant chemotherapy in breast cancer patients: A systematic review', *Eur J Cancer*, 45 (18): 3124–30.
16. American Society of Clinical Oncology (2005), 'ASCO guideline recommendations for sentinel lymph node biopsy in early-stage breast cancer: Guideline summary', *J Clin Oncol*, 1 (4): 134–6.

Section E

1. Halsted, W. S. (1907), 'The results of operations for the cure of carcinoma of the breast', *Ann Surg*, 46: 1–19.
2. Fisher, B. (1981), 'A commentary in the role of the surgeon in primary breast cancer', *Breast Cancer Res Treat*, 1: 17–28.
3. Fisher, B., Fisher, E. R. and Redmond C. (1985), 'Ten-year results of a randomized clinical trial comparing radical mastectomy and total mastectomy with or without radiation', *N Engl J Med*, 312: 674–81.
4. Veronesi, U., Paganelli, G., Viale, G., et al. (2003), 'A randomized

comparison of sentinel-node biopsy with routine axillary dissection in breast cancer', *N Eng J Med*, 349: 546–53.

5. Salhab, M., Al Sarakbi, W. and Mokbel, K. (2005), 'Skin and fat necrosis of the breast following methylene blue dye injection for sentinel node biopsy in a patient with breast cancer', *Int Semi Surg Onco*, 2: 26.

6. Kitai, T., Inomoto, T., Miwa, M. and Shikayama, T. (2005), 'Fluorescence navigation with indocyanine green for detecting sentinel lymph nodes in breast cancer', *Breast Cancer*, 12: 211–15.

7. Benson, J. R., della Rovere, G. Q. and the Axilla Management Consensus Group (2007), 'Management of the axillary in women with breast cancer', *Lancet Oncol*, 8: 331–48.

8. Yi, M., Meric-Bernstam, F., Ross, M. I., et al. (2008), 'How many sentinel lymph nodes are enough during sentinel lymph node dissection for breast cancer?', *Cancer*, 113 (1): 30–7.

9. de Boer, M., van Deurzen, C. H., van Dijck, J. A., et al. (2009), 'Micrometastases or isolated tumor cells and the outcome of breast cancer', *N Eng J Med*, 361: 653–63.

10. Lambert, L. A., Ayers, G. D., Hwang, R. F., et al. (2006), 'Validation of a breast cancer nomogram for predicting nonsentinel lymph node metastases after a positive sentinel node biopsy', *Ann Surg Oncol*, 13: 310–20.

11. Van Zee, K. J., Manasseh, D. M., Bevilacqua, J. L., et al. (2003), 'A nomogram for predicting the likelihood of additional nodal metastases in breast cancer patients with a positive sentinel node biopsy', *Ann Surg Oncol*, 10: 248–54.

12. Mamounas, E. P., Brown, A., Anderson, S., et al. (2005), 'Sentinel node biopsy after neoadjuvant chemotherapy in breast cancer: Results from National Surgical Adjuvant Breast and Bowel Project Protocol B–27', *J Clin Oncol*, 23: 2694–702.

13. Shen, J., Gilcrease, M. Z., Babiera, G. V., et al. (2007), 'Feasibility and accuracy of sentinel lymph node biopsy after preoperative chemotherapy in breast cancer patients with documented axillary metastases', *Cancer*, 109: 1255–63.

14. Lyman, G. H., Giuliano, A. E., Somerfield, M. R., et al. (2005), 'American Society of Clinical Oncology Guideline Recommendations for sentinel lymph node biopsy in early-stage breast cancer', *J Clin Oncol*, 23: 7703–20.

15. Veronesi, P., Intra, M., Vento, A. R., et al. (2005), 'Sentinel lymph node biopsy for localised ductal carcinoma in situ?', *Breast*, 14 (6): 520–2.

16. Thompson, M., Korourian, S., Henry-Tillman, R., et al. (2007), 'Axillary reverse mapping (ARM): A new concept to identify and enhance lymphatic

preservation', *Ann Surg Oncol*, 14: 1890–5.

Chapter 3

Section A

1. Benson, J. R. and Querci della Rovere, G. (2002), 'The biological significance of ipsilateral local recurrence of breast cancer: Determinant or indicator of poor prognosis', *Lancet Oncology*, 3: 45–9.
2. Vicini, F. A., Kestin, L., Huang, R., et al. (2003), 'Does local recurrence affect the rate of distance metastases and survival in patients with early-stage breast carcinoma treated with breast conserving therapy?', *Cancer*, 97: 901–19.
3. Veronesi, U., Marubini, E., Del Vecchio, M., et al. (1995), 'Local recurrences and distant metastases after conservative breast cancer treatments: Partly independent events', *J Natl Cancer Inst*, 87: 19–27.
4. Hellman, S. (1994), 'Natural history of small breast cancers', *J Clin Oncol*, 12: 2229–34.
5. Halsted, W. S. (1894), 'The results of operation for the cure of cancer of the breast performed at the John Hopkins Hospital from June 1889 to January 1894', *Ann Surg*, 20: 497–555.
6. Crile, G. (1965), 'Treatment of breast cancer by local excision', *Am J Surg*, 109: 400–3.
7. Early Breast Cancer Trialists' Collaborative Group (1998), 'Polychemotherapy for early breast cancer: An overview of the randomized trial', *Lancet*, 352: 930–42.
8. Early Breast Cancer Trialists' Collaborative Group (1998), 'Tamoxifen for early breast cancer: An overview of the randomized trials', *Lancet*, 351: 1451–61.
9. Rosen, P. P., Groshen, S., Saigo, P. E., et al. (1989), 'A long-term follow-up study of survival in stage I (T1M0) and stage II (T1N1) breast carcinoma,' *J Clin Oncol*, 7: 355–66.
10. Fisher, B. (1980), 'Laboratory and clinical research in breast cancer – A personal adventure. The David A. Karnofsky Memorial Lecture', *Cancer Res*, 40: 3863–74.
11. Fisher, B. (1992), 'The evolution of paradigms for the management of breast cancer', *Perspectives in Cancer Research*, 52: 2371–83.
12. Fisher, B., et al. (2002), 'Twenty-year follow-up of a randomized trial comparing total mastectomy, lumpectomy and lumpectomy plus irradiation for the treatment of invasive breast cancer', *N Eng J Med*, 347: 1233–41.

13. Baum, M. and Benson, J. R. (1996), 'Current and future roles of adjuvant endocrine therapy in management of early carcinoma of the breast', in H. -J. Senn, R. D. Goldhirsch, R. D. Gelber and B. Thurlimann (eds), *Recent Results in Cancer Research – Adjuvant Therapy of Breast Cancer*, Berlin, Heidelberg, New York, Springer–Verlag: 215–26.

14. Schnitt, S. J. (2003), 'Risk factors for local recurrence in patients with invasive breast cancer and negative surgical margins of excision', *Am J Clin Path*, 120, 485–8.

15. Schnitt, S. J., Abner, A., Gelman, R., et al. (1994), 'The relationship between microscopic margins of resection and the risk of local recurrence in patients with breast cancer treated with breast-conserving surgery and radiation therapy', *Cancer*, 74: 1746–51.

16. Mirza, N. Q., Vlastos, G., Meric, F., et al. (2002), 'Predictors of loco-regional recurrence amongst patients with early-stage breast cancer treated with breast-conserving therapy', *Ann Surg Oncol*, 9: 256–65.

17. Fisher, B., Anderson, S., Fisher, E. R., et al. (1991), 'Significance of ipsilateral breast tumour recurrence after lumpectomy', *Lancet*, 338: 327–31.

18. Haffty, B. G., Reiss, M., Beinfield, M., et al. (1996), 'Ipsilateral breast tumour recurrence as a predictor of distant disease: Implications for systemic therapy at the time of local relapse', *J Clin Oncol*, 14: 52–7.

19. Komoike, Y., Akiyama, F., Iino, Y., et al. (2006), 'Ipsilateral breast tumour recurrence (IBTR) after breast conserving treatment for early breast cancer: Risk factors and impact on distant metastases', *Cancer*, 106: 35–41.

20. Overgaard, M., Hansen, P. S., Overgaard, J., et al. (1997), 'Post-operative radiotherapy in high-risk premenopausal women with breast cancer who receive adjuvant chemotherapy. Danish Breast Cancer Cooperative Group 82b Trial', *N Eng J Med*, 337: 949–55.

21. Ragaz, J., Jackson, S. M., Le, N., et al. (1997), 'Adjuvant radiotherapy and chemotherapy in node positive pre-menopausal women with breast cancer', *N Eng J Med*, 337: 956–62.

22. Vinh-Hung, V. and Verschraegen, C. (2004), 'Breast conserving surgery with or without radiotherapy: Pooled analysis for risks of ipsilateral breast tumour recurrence and mortality', *J Natl Cancer Inst*, 96: 115–12.

23. Early Breast Cancer Trialists' Collaborative Group (2005), 'Effects of radiotherapy and of differences in the extent of surgery for early breast cancer on local recurrence and 15-year survival: An overview of the randomized trials', *Lancet*, 366: 2087–106.

24. Fortin, A., Larochelle, M., Laverdiere, J., et al. (1999), 'Local failure is responsible for the decrease in survival for patients with breast cancer

treated with conservative surgery and post-operative radiotherapy', *J Clin Oncol*, 101: 104–9.

25. Thornton, H. (1997), 'The voice of the breast cancer patient – A lonely cry in the wilderness', *Eur J Cancer*, 33 (6): 825–8.

26. Hellman S. (1997), 'Stopping metastases at their source', *N Eng J Med*, 337: 996–7.

27. MacMillan, R. D., Purushotham, A. D. and George, W. D. (1996), 'Local recurrence after breast-conserving surgery for breast cancer', *Br J Surg*, 83: 149–55.

28. Locker, G., Sainsbury, R. and Cuzick, J. (2002), 'Breast surgery in the ATAC trial: Women in the United States are more likely to have mastectomy', *Breast Cancer Res Treat*, 76: S35.

29. Ryoo, M. C., Kagan, A. T., Wollin, M., et al. (1989), 'Prognostic factors for recurrence and cosmesis in 393 patients after radiation therapy for early mammary carcinoma', *Radiology*, 172: 555–9.

30. Kurtz, J. M., Jacquemir, J., Amalric, R., et al. (1990), 'Risk factors for breast recurrence in premenopausal and postmenopausal patients with ductal cancers treated by conservation therapy', *Cancer*, 65: 1867–78.

31. Boger, J., Kemperman, H., Hart, A., et al. (1994), 'Risk factors in breast conservation therapy', *J Clin Oncol*, 12: 653–60.

32. Di Biase, S., Komarnicky, L. T., Schwartz, G. F., et al. (1988), 'The number of positive margins influences the outcome of women treated with breast preservation for early stage breast carcinoma', *Cancer*, 82: 2212–20.

33. Schmidt-Ulrich, R., Wazer, D., Tercilla, O., et al. (1989), 'Tumour margin assessment as a guide to optimal conservation surgery and irradiation in early-stage breast carcinoma', *Int J Radiat Oncol Biol Phys*, 17: 733–8.

34. Solin, L. J., Fowble, B. L., Schultz, D. J. and Goodman, R. L. (1991), 'The significance of the pathology margins of the tumor excision on the outcome of patients treated with definitive irradiation for early stage breast cancer', *Int J Radiat Oncol Biol Phys*, 21: 279–87.

35. Smitt, M. C., Nowels, K., Carlson, R. W., et al. (2003), 'Predictors of re-excision findings and recurrence after breast conservation', *Int J Rad Oncol Biol Phys*, 57: 979–85.

36. Petersen, M. E., Schultz, D. J., Reynolds, C., et al. (1999), 'Outcomes in breast cancer patients relative to margin status after treatment with breast-conserving surgery and radiation therapy: The University of Pennsylvania experience', *Int J Radiat Oncol Biol Phys*, 43: 1029–35.

37. Wazer, D. E., Schmidt-Ulrich, R. K., Ruthazer, R., et al. (1998), 'Factors determining outcome for breast-conserving irradiation with margin-directed dose escalation to the tumor bed', *Int J Radiat Oncol Biol Phys*, 40: 851–8.

38. Freedman, G., Fowble, B., Hanlon, A., et al. (1999), 'Patients with early stage invasive cancer with close or positive margins treated with conservative surgery and radiation have an increased risk of breast recurrence that is delayed by adjuvant systemic therapy', *Int J Radiat Oncol Biol Phys*, 44: 1005–15.

39. Liau, S. -S., Cariati, M., Noble, D., et al. (2008), 'Local recurrence following breast conservation surgery with 5 mm target margin and 40-Gray breast radiotherapy for invasive breast cancer', *Eur J Cancer*, 6: 204.

40. Morrow, M., Schmidt, R. and Hassett, C. (1995), 'Patient selection for breast conservation therapy with magnification mammography', *Surgery*, 118: 621–6.

41. Forouhi, P., Brahmbhatt, D. H. and Benson, J. R. (2009), 'Breast conservation: Factors predictive of residual disease following reoperation for narrow surgical margins', *Cancer Res*, 69 (suppl.) (2): 355.

42. Singletary, S. E. (2002), 'Surgical margins in patients with early-stage breast cancer treated with breast conservation therapy', *Am J Surg*, 184: 383–93.

43. Morrow, M. and Harris, J. R. (2007), 'Practice guidelines for breast conserving therapy in the management of invasive breast cancer', *J Am Coll Surg*, 205: 362–76.

44. Veronesi, U., Volterrani, F., Luini, A., et al. (1990), 'Quadrantectomy versus lumpectomy for small size breast cancer', *Eu J Cancer*, 26: 671–3.

45. Asgeirsson, K., McCulley, S., Pinder, S. and MacMillan, R. (2003), 'Size of invasive breast cancer and risk of local recurrence after breast conserving therapy', *Eu J Cancer*, 39: 2462–9.

46. Van Dongen, J. A., Bartelink, H., Fentimen, I., et al. (1992), 'Factors influencing local relapse and survival and results of salvage treatment after breast conserving treatment in operable breast cancer: EORTC trial 10801', *Eu J Cancer*, 28A: 808–15.

47. Fisher, B. J., Perera, F. E., Cooke, A. L., et al. (1997), 'Long-term follow-up of axillary node positive breast cancer patients receiving adjuvant systemic therapy alone: Patterns of recurrence', *Int J Radiat Oncol Biol Phy*, 38: 541–50.

Section B

1. Hong Kong Breast Cancer Foundation (2009): <http://www.hkbcf.org>.
2. *Coleman, M. P.* (1999), 'Opinion: Why the variation in breast cancer survival in Europe?', *Breast Cancer Res*, 1 (1): 22–6.
3. American Cancer Society (2007), *Cancer Facts & Figures 2007*, Atlanta, American Cancer Society.

4. Disease Control Priorities Project (2007): <http:// www.dcp2.org>.
5. Neuner, J. M., Gilligan, M. A., Sparapani R., et al. (2004) 'Decentralization of breast cancer surgery in the United States', *Cancer*, 101 (6): 1323–9.
6. Ritchie, W. P. Jr. (2002), 'Invited commentary: Comment from American Board of Surgery', *Surgery*, 131 (2): 212–13.
7. Pass, H. A., Klimberg, S. V. and Copeland III, E. M. (2008) 'Are "breast-focused" surgeons more competent?', *Ann Surg Oncol*, 15 (4): 953–5.
8. Newman, L. A. (2004), 'Locoregional control of breast cancer: Surgical technique does matter', *Ann Surg Oncol*, 11 (1): 11–13.
9. Fields, R. C., Jeffe, D. B., Trinkaus, K., et al. (2007), 'Surgical resection of the primary tumor is associated with increased long-term survival in patients with stage IV breast cancer after controlling for site of metastasis', *Ann Surg Oncol*, 14 (12): 3345–51.
10. Blanchard, D. K., Shetty, P. B., Hilsenbeck, S. G. and Elledge, R. M. (2008), 'Association of surgery with improved survival in stage IV breast cancer patients', *Ann Surg*, 247 (5): 732–8.
11. Halsted, W. S. (1894), 'The results of operations for the cure of cancer of the breast performed at the Johns Hopkins Hospital from June, 1889, to January, 1894'. *Ann Surg*, 20 (5): 487–555.
12. Newman, L. A. and Mamounas, E. P. (2007), 'Review of breast cancer clinical trials conducted by the National Surgical Adjuvant Breast Project', *Surg Clin North Am*, 87 (2): 279–305.
13. Fisher, B. F., Jeong, J., Anderson, S., et al. (2002), 'Twenty-five-year follow-up of a randomized trial comparing radical mastectomy, total mastectomy, and total mastectomy followed by irradiation', *N Engl J Med*, 347 (8): 567–75.
14. Veronisi, U., Luini, A, Del Vecchio, M., et al. (1993), 'Radiotherapy after breast-preserving surgery in women with localized cancer of the breast', *N Engl J Med*, 328 (22): 1587–91.
15. Veronesi, U., Marubini, E., Mariani, L., et al. (2001), 'Radiotherapy after breast-conserving surgery in small breast carcinoma: Long-term results of a randomized trial', *Ann Oncol*, 12 (7): 997–1003.
16. Morrow, M., White, J., Moughan, J., et. al. (2001), 'Factors predicting the use of breast-conserving therapy in stage I and II breast carcinoma', *J Surg Oncol*, 19 (8): 2252–64.
17. Jerome-D'Emilia, B. and Begun, J. W. (2005), 'Diffusion of breast conserving surgery in medical communities', *Social Science and Medicine*, 60 (1): 143–51.
18. Woon, Y. and Chan, M. (2005), 'Breast conservation surgery – The surgeon's factor', *Breast*, 14 (2): 131–5.

19. Golshan, M. (2009), 'Mastectomy', in J. R. Harris, Marc E. Lippman, C. K. Osborne and M. Morrow (eds), *Diseases of the Breast*, 4th edition, Philadelphia, USA, Lippincott Williams & Wilkins.

20. Iglehart, J. D. and Smith, B. L. (2007), 'Diseases of the Breast', in C. M. Townsend, R. D. Beauchamp, B. M. Evers and K. L. Mattox (eds), *Sabiston Textbook of Surgery – 2007*, Philadelphia, USA, Saunders Elsevier.

21. Erickson, V. S., Pearson, M. L., Ganz, P. A., et al. (2001), 'Arm edema in breast cancer patients', *J Natl Cancer Inst*, 93 (2): 96–111.

22. Hladiuk, M., Huchcroft, S., Temple, W. and Schnurr, B. E. (1992), 'Arm function after axillary dissection for breast cancer: A pilot study to provide parameter estimates', *J Surg Oncol*, 50 (1): 47–52.

23. McMasters, K. M., Wong, S. L., Chao, C., et al. (2001) 'Defining the optimal surgeon experience for breast cancer sentinel lymph node biopsy: A model for implementation of new surgical techniques, *Ann Surg*, 234 (2): 292–300.

24. Giuliano, A. E., Kirgan, D. M., Guenther, J. M. and Morton, D. L. (1994), 'Lymphatic mapping and sentinel lymphadenectomy for breast cancer', *Ann Surg*, 220 (3): 391–8.

25. Krag, D. N., Weaver, D. L., Alex, J. C. and Fairbank, J. T. (1993), 'Surgical resection and radiolocalization of the sentinel lymph node in breast cancer using a gamma probe', *Surg Oncol*, 2(6): 335–9.

26. Newman, E. A. and Newman, L. A. (2007), 'Lymphatic mapping techniques and sentinel lymph node biopsy in breast cancer', *Surg Clin North Am*, 87 (2): viii, 353–64.

27. van der Ploeg, I. M., Nieweg, O. E., van Rijk, M. C., et al. (2008), 'Axillary recurrence after a tumour-negative sentinel node biopsy in breast cancer patients: A systematic review and meta-analysis of the literature', *Eur J Surg Oncol*, 34 (12): 1277–84.

28. Coles, C. E., Wilson, C. B., Cumming, J., et al. (2009), 'Titanium clip placement to allow accurate tumour bed localisation following breast conserving surgery: Audit on behalf of the IMPORT Trial Management Group', *Eur J Surg Oncol*, 35 (6): 578–82.

29. Dalberg, K., Johansson, H., Signomklao, T., et al. (2004), 'A randomised study of axillary drainage and pectoral fascia preservation after mastectomy for breast cancer', *Eur J Surg Oncol*, 30 (6): 602–9.

30. Newman, L. A. (2004), 'Lymphatic mapping and sentinel lymph node biopsy in breast cancer patients: A comprehensive review of variations in performance and technique', *J Am Coll Surg*, 199: 804–16.

31. Vitug, A. F. and Newman, L. A. (2007), 'Complications in Breast Surgery', *Surg Clin North Am*, 87 (2): x, 431–51.

32. Platt, R., Zucker, J. R., Zaleznik, D. F., et al. (1993), 'Perioperative antibiotic prophylaxis and wound infection following breast surgery', *J Antimicrob Chemother*, 31 (suppl. B): 43–8.

33. Platt, R., Zaleznick, D. F., Hopkins, C. C., et al. (1990), 'Perioperative antibiotic prophylaxis for herniorrhaphy and breast surgery', *N Engl J Med*, 322 (3): 153–60.

34. McLaughlin, S. A., Wright, M. J., Morris, K. T., et al. (2008), 'Prevalence of lymphedema in women with breast cancer 5 years after sentinel lymph node biopsy or axillary dissection: objective measurements', *J Clin Oncol*, 26 (32): 5213–19.

35. Laurie, S. A., Khan, D. A., Gruchalla, R. S., et al. (2002), 'Anaphylaxis to isosulfan blue', *Ann Allergy Asthma Immunol*, 88 (1): 64–6.

Section C

1. Fisher, B., Redmond, C., Poisson, R., et al. (1989), 'Eight-year results of a randomized clinical trial comparing total mastectomy and lumpectomy with or without radiation in the treatment of breast cancer', *N Engl J Med*, 320: 822–8.

2. Fisher, B., Constantino, J., Redmond, C., et al. (1993), 'Initial results from a randomized trial evaluating lumpectomy and radiation therapy for the treatment of intraductal breast cancer', *N Engl J Med*, 328: 1581–6.

3. Fisher, B., Wolmark, N., Fisher, E. R., et al. (1985), 'Lumpectomy and axillary dissection for breast cancer: Surgical, pathological and radiation considerations', *World J Surg*, 9: 692–8.

4. Morton, D. L., Wen, D. -R., Wong, J. H., et al. (1992), *Arch Surg*, 27: 392–9.

5. Giuliano, A. E., Jones, R. C., Brennan, M., et al. (1997), *J Clin Oncol*, 15: 2345–50.

6. Krag, D. N., Weaver, D. L., Ashkaga T., et al. (1998), *New Engl J Med*, 339: 941–946.

7. American College of Surgeons Oncology Group (ACOSOG), Z10/Z11 trial: Axillary lymphadenectomy vs observation after ositive sentinel node biopsy.

8. ACOSOG/CTSU Z1031 trial (2009): A randomized phase III trial comparing 16 to 18 weeks of neo-adjuvant exemestane, letrozole or anastrozole in post-menopausal women with clinical stage II and III and estrogen receptor positive breast cancer (active study).

9. Fisher, B., Jeong, G. H., Anderson, S., et al. (2002) 'Twenty-five year follow-up of a randomized trial comparing radical mastectomy and total mastectomy followed by irradiation', *N Engl J Med*, 347: 567–75.

10. Fisher, B., Anderson, S., Bryant, J., et al. (2002), 'Twenty-year follow-

up of a randomized trial comparing total mastectomy, lumpectomy and lumpectomy plus irradiation for the treatment of invasive breast cancer', *N Engl J Med*, 347: 1233–41.

11. Nielsen, H. M., Overgaard, M., Grau, C., et al. (2006), 'Study of failure pattern among high-risk breast cancer patients with or without postmastectomy radiotherapy in addition to adjuvant systemic therapy: Long-term results from the Danish Breast Cancer Cooperative Group DBCG 82 b and c randomized studies', *J Clin Oncol*, 24: 2268–75.

12. Fisher, B., Dignam, J., Bryant, J., et al. (1996), 'Five versus more than five years of Tamoxifen therapy for breast cancer patients with negative lymph nodes and estrogen receptor positive tumors', *J Natl Cancer Inst*, 88: 1529–42.

13. Clarke, M., Collins, R., Darby, S., et al. (2005), 'Effect of radiotherapy and of differences in the extent of surgery for early breast cancer on local recurrence and 15-year survival: An overview of the randomized trials', *Lancet*, 366: 2087–106.

14. Doyle, B., Al-Mudhaffer, M., Kennedy, M. M., et al. (2009), 'Sentinel lymph node biopsy in patients with a needle core biopsy diagnosis of DCIS – Is it justified?', *J Clin Pathol*, Feb. 9 (e-publ).

15. Grin, A., Horne, G., Ennis, M., et al. (2009), 'Measuring extent of ductal carcinoma in-situ in breast excision specimens: A comparison of 4 methods', *Arch Pathol Lab Med*, 133 (1): 31–7.

16. Rudloff, U., Brockway, J. P., Goldberg, J. I., et al. (2009), 'Concurrent lobular neoplasia increases the risk of ipsilateral breast cancer recurrence in patients with ductal carcinoma in-situ treated with breast conserving therapy', *Cancer*, 115 (6): 1203–14.

17. Fisher, B., Land, S., Mamounas, E., et al. (2001), 'Prevention of invasive breast cancer in young women with ductal carcinoma in-situ: An update of the National Surgical Adjuvant Breast and Bowel Project experience', *Semin Oncol*, 28: 400–18.

18. Julien, J. P., Bijker, N., Fentiman, I. S., et al. (2000), 'Radiotherapy in breast-conserving treatment for ductal carcinoma in-situ: First results of the EORTC randomised phase III trial 10853', *Lancet*, 355: 528–33.

19. Wagoner, M. J., Laronga, C., and Acs, G. (2009), 'Extent and histologic pattern of atypical ductal hyperplasia present on core needle biopsy specimens of the breast can predict ductal carcinoma in-situ in subsequent excision', *Am J Clinical Pathol*, 131 (1): 112–21.

20. Arora, S., Menes, T. S., Moung, C., et al. (2008), 'Atypical ductal hyperplasia at margin of breast biopsy – Is re-excision indicated?', *Ann Surg Oncol*, 3: 843–7.

21. Hu, M., Peluffo, G., Chen, H., Gelman, R., et al. (2009), 'Role of COX–2 in epithelial-stromal cell interactions and progression of ductal carcinoma in-situ of the breast. *Proc Natl Acad Scie USA*, 106 (9): 3372–7.
22. Dunne, B., Burke, J., Morrow, M., et al. (2009), 'Margins for DCIS resection', *J Clin Oncol*, (e-publ).
23. Krag, D. N., Anderson, S. J., Julian, T. B., et al. (2007), 'Technical outcomes of sentinel lymph node resection and conventional axillary lymphnode dissection in patients with clinically node-negative breast cancer: Results from the NSABP–32 randomized phase III trial', *Lancet Oncol*, 8: 881–8.
24. Mabry, H. and Giuliano, A. E. (2007), 'Sentinel node mapping for breast cancer: Progress to date and prospects for the future', *Sur Oncol Clin N Am*, 16 (1): 55–70.
25. Gimbergues, P., Abrial, C., Durando, X., et al. (2008), 'Sentinel lymph node biopsy after neoadjuvant chemotherapy is accurate in breast cancer patients with a clinically negative axillary nodal status at presentation', *Ann Surg Oncol*, 15: 1316–21.
26. Chagpar, A. B, McMasters, K. M., Edwards, M. J., et al. (2009) 'Can sentinel node biopsy be avoided in some elderly breast cancer patients?', *Ann Surg*, 249 (3): 445–60.
27. Vanderveen, K. A., Ramsamooj, R., Bold, R. J., et al. (2008), 'A prospective, blinded trial of touch prep analysis versus frozen section for intraoperative evaluation of sentinel lymph nodes in breast cancer', *Ann Surg Oncol*, 15 (7): 2006–11.
28. Veronesi, U. et al (2009), 'Axillary metastases after negative sentinel nodes', *Eur J Canc*, Jan. 15 (e-publ).
29. Ramjeesingh, R., Quan, M. L., Gardner, S., et al. (2009), 'Prediction of involvement of sentinel and nonsentinel lymph nodes in a Candian population with breast cancer', *Can J Surg*, 52 (1): 23–30.
30. Krynickyi, B., Shafir, M., Kim, S. C., et al. (2005), 'Lymphoscintigraphy and triangulated body marking for morbidity reduction during sentinel node biopsy in cancer', *Internatl Semin Surg Oncol*, 2: 25–35.
31. Krynickyi, B., Shafir, M., Travis, A., et al. (2006), 'The current state of the art in lymphoscintigraphy', *Breast Dis*, 17 (2): 127–31.
32. Bines, S., Kopkash, K., Ali, A., et al. (2008), 'The use of radioisotope combined with isosulfan blue dye is not superior to radioisotope alone for the identification of sentinel lymph nodes in patients with breast cancer', *Surgery*, 144 (4): 606–10.
33. Hartmann, L. C., Sellers, T. A., Schaid, T. J., et al. (2001), 'Efficacy of bilateral prophylactic mastectomy in BRCA1 and BRCA2 gene mutations

carriers', *J Natl Cancer Inst*, 93 (21): 1633–7.

34. Batista, L. I., et al. (2008), 'Simultaneous operations feasible for hereditary breast-ovarian cancer syndrome', *BMC Cancer*, (e-publ).

35. Tuttle, T. M., Jarosek, S., Habermann, E. B., et al. (2009), 'Increasing rates of contralateal prophylactic mastectomy among patients with ductal carcinoma in situ', *J Clin Oncol*, Feb. 17 (e-publ).

36. Ken-ichi Ito, et al. (2008), 'Endoscopic surgery for early breast cancer may improve aesthetic results,' *ANZ J Surg*.

37. Huemer, G. M., Schrenk, P., Moser, F., et al. (2007), 'Oncoplastic techniques allow breast-conserving treatment in centrally located breast cancers', *Plast Reconstr Surg*, 120: 390–8.

38. Sahoo, S., Talwalkar, S. S., Martin, A. W., et al. (2007), 'Pathologic evaluation of cryoprobe-assisted lumpectomy for breast cancer', *Am J Clin Pathol*, 9/10 (e-publ).

39. James, T. A., Harlow, S., Sheehey-Jones, J, et al. (2009) 'Intraoperative ultrasound versus mammographic needle localization for ductal carcinoma in situ', *Ann Surg Oncol*, March 7 (e-publ).

40. Krynyckyi, B., Kim, C. K., Shafir, M., et al. (2003), 'Breast cancer and its management – The utility and technique of lymphoscintigraphy', in Leonard M. Freeman, Lippincott Williams, and Wilkins (eds), *Nuclear Medicine Annual*, 131–69.

41. Thompson, M., Henry-Tillman, R., Margulies, A., et al. (2007), 'Hematoma-directed ultrasound-guided breast lumpectomy', *Ann Surg Oncol*, 14: 148–56.

42. Hughes, H. G., Mason, M. C., Gray, R. J., et al. (2008), 'A multicenter validation trial of radioactive seed localization as an alternative to wire localization', *Breast J*, 14 (2): 153–7.

43. Sofocleus, C. T., Nascimento, R. G., Gonen, M., et al. (2007), 'Radiofrequency ablation in the management of liver metastases from breast cancer', *Am J Roentegonol*, 189 (4): 883–9.

44. Adam, R., Krissat, A. T., et al. (2006), 'Is liver resection justified for patients with hepatic metastases from breast cancer?', *Ann Surg*, 244: 897–908.

45. Khan, S. (2007), 'Does resection of an intact breat primary improve survival in metastatic breast cancer?', *Oncology* (Williston Park), 21: 1375–81.

46. Le Scodan, R., Stevens, D., Brain, E., et al. (2009), 'Breast cancer with synchronous metastatases: Survival impact of exclusive loco-regional radiotherapy', *J Clin Oncol*, 27: 1375–81.

Section D

1. Crile, G. (1965), 'Treatment of breast cancer by local excision', *Am J Surg*, 109 (4): 400–3.
2. Fisher, B. (1980), 'Laboratory and clinical research in breast cancer – A personal adventure. The David A. Karnofsky Memorial Lecture', *Cancer Res*, 40: 3863–74.
3. Fisher, B., Anderson, S., Bryant, J., et al. (2002), 'Twenty-year follow-up of a randomized trial comparing total mastectomy, lumpectomy, and lumpectomy plus irradiation for the treatment of invasive breast cancer', *N Eng J Med*, 347 (16): 1233–41.
4. Levine, D. A. and Gemignani, M. L. (2003), 'Prophylactic surgery in hereditary breast/ovarian cancer syndrome', *Oncology*, 17 (7): 932–41.
5. Kirova, Y. M., Stoppa-Lyonnet, D., Savignoni, A., et al., for the Institut Curie Breast Cancer Study Group (2005), 'Risk of breast cancer recurrence and contralateral breast cancer in relation to BRCA1 and BRCA2 mutation status following breast-conserving surgery and radiotherapy', *Eur J Cancer*, 41 (15): 2304–11.
6. Seynaeve, C., Verhoog, L. C., van de Bosch, L. M., et al. (2004), 'Ipsilateral breast tumour recurrence in hereditary breast cancer following breast-conserving therapy', *Eur J Cancer*, 40 (8): 1150–8.
7. Editorial (1993), 'Breast cancer: Have we lost our way?', *Lancet*, 341: 343–4.
8. Evans, I. (1994), 'The challenge of breast cancer', *Lancet*, 343: 1085–6.

Chapter 4

1. Fisher, B., Bauer, M., Wickerham, D. L., et al. (1983), 'Relation of number of positive axillary nodes to the prognosis of patients with primary breast cancer. An NSABP update', *Cancer*, 52 (9): 1551–7.
2. Rosen, P. P., Saigo, P. E., Braun, D. W., Jr., et al. (1981), 'Predictors of recurrence in stage I (T1N0M0) breast carcinoma', *Ann Surg*, 193 (1): 15–25.
3. Fitzgibbons, P. L. (2001), 'Breast Cancer', in: M. K. Gospodarowicz, D. E. Henson, R. V. P. Hutter, B. O'Sullivan, L. H. Sobin and C. Wittekind (eds), *Prognostic Factors in Cancer*, 2nd ed. New York: Wiley-Liss, 465–86.
4. Fisher, E. R., Anderson, S., Redmond, C. and Fisher, B. (1993), 'Pathologic findings from the National Surgical Adjuvant Breast Project protocol B–06. 10-year pathologic and clinical prognostic discriminants', *Cancer*, 71 (8):

2507–14.

5. Russo, J., Frederick, J., Ownby, H. E., et al. (1987), 'Predictors of recurrence and survival of patients with breast cancer', *Am J Clin Pathol*, 88 (2): 123–31.

6. Smith J. A., 3rd, Gamez-Araujo, J. J., Gallager, H. S., White, E. C. and McBride, C. M. (1977), 'Carcinoma of the breast: Analysis of total lymph node involvement versus level of metastasis', *Cancer*, 39 (2): 527–32.

7. Fitzgibbons, P. L., Page, D. L., Weaver, D., et al. (2000), 'Prognostic factors in breast cancer. College of American Pathologists Consensus Statement 1999', *Arch Pathol Lab Med*, 124 (7): 966–78.

8. Mambo, N. C. and Gallager, H. S. (1977), 'Carcinoma of the breast: The prognostic significance of extranodal extension of axillary disease', *Cancer*, 39 (5): 2280–5.

9. Fisher, E. R., Gregorio, R. M., Redmond, C., et al. (1976), 'Pathologic findings from the national surgical adjuvant breast project (protocol no. 4). III. The significance of extranodal extension of axillary metastases', *Am J Clin Pathol*, 65 (4): 439–44.

10. Donegan, W. L., Stine, S. B. and Samter, T. G. (1993), 'Implications of extracapsular nodal metastases for treatment and prognosis of breast cancer', *Cancer*, 72 (3): 778–82.

11. American Joint Committee on Cancer (AJCC) (2002), *AJCC Cancer Staging Manual*, 6th ed. New York: Springer Verlag.

12. Union Internationale Contre le Cancer (UICC) (2002), *TNM Classification of Malignant Tumours*, 6th ed., New York: Wiley-Liss.

13. Kahn, H. J., Hanna, W. M., Chapman, J. A. et al. (2006), 'Biological significance of occult micrometastases in histologically negative axillary lymph nodes in breast cancer patients using the recent American Joint Committee on Cancer breast cancer staging system', *Breast J*, 12 (4): 294–301.

14. Schwartz, G. F., Giuliano, A. E. and Veronesi, U. (2002), 'Proceedings of the consensus conference on the role of sentinel lymph node biopsy in carcinoma of the breast, April 19–22, 2001', Philadelphia, Pennsylvania, *Cancer*, 94 (10): 2542–51.

15. Weaver, D. L. (2003), 'Sentinel lymph nodes and breast carcinoma: Which micrometastases are clinically significant?', *Am J Surg Pathol*, 27 (6): 842–5.

16. Lyman, G. H., Giuliano, A. E., Somerfield, M. R., et al. (2005), 'American Society of Clinical Oncology guideline recommendations for sentinel lymph node biopsy in early-stage breast cancer', *J Clin Oncol*, 23 (30): 7703–20.

17. Chen, S. L., Hoehne, F. M., Giuliano, A. E. (2007), 'The prognostic significance of micrometastases in breast cancer: A SEER population-based analysis', *Ann Surg Oncol.*, 14 (12): 3378–84.

18. de Boer, M., van Deurzen, C. H., van Dijck, J. A., et al. (2009), 'Micrometastases or isolated tumor cells and the outcome of breast cancer', *N Engl J Med*, 361 (7): 653–63.

19. Sahin, A. A., Guray, M. and Hunt, K. K. (2009), 'Identification and biologic significance of micrometastases in axillary lymph nodes in patients with invasive breast cancer', *Arch Pathol Lab Med*, 133 (6): 869–78.

20. Carter, C. L., Allen, C. and Henson, D. E. (1989), 'Relation of tumor size, lymph node status, and survival in 24,740 breast cancer cases', *Cancer*, 63 (1): 181–7.

21. Rosen, P. P., Groshen, S., Kinne, D. W. and Norton, L. (1993), 'Factors influencing prognosis in node-negative breast carcinoma: Analysis of 767 T1N0M0/T2N0M0 patients with long-term follow-up', *J Clin Oncol*, 11 (11): 2090–100.

22. Seidman, J. D., Schnaper, L. A. and Aisner, S. C. (1995), 'Relationship of the size of the invasive component of the primary breast carcinoma to axillary lymph node metastasis', *Cancer*, 75 (1): 65–71.

23. Kollias, J., Elston, C. W., Ellis, I. O., Robertson, J. F. and Blamey, R. W. (1997), 'Early-onset breast cancer – Histopathological and prognostic considerations', *Br J Cancer*, 75 (9): 1318–23.

24. Hanrahan, E. O., Valero, V., Gonzalez-Angulo, A. M. and Hortobagyi, G. N. (2006), 'Prognosis and management of patients with node-negative invasive breast carcinoma that is 1 cm or smaller in size (stage 1; T1a, bN0M0): A review of the literature', *J Clin Oncol*, 24 (13): 2113–22.

25. Silverstein, M. J., Gierson, E. D., Waisman, J. R., et al. (1994), 'Axillary lymph node dissection for T1a breast carcinoma. Is it indicated?', *Cancer*, 73 (3): 664–7.

26. McGuire, W. L. and Clark, G. M. (1992), 'Prognostic factors and treatment decisions in axillary-node-negative breast cancer', *N Engl J Med*, 326 (26): 1756–61.

27. Abner, A. L., Collins, L., Peiro, G., et al. (1998), 'Correlation of tumor size and axillary lymph node involvement with prognosis in patients with T1 breast carcinoma', *Cancer*, 83(12): 2502–8.

28. Coombs, N. J. and Boyages, J. (2005), 'Multifocal and multicentric breast cancer: Does each focus matter?', *J Clin Oncol*, 23(30): 7497–502.

29. Andea, A. A., Bouwman, D., Wallis, T. and Visscher, D. W. (2004), 'Correlation of tumor volume and surface area with lymph node status in patients with multifocal/multicentric breast carcinoma', *Cancer*, 100 (1):

20-7.

30. Bloom, H. J., Richardson, W. W. and Harries, E. J. (1962), 'Natural history of untreated breast cancer (1805–1933). Comparison of untreated and treated cases according to histological grade of malignancy', *Br Med J*, 2 (5299): 213–21.

31. Bloom, H. J. (1965), 'The influence of tumour grade on radiotherapy results', *Br J Radiol*, 38: 227–40.

32. Bloom, H. J. and Field, J. R. (1971), 'Impact of tumor grade and host resistance on survival of women with breast cancer', *Cancer*, 28 (6): 1580–9.

33. Elston, C. W. (1984), 'The assessment of histological differentiation in breast cancer', *Aust NZ J Surg*, 54 (1): 11–15.

34. Contesso, G., Mouriesse, H., Friedman, S., et al. (1987), 'The importance of histologic grade in long-term prognosis of breast cancer: A study of 1,010 patients, uniformly treated at the Institut Gustave-Roussy', *J Clin Oncol*, 5 (9): 1378–86.

35. Davis, B. W., Gelber, R. D., Goldhirsch, A., et al. (1986), 'Prognostic significance of tumor grade in clinical trials of adjuvant therapy for breast cancer with axillary lymph node metastasis', *Cancer*, 58 (12): 2662–70.

36. Le Doussal, V., Tubiana-Hulin, M., Friedman, S., et al. (1989), 'Prognostic value of histologic grade nuclear components of Scarff-Bloom-Richardson (SBR). An improved score modification based on a multivariate analysis of 1,262 invasive ductal breast carcinomas', *Cancer*, 64 (9): 1914–21.

37. Clayton, F. and Hopkins, C. L. (1993), 'Pathologic correlates of prognosis in lymph node-positive breast carcinomas', *Cancer*, 71 (5): 1780–90.

38. Pereira, H., Pinder, S. E., Sibbering, D. M., et al. (1995), 'Pathological prognostic factors in breast cancer. IV: Should you be a typer or a grader? A comparative study of two histological prognostic features in operable breast carcinoma', *Histopathology*, 27 (3): 219–26.

39. Frierson, H. F., Jr., Wolber, R. A., Berean, K. W., et al. (1995), 'Interobserver reproducibility of the Nottingham modification of the Bloom and Richardson histologic grading scheme for infiltrating ductal carcinoma', *Am J Clin Pathol*, 103 (2): 195–8.

40. Dalton, L. W., Page, D. L. and Dupont, W. D. (1994), 'Histologic grading of breast carcinoma. A reproducibility study', *Cancer*, 73 (11): 2765–70.

41. Robbins, P., Pinder, S., de Klerk, N., et al. (1995), 'Histological grading of breast carcinomas: A study of interobserver agreement', *Hum Pathol*, 26 (8): 873–9.

42. Harvey, J. M., Clark, G. M., Osborne, C. K. and Allred, D. C. (1999), 'Estrogen receptor status by immunohistochemistry is superior to the

ligand-binding assay for predicting response to adjuvant endocrine therapy in breast cancer', *J Clin Oncol*, 17 (5): 1474–81.

43. Sotiriou, C., Wirapati, P., Loi, S., et al. (2006), 'Gene expression profiling in breast cancer: Understanding the molecular basis of histologic grade to improve prognosis', *J Natl Cancer Inst*, 98 (4): 262–72.

44. Goldhirsch, A., Ingle, J. N., Gelber, R. D., et al. (2009), 'Thresholds for therapies: Highlights of the St Gallen International Expert Consensus on the primary therapy of early breast cancer 2009', *Ann Oncol*, 20 (8): 1319–29.

45. Ellis, I. O., Galea, M., Broughton, N., et al. (1992), 'Pathological prognostic factors in breast cancer. II. Histological type. Relationship with survival in a large study with long-term follow-up', *Histopathology*, 20 (6): 479–89.

46. World Health Organization (2003), *Classification of Tumours. Pathology and Genetics of Tumours of the Breast and Female Genital Organs*, IARC Press: Lyon.

47. Orbo, A., Stalsberg, H. and Kunde, D. (1990), 'Topographic criteria in the diagnosis of tumor emboli in intramammary lymphatics', *Cancer*, 66 (5): 972–7.

48. Davis, B. W., Gelber, R. and Goldhirsch, A., et al. (1985), 'Prognostic significance of peritumoral vessel invasion in clinical trials of adjuvant therapy for breast cancer with axillary lymph node metastasis', *Hum Pathol*, 16 (12): 1212–18.

49. Leitner, S. P., Swern, A. S., Weinberger, D., et al. (1995), 'Predictors of recurrence for patients with small (one centimeter or less) localized breast cancer (T1a, b N0 M0)', *Cancer*, 76 (11): 2266–74.

50. Budrukkar, A. N., Sarin, R., Chinoy, R. F., et al. (2008), 'Prognostic factors in node negative premenopausal women treated with breast conserving therapy without adjuvant systemic therapy', *Breast*, 17 (3): 263–9.

51. Nime, F. A., Rosen, P. P., Thaler, H. T., et al. (1977), 'Prognostic significance of tumor emboli in intramammary lymphatics in patients with mammary carcinoma', *Am J Surg Pathol*, 1 (1): 25–30.

52. Pinder, S. E., Ellis, I. O., Galea, M., et al. (1994), 'Pathological prognostic factors in breast cancer. III. Vascular invasion: Relationship with recurrence and survival in a large study with long-term follow-up', *Histopathology*, 24 (1): 41–7.

53. Mohammed, R. A., Martin, S. G., Gill, M. S., et al. (2007), 'Improved methods of detection of lymphovascular invasion demonstrate that it is the predominant method of vascular invasion in breast cancer and has important clinical consequences', *Am J Surg Pathol*, 31 (12): 1825–33.

54. Maiorano, E., Regan, M. M., Viale, G., et al. (2009), 'Prognostic and predictive impact of central necrosis and fibrosis in early breast cancer: Results from two International Breast Cancer Study Group randomized trials of chemoendocrine adjuvant therapy', *Breast Cancer Res Treat* (in press).

55. Hasebe, T., Tsuda, H., Hirohashi, S., et al. (1996), 'Fibrotic focus in invasive ductal carcinoma: An indicator of high tumor aggressiveness', *Jpn J Cancer Res*, 87 (4): 385–94.

56. Shimokawara, I., Imamura, M., Yamanaka, N., et al. (1982), 'Identification of lymphocyte subpopulations in human breast cancer tissue and its significance: An immunoperoxidase study with anti-human T- and B-cell sera', *Cancer*, 49 (7): 1456–64.

57. Tamiolakis, D., Simopoulos, C., Cheva, A., et al. (2002), 'Immunophenotypic profile of tumor infiltrating lymphocytes in medullary carcinoma of the breast', *Eur J Gynaecol Oncol*, 23: 433–6.

58. Aaltomaa, S., Lipponen, P., Eskelinen, M., et al. (1992), 'Lymphocyte infiltrates as a prognostic variable in female breast cancer', *Eur J Cancer*, 28A (4–5): 859–64.

59. Lucin, K., Iternicka, Z. and Jonjic, N. (1994), 'Prognostic significance of T-cell infiltrates, expression of beta 2-microglobulin and HLA-DR antigens in breast carcinoma', *Pathol Res Pract*, 190 (12): 1134–40.

60. Menard, S., Tomasic, G., Casalini, P., et al. (1997), 'Lymphoid infiltration as a prognostic variable for early-onset breast carcinomas', *Clin Cancer Res*, 3 (5): 817–19.

61. Allred, D. C., Harvey, J. M., Berardo, M. and Clark, G. M. (1998), 'Prognostic and predictive factors in breast cancer by immunohistochemical analysis', *Mod Pathol*, 11 (2): 155–68.

62. Pertschuk, L. P., Feldman, J. G., Kim, Y. D., et al. (1996), 'Estrogen receptor immunocytochemistry in paraffin embedded tissues with ER1D5 predicts breast cancer endocrine response more accurately than H222Sp gamma in frozen sections or cytosol-based ligand-binding assays', *Cancer*, 77 (12): 2514–19.

63. Andersen, J. and Poulsen, H. S. (1989), 'Immunohistochemical estrogen receptor determination in paraffin-embedded tissue. Prediction of response to hormonal treatment in advanced breast cancer', *Cancer*, 64 (9): 1901–8.

64. Schnitt, S. J. (2006), 'Estrogen receptor testing of breast cancer in current clinical practice: What's the question?', *J Clin Oncol*, 24 (12): 1797–9.

65. Layfield, L. J., Gupta, D. and Mooney, E. E. (2000), 'Assessment of tissue estrogen and progesterone receptor levels: A survey of current practice, techniques, and quantitation methods', *Breast J*, 6 (3): 189–96.

66. Eifel, P., Axelson, J. A., Costa, J., et al. (2001), 'National Institutes of Health Consensus Development Conference Statement: Adjuvant therapy for breast cancer, November 1–3, 2000', *J Natl Cancer Inst*, 93 (13): 979–89.

67. Albain, K. S. (2004), 'Adjuvant chemotherapy for lymph node-negative, estrogen receptor-negative breast cancer: A tale of three trials', *J Natl Cancer Inst*, 96 (24): 1801–4.

68. Wolff, A. C., Hammond, M. E., Schwartz, J. N., et al. (2007), 'American Society of Clinical Oncology/College of American Pathologists guideline recommendations for human epidermal growth factor receptor 2 testing in breast cancer', *Arch Pathol Lab Med*, 131 (1): 18–43.

69. Sauter, G., Lee, J., Bartlett, J. M., et al. (2009), 'Guidelines for human epidermal growth factor receptor 2 testing: biologic and methodologic considerations', *J Clin Oncol*, 27 (8): 1323–33.

70. Abboud, P., Lorenzato, M., Joly, D., et al. (2008), 'Prognostic value of a proliferation index including MIB1 and argyrophilic nucleolar organizer regions proteins in node-negative breast cancer', *Am J Obstet Gynecol*, 199 (2): 146 e1–7.

71. Ahlin, C., Aaltonen, K., Amini, R. M., et al. (2007), 'Ki67 and cyclin A as prognostic factors in early breast cancer. What are the optimal cut-off values?', *Histopathology*, 51 (4): 491–8.

72. Guarneri, V., Piacentini, F., Ficarra, G., et al. (2009), 'A prognostic model based on nodal status and Ki–67 predicts the risk of recurrence and death in breast cancer patients with residual disease after preoperative chemotherapy', *Ann Oncol*, 20 (7): 1193–8.

73. Lee, J., Im, Y. H., Lee, S. H., et al. (2008), 'Evaluation of ER and Ki–67 proliferation index as prognostic factors for survival following neoadjuvant chemotherapy with doxorubicin/docetaxel for locally advanced breast cancer', *Cancer Chemother Pharmacol*, 61 (4): 569–77.

74. Jones, R. L., Salter, J., A'Hern, R., et al. (2009), 'The prognostic significance of Ki67 before and after neoadjuvant chemotherapy in breast cancer', *Breast Cancer Res Treat*, 116 (1): 53–68.

75. Dowsett, M., Smith, I. E., Ebbs, S. R., et al. (2007), 'Prognostic value of Ki67 expression after short-term presurgical endocrine therapy for primary breast cancer', *J Natl Cancer Inst*, 99 (2): 167–70.

76. Fernandez-Sanchez, M., Gamboa-Dominguez, A., Uribe, N., et al. (2006), 'Clinical and pathological predictors of the response to neoadjuvant anthracycline chemotherapy in locally advanced breast cancer', *Med Oncol*, 23 (2): 171–83.

77. Vincent-Salomon, A., Rousseau, A., Jouve, M., et al. (2004), 'Proliferation

markers predictive of the pathological response and disease outcome of patients with breast carcinomas treated by anthracycline-based preoperative chemotherapy', *Eur J Cancer*, 40 (10): 1502–8.

78. Sharma, S., Saboorian, H. M., Frawley, W. H., et al. (2004), 'MIB1 labeling index as an indicator of chemoresponse in carcinoma of the breast', *Appl Immunohistochem Mol Morphol*, 12 (4): 290–5.

79. Dowsett, M., Smith, I. E., Ebbs, S. R., et al. (2006), 'Proliferation and apoptosis as markers of benefit in neoadjuvant endocrine therapy of breast cancer', *Clin Cancer Res*, 12 (3 Pt 2): 1024s–30s.

80. Dowsett, M., Smith, I. E., Ebbs, S. R., et al. (2005), 'Short-term changes in Ki–67 during neoadjuvant treatment of primary breast cancer with anastrozole or tamoxifen alone or combined correlate with recurrence-free survival', *Clin Cancer Res*, 11 (2 Pt 2): 951s–8s.

81. Burcombe, R. J., Makris, A., Richman, P. I., et al. (2005), 'Evaluation of ER, PgR, HER–2 and Ki–67 as predictors of response to neoadjuvant anthracycline chemotherapy for operable breast cancer', *Br J Cancer*, 92 (1): 147–55.

82. Jones, R. L., Salter, J., A'Hern, R., et al. (2010), 'Relationship between oestrogen receptor status and proliferation in predicting response and long-term outcome to neoadjuvant chemotherapy for breast cancer', *Breast Cancer Res Treat*, 119 (2): 315–23.

83. Viale, G., Regan, M. M., Mastropasqua, M. G., et al. (2008), 'Predictive value of tumor Ki–67 expression in two randomized trials of adjuvant chemoendocrine therapy for node-negative breast cancer', *J Natl Cancer Inst*, 100 (3): 207–12.

84. Potemski, P., Pluciennik, E., Bednarek, A. K., et al. (2006), 'Ki–67 expression in operable breast cancer: A comparative study of immunostaining and a real-time RT-PCR assay', *Pathol Res Pract*, 202 (7): 491–5.

85. Urruticoechea, A., Smith, I. E. and Dowsett, M. (2005), 'Proliferation marker Ki–67 in early breast cancer', *J Clin Oncol*, 23 (28): 7212–20.

86. Perou, C. M., Sorlie, T., Eisen, M. B., et al. (2000), 'Molecular portraits of human breast tumours', *Nature*, 406 (6797): 747–52.

87. Livasy, C. A., Perou, C. M., Karaca, G., et al. (2007), 'Identification of a basal-like subtype of breast ductal carcinoma in situ', *Hum Pathol*, 38 (2): 197–204.

88. Sorlie, T., Tibshirani, R., Parker, J., et al. (2003), 'Repeated observation of breast tumor subtypes in independent gene expression data sets', *Proc Natl Acad Sci USA*, 100 (14): 8418–23.

89. Sorlie, T., Perou, C. M., Tibshirani, R., et al. (2001), 'Gene expression

patterns of breast carcinomas distinguish tumor subclasses with clinical implications', *Proc Natl Acad Sci USA*, 98 (19): 10869–74.

90. Evans, A. J., Rakha, E. A., Pinder, S. E., et al. (2007), 'Basal phenotype: A powerful prognostic factor in small screen-detected invasive breast cancer with long-term follow-up', *J Med Screen*, 14 (4): 210–14.

91. Domagala, W., Wozniak, L., Lasota, J., et al. (1990), 'Vimentin is preferentially expressed in high-grade ductal and medullary, but not in lobular breast carcinomas', *Am J Pathol*, 137 (5): 1059–64.

92. Fisher, E. R., Wang, J., Bryant, J., et al. (2002), 'Pathobiology of preoperative chemotherapy: Findings from the National Surgical Adjuvant Breast and Bowel (NSABP) protocol B–18', *Cancer*, 95 (4): 681–95.

93. Chevallier, B., Roche, H., Olivier, J. P., et al. (1993), 'Inflammatory breast cancer. Pilot study of intensive induction chemotherapy (FEC-HD) results in a high histologic response rate', *Am J Clin Oncol*, 16 (3): 223–8.

94. Sataloff, D. M., Mason, B. A., Prestipino, A. J., et al. (1995), 'Pathologic response to induction chemotherapy in locally advanced carcinoma of the breast: A determinant of outcome', *J Am Coll Surg*, 180 (3): 297–306.

95. Ogston, K. N., Miller, I. D., Payne, S., et al. (2003), 'A new histological grading system to assess response of breast cancers to primary chemotherapy: Prognostic significance and survival', *Breast*, 12 (5): 320–7.

96. Symmans, W. F., Peintinger, F., Hatzis, C., et al. (2007), 'Measurement of residual breast cancer burden to predict survival after neoadjuvant chemotherapy', *J Clin Oncol*, 25 (28): 4414–22.

97. Carey, L. A., Metzger, R., Dees, E. C., et al. (2005), 'American Joint Committee on Cancer tumor-node-metastasis stage after neoadjuvant chemotherapy and breast cancer outcome', *J Natl Cancer Inst*, 97 (15): 1137–42.

98. Rouzier, R., Pusztai, L., Delaloge, S., et al. (2005), 'Nomograms to predict pathologic complete response and metastasis-free survival after preoperative chemotherapy for breast cancer', *J Clin Oncol*, 23 (33): 8331–9.

99. Abrial, S. C., Penault-Llorca, F., Delva, R., et al. (2005), 'High prognostic significance of residual disease after neoadjuvant chemotherapy: A retrospective study in 710 patients with operable breast cancer', *Breast Cancer Res Treat*, 94 (3): 255–63.

100. Rajan, R., Poniecka, A., Smith, T. L., et al. (2004), 'Change in tumor cellularity of breast carcinoma after neoadjuvant chemotherapy as a variable in the pathologic assessment of response', *Cancer*, 100 (7): 1365–73.

101. Galea, M. H., Blamey, R. W., Elston, C. E. and Ellis, I. O. (1992), 'The

Nottingham Prognostic Index in primary breast cancer', *Breast Cancer Res Treat*, 22 (3): 207–19.

Chapter 5

1. Jemal, A., Siegel, R., Ward, E., et al. (2008), 'Cancer Statistics', *CA Cancer J. Clin*, 58 (2): 71–96.
2. Roukos, D. H. and Briasoulis, E. (2007), 'Individualized preventive and therapeutic management of hereditary breast ovarian cancer', *Nat Clin Pract Oncol*, 4 (10): 578–90.
3. Roukos, D. H. (2007), 'Prognosis of breast cancer in carriers of BRCA1 and BRCA2 mutations', *N Engl J Med*, 357 (15): 1555–6.
4. Fisher, B. (1977), 'Biological and clinical considerations regarding the use of surgery and chemotherapy in the treatment of primary breast cancer', *Cancer*, 40 (suppl. 1): 574–87.
5. Clarke, M., Collins, R., Darby, S., et al. (2005), 'Effects of radiotherapy and of differences in the extent of surgery for early breast cancer on local recurrence and 15-year survival: An overview of the randomized trials', *Lancet*, 366: 2087–106.
6. Punglia, R. S., Morrow, M., Winer, E. P. and Harris, J. R. (2007), 'Local therapy and survival in breast cancer', *N Engl J Med*, 356 (23): 2399–405.
7. Arimidex, Tamoxifen, Alone or in Combination (ATAC) Trialists' Group, Forbes, J. F., Cuzick, J., et al. (2008), 'Effect of anastrozole and tamoxifen as adjuvant treatment for early-stage breast cancer: 100-month analysis of the ATAC trial', *Lancet Oncol*, 9 (1): 45–53.
8. Piccart-Gebhart, M. J., Procter, M., Leyland-Jones, B., et al. (2005), 'Trastuzumab after adjuvant chemotherapy in HER–2-positive breast cancer', *N Engl J Med*, 353: 1659–72.
9. Romond, E. H., Perez, E. A, Bryant, J., et al. (2005), 'Trastuzumab plus adjuvant chemotherapy for operable HER–2-positive breast cancer', *N Engl J Med*, 353: 1673–1684.
10. Wapnir, I. L., Aebi, S., Gelber, S., et al. (2008), 'Progress on BIG 1–02/IBCSG 27–02/NSABP B–37, a prospective randomized trial evaluating chemotherapy after local therapy for isolated locoregional recurrences of breast cancer', *Ann Surg Oncol*, 11: 3227–31.
11. Tuttle, T. M., Habermann, E. B., Grund, E. H., et al. (2007), 'Increasing use of contralateral prophylactic mastectomy for breast cancer patients: A trend toward more aggressive surgical treatment', *J Clin Oncol*, 25: 5203–9.
12. Roukos, D. H. (2008), 'Linking contralateral breast cancer with genetics',

Radiother Oncol, 86: 139–141.

13. Goldhirsch, A., Wood, W. C., Gelber, R. D., et al. (2007), 'Progress and promise: Highlights of the international expert consensus on the primary therapy of early breast cancer 2007', *Ann Oncol*, 18 (7): 1133–44.

14. Roukos, D. H., Murray S., Briasoulis, E. (2007), 'Molecular genetic tools shape a roadmap towards a more accurate prognostic prediction and personalized management of cancer', *Cancer Biol Ther*, 6 (3): 308–12.

15. Wood, L. D., Parsons, D. W., Jones, S., et al. (2007), 'The genomic landscapes of human breast and colorectal cancers', *Science*, 318 (5853): 1108–113.

16. International HapMap Consortium, Frazer, K. A., Ballinger, D. G., et al. (2007), 'A second generation human haplotype map of over 3.1 million SNPs', *Nature*, 449 (7164): 851–61.

17. Lee, C., Morton, C. C. (2008), 'Structural genomic variation and personalized medicine', *N Engl J Med*, 358 (7): 740–1.

18. Korbel, J. O., Urban, A. E., Affourtit, J. P., et al. (2007), 'Paired-end mapping reveals extensive structural variation in the human genome', *Science*, 318: 420–6.

19. Pennisi, E. (2007), 'Breakthrough of the year. Human genetic variation', *Science*, 318 (5858): 1842–3.

20. Easton, D. F., Pooley, K. A., Dunning, A. M. (2007), 'Genome-wide association study identifies novel breast cancer susceptibility loci', *Nature*, 447 (7148): 1087–1093.

21. Gold, B., Kirchhoff, T., Stefanov, S., et al. (2008), 'Genome-wide association study provides evidence for a breast cancer risk locus at 6q22.33', *Proc Natl Acad Sci USA*, 105 (11): 4340–5.

22. Hunter, D. J., Kraft, P., Jacobs, K. B., et al. (2007), 'A genome-wide association study identifies alleles in FGFR2 associated with risk of sporadic postmenopausal breast cancer', *Nat Genet*, 39: 870–4.

23. Weir, B. A., Woo, M. S., Getz, G., et al. (2007), 'Characterizing the cancer genome in lung adenocarcinoma', *Nature*, 450 (7171): 893–8.

24. Zheng, S. L., Sun, J., Wiklund, F., et al. (2008), 'Cumulative association of five genetic variants with prostate cancer', *N Engl J Med*, 358 (9): 910–19.

25. Nguyen, P. L., Taghian, A. G., Katz, M. S., et al. (2008), 'Breast cancer subtype approximated by estrogen receptor, progesterone receptor, and HER–2 is associated with local and distant recurrence after breast-conserving therapy', *J Clin Oncol*, 26 (14): 2373–8.

26. Kyndi, M., Sorensen, F. B., Knudsen, H., et al. (2008), 'Estrogen receptor, progesterone receptor, HER–2, and response to postmastectomy radiotherapy in high-risk breast cancer: The Danish Breast Cancer

Cooperative Group', *J Clin Oncol*, 26: 1419–26.

27. Hooning, M. J., Aleman, B. M., Hauptmann, M., et al. (2008), 'Roles of radiotherapy and chemotherapy in the development of contralateral breast cancer', *J Clin Oncol*, 26: 5561–8.

28. Offersen, B. V., Overgaard, M., Kroman, N. and Overgaard, J. (2009), 'Accelerated partial breast irradiation as part of breast conserving therapy of early breast carcinoma: A systematic review', *Radiother Oncol*, 90 (1): 1–13.

29. Goss, P. E., Ingle, J. N., Pater, J. L., et al. (2008), 'Late extended adjuvant treatment with letrozole improves outcome in women with early-stage breast cancer who complete 5 years of tamoxifen', *J Clin Oncol*, 26 (12): 1948–55 (E-pub: March 10, 2008. Erratum in: *J Clin Oncol*, July 20, 2008, 26 (21): 3659).

30. Muss, H. B., Tu, D., Ingle, J. N., et al. (2008), 'Efficacy, toxicity, and quality of life in older women with early-stage breast cancer treated with letrozole or placebo after 5 years of tamoxifen: NCIC CTG intergroup trial MA. 17', *J Clin Oncol*, 26 (12): 1956–64.

31. Perou, C. M., Sørlie, T., Eisen, M. B., et al. (2000), 'Molecular portraits of human breast tumors', *Nature*, 406 (6797): 747–52.

32. Sorlie, T., Tibshirani, R., Parker, J., et al. (2003), 'Repeated observation of breast tumor subtypes in independent gene expression data sets', *Proc Natl Acad Sci USA*, 100 (14): 8418–23.

33. Sotiriou, C. and Piccart, M. J., (2007), 'Taking gene-expression profiling to the clinic: When will molecular signatures become relevant to patient care?', *Nat Rev Cancer*, 7 (7): 545–53.

34. Roukos, D. H., Lykoudis, E., Liakakos, T. (2008), 'Genomics and challenges toward personalized breast cancer local control', *J Clin Oncol*, 26 (26): 4360–1 (author reply: 4361–2).

35. Rakha, E. A., Reis-Filho, J. S, Ellis, I. O. (2008), 'Basal-like breast cancer: A critical review', *J Clin Oncol*, 26: 2568–81.

36. van de Vijver, M. J., He, Y. D., van't Veer, L. J., et al. (2002), 'A gene-expression signature as a predictor of survival in breast cancer', *N Engl J Med*, 347 (25): 1999–2009.

37. Paik, S., Tang, G., Shak, S., et al. (2006), 'Gene expression and benefit of chemotherapy in women with node-negative, estrogen receptor-positive breast cancer', *J Clin Oncol*, 24: 3726–34.

38. Huang, C. C. and Bredel, M. (2008), 'Use of gene signatures to improve risk estimation in cancer', *JAMA*, 299 (13): 1605–6.

39. Roukos, D. H. (2009), '21-gene assay: Challenges and promises in translating personal genomics and whole genome scans into personalized

treatment of breast cancer', *J Clin Oncol,* 27 (8): 1337–8 (author reply: 1338–9).

40. Hayes, D. F., Stearns, V., Rae, J., Flockhart, D., Consortium on Breast Cancer Pharmacogenomics (2008), 'A model citizen? Is tamoxifen more effective than aromatase inhibitors if we pick the right patients?', *J Natl Cancer Inst,* 100 (9): 610–13.

41. Fisher, B, Anderson, S, Bryant, J., et al (2002), 'Twenty-year follow-up of a randomized trial comparing total mastectomy, lumpectomy, and lumpectomy plus irradiation for the treatment of invasive breast cancer', *N Engl J Med,* 347: 1233–41.

42. Metcalfe, K., Lynch, H. T., Ghadirian, P., et al. (2004), 'Contralateral breast cancer in BRCA1 and BRCA2 mutation carriers', *J Clin Oncol,* 22 (12): 2328–35.

43. Pierce, L. J., Levin, A. M., Rebbeck, T. R., et al. (2006), 'Ten-year multiinstitutional results of breast-conserving surgery and radiotherapy in BRCA1/2-associated stage I/II breast cancer', *J Clin Oncol,* 24, 2437–43.

44. Metcalfe, K. A., Lubinski, J., Ghadirian, P., et al. (2008), 'Predictors of contralateral prophylactic mastectomy in women with a BRCA1 or BRCA2 mutation: The Hereditary Breast Cancer Clinical Study Group', *J Clin Oncol,* 26 (7): 1093–7.

45. Fatouros, M., Baltoyiannis, G. and Roukos, D. H. (2008), 'The predominant role of surgery in the prevention and new trends in the surgical treatment of women with BRCA1/2 mutations', *Ann Surg Oncol,* 15, 21–33.

46. Narod, S. A. and Offit, K. (2005), 'Prevention and management of hereditary breast cancer', *J Clin Oncol,* 23: 1656–63.

47. Farmer, H., McCabe, N., Lord, C. J., et al. (2005), 'Targeting the DNA repair defect in BRCA mutant cells as a therapeutic strategy', *Nature,* 434: 917–21.

48. Venkitaraman, A. R. (2002), 'Cancer susceptibility and the functions of BRCA1 and BRCA2', *Cell,* 108: 171–82.

49. Roukos, D. H., Kappas, A. M., Tsianos, E. (2002), 'Role of surgery in the prophylaxis of hereditary cancer syndromes', *Ann Surg Oncol,* 9 (7): 607–9.

50. Barnett, G. C., Shah, M., Redman, K., et al. (2008), 'Risk factors for the incidence of breast cancer: Do they affect survival from the disease?', *J Clin Oncol,* 26 (20): 3310–6.

51. Pharoah, P. D., Antoniou, A., Bobrow, M., et al. (2002), 'Polygenic susceptibility to breast cancer and implications for prevention', *Nat. Genet,* 31: 33–6.

52. Miki, Y., Swensen, J., Shattuck-Eidens, D., et al. (1994), 'A strong candidate for the breast and ovarian cancer susceptibility gene BRCA1',

Science, 266: 66–71.

53. Wooster, R., Bignell, G., Lancaster, J., et al. (1995), 'Identification of the breast cancer susceptibility gene BRCA2', *Nature*, 378: 789–92.

54. Smith, P., McGuffog, L., Easton, D. F., et al. (2006), 'A genome wide linkage search for breast cancer susceptibility genes', *Genes Chromosomes Cancer*, 45: 646–55.

55. Antoniou, A. C., Sinilnikova, O. M., Simard, J., et al. (2007), 'RAD51 135GC modifies breast cancer risk among BRCA2 mutation carriers: Results from a combined analysis of 19 studies', *Am J Hum Genet*, 81 (6): 1186–200.

56. Antoniou, A. C., Spurdle, A. B. and Sinilnikova, O. M. (2008), 'Common breast cancer-predisposition alleles are associated with breast cancer risk in BRCA1 and BRCA2 mutation carriers', *Am J Hum Genet*, 82 (4): 937–948.

57. Offit, K. and Garber, J. E. (2008), 'Time to check CHEK2 in families with breast cancer?', *J Clin Oncol*, 26: 519–520.

58. Friedman, A. and Perrimon, N. (2007), 'Genetic screening for signal transduction in the era of network biology', *Cell*, 128 (2), 225–231.

59. Lobo, N. A., Shimono, Y., Qian, D. and Clarke, M. F. (2007), 'The biology of cancer stem cells, *Ann Rev Cell Dev Biol*, 23: 675–699.

60. Jain, R. K., Duda, D. G., Clark, J. W. and Loeffler, J. S. (2006), 'Lessons from phase III clinical trials on anti-VEGF therapy for cancer', *Nat Clin Pract Oncol*, 3 (1), 24–40.

61. Miller, K., Wang, M., Gralow, J., et al. (2007), 'Paclitaxel plus bevacizumab versus paclitaxel alone for metastatic breast cancer', *N Engl J Med*, 357 (26): 2666–76.

62. Patocs, A., Zhang, L., Xu, Y., et al. (2007), 'Breast-cancer stromal cells with TP53 mutations and nodal metastases', *N. Engl J Med*, 357: 2543–51.

63. Roukos, D. H. (2008), 'Breast-cancer stromal cells with TP53 mutations', *N Engl J Med*, 358 (15): 1636.

64. Aguirre-Ghiso, J. A. (2007), 'Models, mechanisms and clinical evidence for cancer dormancy', *Nat Rev Cancer*, 7 (11): 834–46.

65. Roukos, D. H. (2008), 'HER2 and response to paclitaxel in node-positive breast cancer', *N Engl J Med*, 358: 197.

66. ENCODE Project Consortium, Birney, E., Stamatoyannopoulos, J. A., et al. (2007), 'Identification and analysis of functional elements in 1% of the human genome by the ENCODE pilot project', *Nature*, 447 (7146): 799–816.

67. Kaiser, J. (2007), 'Breakthrough of the year. It's all about me', *Science*, 318 (5858): 1843.

68. Hunter, D. J., Khoury, M. J. and Drazen, J. M. (2008), 'Letting the genome out of the bottle – Will we get our wish?', *N Engl J Med*, 358 (2): 105–7.
69. Lakhani, S. R., Van De Vijver, M. J., Jacquemier, J., et al. (2002), 'The pathology of familial breast cancer: Predictive value of immunohistochemical markers estrogen receptor, progesterone receptor, HER–2, 59, 60 and p53 in patients with mutations in BRCA1 and BRCA2', *J Clin Oncol*, 20: 2310–18.
70. Foulkes, W. D., Kelly Metcalfe, K., Sun, P., et al. (2004), 'Estrogen receptor status in BRCA1- and BRCA2-related breast cancer: The influence of age, grade, and histological type', *Clin Cancer Res*, 10: 2029–34.
71. Kauff, N. D., Domchek, S. M., Friebel, T. M., et al. (2008), 'Risk-reducing salpingo-oophorectomy for the prevention of BRCA1- and BRCA2-associated breast and gynecologic cancer: A multicenter, prospective study', *J Clin Oncol*, 26 (8), 1331–7.
72. Manolio, T. A., Brooks, L. D. and Collins, F. S. (2008), 'A HapMap harvest of insights into the genetics of common disease', *J Clin Invest*, 18: 1590–605.
73. Esteller, M. (2008), 'Epigenetics in Cancer', *N Engl J Med*, 358: 1148–59.
74. Herman, J. G. and Baylin, S. B. (2003), 'Gene silencing in cancer in association with promoter hypermethylation', *N Engl J Med*, 349: 2042–54.
75. Esteller, M., Silva, J. M., Dominguez, G., et al. (2000), 'Promoter hypermethylation and BRCA1 inactivation in sporadic breast and ovarian tumors', *J Natl Cancer Inst*, 92: 564–9.
76. Saito, Y., Liang, G., Egger, G., et al. (2006), 'Specific activation of microRNA–127 with downregulation of the proto-oncogene BCL6 by chromatin-modifying drugs in human cancer cells', *Cancer Cell*, 9: 435–43.
77. Lujambio, A., Ropero, S., Ballestar, E., et al. (2007), 'Genetic unmasking of an epigenetically silenced microRNA in human cancer cells', *Cancer Res*, 67: 1424–9 (Erratum: Cancer Res, 67: 3492).
78. Roukos, D. H. (2008), 'Innovative genomic-based model for personalized treatment of gastric cancer: integrating current standards and new technologies', *Expert Rev Mol Diagn*, 8 (1): 29–39.

Chapter 6

Section A

1. Early Breast Cancer Trialists' Collaborative Group (2000), 'Favourable and

unfavourable effects on long-term survival of radiotherapy for early breast cancer: An overview of the randomised trials', *Lancet*, 355: 1757–70.

2. Early Breast Cancer Trialists' Collaborative Group (2005), 'Effects of chemotherapy and hormonal therapy for early breast cancer on recurrence and 15-year survival: An overview of the randomized trials', *Lancet*, 365: 1687–717.

3. Arriagada, R., Rutqvist, L. E., Mattsson, A., et al. (1995), 'Adequate locoregional treatment for early breast cancer may prevent secondary dissemination', *J Clin Oncol*, 13: 2869–78.

4. Arriagada, R., Mouriesse, H., Sarrazin, D., et al. (1985), 'Radiotherapy alone in breast cancer. I. Analysis of tumor parameters, tumor dose and local control: The experience of the Gustave-Roussy Institute and The Princess Margaret Hospital', *Int J Radiat Oncol Biol Phys*, 11: 1751–7.

5. Dutreix, J., Tubiana, M. and Dutreix, A. (1988), 'An approach to the interpretation of clinical data on the tumour control probability dose relationship', *Radiother Oncol*, 11: 239–48.

6. Romestaing, P., Lehingue, Y., Carrie, C., et al. (1997), 'Role of a 10-Gy boost in the conservative treatment of early breast cancer: Results of a randomized clinical trial in Lyon, France', *J Clin Oncol*, 15: 963–8.

7. Bartelink, H., Horiot, J. C., Poortmans, P., et al. for the EORTC radiotherapy and breast Cancer Groups (2001), 'Recurrence rates after treatment of breast cancer with standard radiotherapy or without additional radiation', *N Engl J Med*, 345: 1378–87.

8. Bartelink, H., Horiot, J. C., Poortmans, P. M., et al. (2007), 'Impact of a higher radiation dose on local control and survival in breast-conserving therapy of early breast cancer: 10-year results of the randomized boost versus no boost EORTC 22881–10882 trial', *J Clin Oncol*, 25: 3259–65.

9. Arriagada, R. and Bourgier, C. (2008), 'Effect of radiation dose on local control in breast cancer', *Radiother Oncol*, 86: 285–6.

10. Fisher, B. (1980), 'Laboratory and clinical research in breast cancer: A personal adventure. The David A. Karnovsky Memorial Lecture', *Cancer Res*, 40: 3863–74.

11. Dewar, J. A., Sarrazin, D., Benhamou, S., et al. (1987), 'Management of the axilla in conservatively-treated breast cancer: 592 patients treated at the Institut Gustave-Roussy', *Int J Radiat Oncol Biol Phys*, 13: 475–781.

12. Lacour, J., Lê, M. G., Caceres, E., et al. (1983), 'Radical mastectomy versus radical mastectomy plus internal mammary dissection. Ten-year results of an international cooperative trial in breast cancer', *Cancer*, 51: 1941–3.

13. Lacour, J., Lê, M. G., Hill, C., et al. (1987), 'Is it useful to remove internal

mammary nodes in operable breast cancer?', *Eur J Surg Oncol*, 13: 309–14.

14. Arriagada, R., Lê, M. G., Mouriesse, H., et al. (1988), 'Long-term effect of internal mammary chain treatment. Results of a multivariate analysis of 1195 patients with operable breast cancer and positive nodes', *Radiother Oncol*, 11: 213–22.

15. Veronesi, U., Arnone, P., Veronesi, P., et al. (2008), 'The value of radiotherapy on metastatic internal mammary nodes in breast cancer. Results on a large series', *Ann Oncol*, 19: 1553–60.

16. Romestaing, P., Belot, A., Hennequin, C. et al., 'Ten year results of a randomized trial of internal mammary chain irradiation (IMC-RT) after mastectomy', ASTRO plenary session 2009, *Int J Radiat Oncol Biol Phys* (abstract in press)

17. Musat, E., Poortmans, P., Van den Bogaert, W., et al. (2007), 'Quality assurance in breast cancer: EORTC experience in the phase III trial on irradiation of the internal mammary nodes', *Eur J Cancer*, 43: 718–24.

18. Holmes, D. R., Baum, M., Joseph, D., et al. (2007), 'The TARGIT trial: Targeted intraoperative radiation therapy versus conventional postoperative whole-breast radiotherapy after breast-conserving surgery for the management of early-stage invasive breast cancer (a trial update)', *Am J Surg*, 194: 507–10.

19. Veronesi, U., Orecchia, R., Luini, A., et al. (2005), 'Full-dose intraoperative radiotherapy with electrons during breast-conserving surgery: Experience with 590 cases', *Ann Surg*, 242: 101–6.

20. Niehoff, P., Polgar, C., Ostertag, H., et al. (2006), 'Clinical experience with the MammoSite radiation therapy system for brachytherapy of breast cancer: Results from an international phase II trial', *Radiother Oncol*, 79: 316–20.

21. Vicini, F. A., Chen, P., Wallace, M., et al. (2007), 'Interim cosmetic results and toxicity using 3D conformal external beam radiotherapy to deliver accelerated partial breast irradiation in patients with early-stage breast cancer treated with breast-conserving therapy', *Int J Radiat Oncol Biol Phys*, 69: 1124–30.

22. Formenti, S. C., Truong, M. T., Goldberg, J. D., et al. (2004), 'Prone accelerated partial breast irradiation after breast-conserving surgery: Preliminary results and dose-volume histogram analysis', *Int J Radiat Oncol Biol Phys*, 60: 493–504.

23. Taghian, A., Kozak, K. R., Doppke, K. P., et al. (2006), 'Initial dosimetric experience using simple three-dimensional conformal external-beam accelerated partial-breast irradiation', *Int J Radiat Oncol Biol Phys*, 64:

1092–9.

24. Ribeiro, G. G., Magee, B., Swindell, R., et al. (1993), 'The Christie Hospital breast conservation trial: An update at 8 years from inception', *Clin Oncol (R Coll Radiol)*, 5: 278–83.

25. Dodwell, D. J., Dyker, K., Brown, J., et al. (2005), 'A randomised study of whole-breast vs tumour-bed irradiation after local excision and axillary dissection for early breast cancer', *Clin Oncol (R Coll Radiol)*, 17: 618–22.

26. McCormick, B. (2005), 'Partial-breast radiation for early staged breast cancers: hypothesis, existing data, and a planned phase III trial', *JNCCN*, 3: 301–7.

27. Polgar, C., Strnad, V. and Major, T. (2005), 'Brachytherapy for partial breast irradiation: The European experience', *Semin Radiat Oncol*, 15: 116–22.

28. Orecchia, R., Ciocca, M., Tossi, G., et al. (2005), 'Intraoperative electron beam radiotherapy (ELIOT) to the breast: A need for a quality assurance programme', *Breast*, 14: 541–6.

29. Vaidyia, J. S. (2007), 'Partial breast irradiation using targeted intraoperative radiotherapy (Targit)', *Nat Clin Pract Oncol*, 4: 384–5.

30. Smith, B. D., Arthur, D. W., Buchholz, T., et al. (2009), 'Accelerated partial breast irradiation consensus statement from the American Society for Radiation Oncology (ASTRO)', *Int J Radiat Oncol Biol Phys*, 74: 987–1001.

31. Offersen, B. V., Overgaard, M., Kroman, N., et al. (2009), 'Accelerated partial breast irradiation as part of breast conserving therapy of early breast carcinoma: A systematic review', *Radiother Oncol*, 90: 1–13.

32. Goldhirsch, A., Ingle, J. N., Gelber, R. D., et al. (2009), 'Thresholds for therapies: Highlights of the St Gallen International Expert Consensus on the primary therapy of early breast cancer 2009', *Ann Oncol*, 20: 1319–29.

33. Arriagada, R., Lê, M. G., Guinebretière, J. M., et al. (2003), 'Late local recurrences in a randomised trial comparing conservative treatment with total mastectomy in early breast cancer', *Ann Oncol*, 14: 1617–22.

34. Bourhis, J., Overgaard, J., Audry, H., et al. (2006), 'Hyperfractionated or accelerated radiotherapy in head and neck cancer: A meta-analysis', *Lancet*, 368: 843–54.

35. Turrisi, A., Kim, K., Blum, R. et al. (1999), 'Twice-daily compared with once-daily thoracic radiotherapy in limited small cell lung cancer treated concurrently with cisplatin and etoposide', *N Engl J Med*, 340: 265–71.

36. Fowler, J. F. (1989), 'The linear-quadratic formula and progress in fractionated radiotherapy', *Br J Radiol*, 62: 679–94.

37. Whelan, T., MacKenzie, R., Julian, J., et al. (2002), 'Randomized trial of

breast irradiation schedules after lumpectomy for women with lymph node-negative breast cancer', *J Natl Cancer Inst*, 94: 1143–50.

38. Whelan, T., Pignol, J. P., Julian, J., et al. (2008), 'Long-term results of a randomized trial of accelerated hypofractionated whole breast irradiation following breast conserving surgery (ASTRO Plenary)', *Int J Radiat Oncol Biol Phys*, 72: Suppl. S28, abstr. 60.

39. Owen, J. R., Ashton, A., Bliss, J. M., et al. (2006), 'Effect of radiotherapy fraction size on tumour control in patients with early-stage breast cancer after local tumour excision: Long-term results of a randomised trial', *Lancet Oncol*, 7: 467–71.

40. The START Trialists' Group (2008), 'The UK Standardisation of Breast Radiotherapy (START) Trial A of radiotherapy hypofractionation for treatment of early breast cancer: A randomised trial', *Lancet Oncol*, 9: 331–41.

41. The START Trialists' Group (2008), 'The UK Standardisation of Breast Radiotherapy (START) Trial B of radiotherapy hypofractionation for treatment of early breast cancer: A randomised trial', *Lancet*, 371: 1098–107.

42. Brunt, A. M., Sydenham, M., Bliss, J., et al. (2009), 'A 5-fraction regimen on adjuvant radiotherapy for women with early breast cancer: First analysis of the randomised UK FAST trial', *Eur J Cancer*, 7: Suppl. Presidential Sessions, abstr. 7LBA.

43. Bartelink, H. and Arriagada, R. (2008), 'Hypofractionation in radiotherapy for breast cancer', *Lancet*, 371: 1050–2.

44. Arriagada, R., Averbeck, D., Dahl, A. A., et al. (2009), 'OECI Workshop on late side-effects of cancer treatments', *Eur J Cancer*, 45: 354–9.

Section B

1. Recht, A., Gray, R., Davidson, N. E., et al. (1999), 'Loco-regional failure ten years after mastectomy and adjuvant chemotherapy with or without tamoxifen without irradiation. Experience of the Eastern Cooperative Oncology Group', *J Clin Oncol*, 17: 1689–700.

2. Overgaard, M., Hansen, P. S., Overgaard, J., et al. (1997), 'Postoperative radiotherapy in high-risk premenopausal women with breast cancer who receive adjuvant chemotherapy. Danish Breast Cancer Cooperative Group 82b Trial', *N Engl J Med*, 337: 949–55.

3. Ragaz, J., Jackson, S. M., Le, N., et al. (1997), 'Adjuvant radiotherapy and chemotherapy in node-positive premenopausal women with breast cancer', *N Engl J Med*, 337: 956–62.

4. Overgaard, M., Jensen, M. B., Overgaard, J., et al. (1999), 'Randomised

trial evaluating postoperative radiotherapy in high risk postmenopausal breast cancer patients given adjuvant tamoxifen. Results of the DBCG 82c trial', *Lancet*, 353: 1043–8.

5. Van der Steene, J., Soete, G. and Storme, G. (2000), 'Adjuvant radiotherapy for breast cancer significantly improves overall survival: The missing link', *Radiother Oncol*, 55: 263–72.

6. Early Breast Cancer Trialists' Collaborative Group (1995), 'Effects of radiotherapy and surgery in early breast cancer: An overview of the randomized trials', *N Engl J Med*, 333: 1444–55.

7. Early Breast Cancer Trialists' Collaborative Group (2000), 'Favourable and unfavourable effects on long-term survival of radiotherapy for early breast cancer: An overview of the randomised trials', *Lancet*, 355: 1757–70.

8. Early Breast Cancer Trialists' Collaborative Group (2005), 'Effects of radiotherapy and of differences in the extent of surgery for early breast cancer on local recurrence and 15-year survival: An overview of the randomised trials', *Lancet*, 366: 2087–106.

9. Strom, E. A., Woodward, W. A., Katz, A., et al. (2005), 'Clinical investigation: Regional nodal failure patterns in breast cancer patients treated with mastectomy without radiotherapy', *Int J Rad Oncol Biol Phys*, 63: 1508–13.

10. Fu, K. K. (1985), 'Biological basis for interaction of chemotherapeutic agents and radiation therapy', *Cancer*, 55: Suppl. 2123–30.

11. Arriagada, R., Rutqvist, L. E., Mattson, A., et al. (1995), 'Adequate loco-regional treatment for early breast cancer may prevent secondary dissemination', *J Clin Oncol*, 14: 2869–78.

12. Cuzick, J., Stewart, H. J., Peto, R., et al. (1987), 'Overview of randomised trials of postoperative radiotherapy in breast cancer', *Canc Treat Rep*, 71: 15–29.

13. Kuske, R. R. (1999), 'The role of postmastectomy radiation in the treatment of early-stage breast cancer: Taps or a call to arms?', *J Clin Oncol Educational Handbook*, American Society of Clinical Oncology (ASCO): 629–34.

14. Levitt, S. H. and Fletcher, G. H. (1991), 'Trials and tribulations: Do clinical trials prove that irradiation increases cardiac and secondary cancer mortality in the breast cancer patient?', *Int J Rad Oncol Biol Phys*, 20: 523–527.

15. Fowble, B. (1997), 'Postmastectomy radiation. Then and now', *Oncology*, 11: 213–39.

16. Cuzick, J., Stewart, H. J., Rutqvist, I., et al. (1994), 'Cause-specific mortality in long-term survivors of breast cancer who participated in trials

of radiotherapy', *J Clin Oncol*, 12: 1444–55.

17. Goldhirsch, A., Glick, J. H., Gelber, R., et al. (1998), 'Meeting highlights: International Consensus Panel on the Treatment of Primary Breast Cancer', *J Nat Cancer Inst*, 90: 1601–8.

18. Recht, A., Bartelink, H., Fourquet, A., et al. (1998), 'Postmastectomy radiotherapy: Questions for the twenty-first century', *J Clin Oncol*, 16: 2886–9.

19. Harris, J. R., Halpin-Murphy, P., McNeese, M., et al. (1999), 'Consensus statement on postmastectomy radiation therapy', *Int J Rad Oncol Biol Phys*, 44: 989–90.

20. Whelan, T. J., Julian, J., Wright, J., et al. (2000), 'Does loco-regional radiation therapy improve survival in breast cancer? A meta-analysis', *J Clin Oncol*, 18: 1220–9.

21. National Collaborating Centre for Cancer (CGSO) (2009), *Early and locally advanced breast cancer: Diagnosis and treatment*, National Institute for Health and Clinical Excellence (NICE), May, London, UK: 75.

22. Goldhirsch, A., Wood, W. C., Gelver, R. D., et al. (2007), '10th St Gallen Conference. Progress and promise: Highlights of the international expert consensus on the primary therapy of early breast cancer', *Ann Oncol*, 18: 1133–44.

23. Goldhirsch, A., Ingle, J. M., Gelber, R. D., et al. (2009), 'Thresholds for therapies: Highlights of the St Gallen international expert consensus on the primary therapy of early breast cancer', *Ann Oncol*, 20: 1319–29.

24. Ceilley, E., Jagsi, R., Goldberg, S., et al. (2005), 'Radiotherapy for invasive breast cancer in North America and Europe: Results of a survey', *Int J Rad Oncol Biol Phys*, 61: 365–73.

25. Russell, N. S., Kunkler, I. H. and Van Tienhoven, G. (2009), 'Postmastectomy radiotherapy: Will the selective use of postmastectomy radiotherapy study end the debate?', *J Clin Oncol*, 6: 996–997.

26. Overgaard, M., Nielsen, H. M. and Overgaard, J. (2007), 'Is the benefit of postmastectomy irradiation limited to patients with four or more positive nodes, as recommended in international consensus reports? A subgroup analysis of the DBCG 82 b&c randomized trials', *Radiother Oncol*, 84: 102–3.

27. Poortmans, P. (2007), 'Evidence based radiation oncology: Breast cancer', *Radiother Oncol*, 84: 84–101.

28. Kunkler, I. H., Canney, P., van Tienhoven, G., Russell, N. S. on behalf of the MRC/EORTC (BIG 2–04) SUPREMO Trial Management Group 2007 (2008), 'Elucidating the Role of Chest Wall Irradiation in "Intermediate-risk" Breast Cancer: The MRC/EORTC SUPREMO Trial', *Clin Oncol*, 20:

31–34.
29. Kyndi, M., Overgaard, M., Nielsen, H. M., et al. (2009), 'High local recurrence risk is not associated with large survival reduction after postmastectomy radiotherapy in high-risk breast cancer. A subgroup analysis of DBCG 82 b&c', *Radiother Oncol*, 90: 74–79.
30. Van der Hage, J. A., Putter, H., Bonnema, H., et al. (2003), 'Impact of locoregional treatment on early-stage breast cancer patients: A retrospective analysis', *Eur J Cancer*, 39: 2192–99.
31. Ragaz, J., Olivotto, I. A., Spinelli, J., et al. (2005), 'Locoregional radiation therapy in patients with high-risk breast cancer receiving adjuvant chemotherapy: 20-year results of the British Columbia randomized trial', *J. Natl Cancer Inst*, 97: 116–26.
32. Fourquet, A., Cutuli, B., Luporsi, E., et al. (2002), '"Standards, Options and Recommendations 2001" for radiotherapy in patients with non-metastastic infiltrating breast cancer. Update. National Federation of Cancer Campaign Centers (FNCLCC)', *Cancer Radiother*, 4: 238–58.
33. Kyndi, M., Sorensen, F. B., Knudsen, H., et al. (2008), 'Estrogen receptor, progesterone receptor, HER–2 and response to postmastectomy radiotherapy in high-risk breast cancer: The Danish Breast Cancer Cooperative Group', *J Clin Oncol*, 26: 1419–1426.
34. Marks, L. B., Zeng, J. and Prosnitz, L. R. (2008), 'One to three versus four or more positive nodes and postmastectomy radiotherapy: Time to end the debate', *J Clin Oncol*, 26: 2075–77.
35. Gebski, V., Lagleva, M., Keach, A., et al. (2006) 'Survival effects of postmastectomy adjuvant radiation therapy using biologically equivalent doses: A clinical perspective', *J. Natl Cancer Inst*, 98: 26–38.
36. National Institutes for Health (NIH) (2000), 'NIH consensus statement: Adjuvant therapy for breast cancer', Nov. 1–3, 17: 1–35.
37. Poole, C. J., Earl, H. M., Hiller, L., et al. (2006), 'NEAT [National Epirubicin Adjuvant Trial] Investigators and the SCTBG [Scottish Cancer Trials Breast Group]. Epirubicin and cyclophosphamide, methotrexate, and fluorouracil as adjuvant therapy for early breast cancer', *N Engl J Med*, 355: 1851–62.
38. Recht, A., Edge, S. B., Solin, L. J., et al. (2001), 'Postmastectomy radiotherapy: Guidelines of the American Society of Clinical Oncology', *J Clin Oncol*, 19: 1539–69.
39. Harris, J. R. and Morrow, M. (1996), 'Local management of invasive breast cancer', in J. R. Harris, M. E. Lippmann, M. Morrow and S. Hellman (eds), *Diseases of the breast*, Lippincott-Raven, Philadelphia, New York: 487–547.

40. Mansel, R. E. and Goyal, A. (2004), 'European studies on breast lymphatic mapping', *Sem Oncol*, 31: 304–10.
41. Chetty, U., Jack, W., Prescott, R. J., et al. (2000), 'Management of the axilla in operable breast cancer treated by breast conservation: A randomized clinical trial', *Br J Surg*, 87: 163–9.
42. MacDonald, S. M., Ahi-Raad, R. F., Alm, El-Din, et al. (2009), 'Chest wall radiotherapy: Middle ground for treatment of patients with one to three positive lymph nodes after mastectomy', *Int J Rad Oncol Biol Phys* (E-pub ahead of print).
43. Kurtz, J. (2002), 'The curative role of radiotherapy in the treatment of operable breast cancer', *Eur J Cancer*, 36: 1961–74.
44. Freedman, G. M., Fowble, B., Hoffman, J., et al. (2000), 'Should internal mammary lymph nodes in breast cancer be a target for the radiation oncologist?', *Int J Rad Oncol Biol Phys*, 48: 805–14.
45. Chen, R. C., Lin, N. U., Golshan, M., et al. (2008), 'Internal mammary nodes in breast cancer: Diagnosis and implications for patient management – A systematic review', *J Clin Oncol*, 26: 4981–9.
46. Poortmans, P., Kouloudias, V., Venselaar, J. L., et al. (2003), 'Quality assurance in the EORTC randomized trial 22922/10925 investigating the role of irradiation of the internal mammary – Medial supraclavicular irradiation in stage I–III breast cancer: The individual case review', *Eur J Cancer*, 39: 2035–42.
47. Paszat, L. F., Vallis, K. A., Benk, V. M. A., et al. (2007), 'A population-based case-cohort study of the risk of myocardial infarction following radiation therapy for breast cancer', *Radiother Oncol*, 82: 294–300.
48. Rutqvist, L. E., Lax, I., Fornander, T., et al. (1992), 'Cardiovascular mortality in a randomised trial of adjuvant radiation therapy versus surgery alone in primary breast cancer', *Int J Rad Oncol Biol Phys*, 22: 887–96.
49. Giordano, S. H., Kuo, Y. F., Freeman, J. L., Buchholz, T. A., et al. (2005), 'Risk of cardiac death after adjuvant radiotherapy for breast cancer', *J Natl Cancer Inst*, 97: 419–24.
50. Hojris, I., Overgaard, M., Christensen, J. J., et al. (1999), 'Morbidity and mortality of ischaemic heart disease in high-risk breast cancer patients after adjuvant postmastectomy systemic treatment with or without radiotherapy: Analysis of DBCG 82b and 82c randomised trials', *Lancet*, 354: 1425–1430.
51. Hanna, Y. M., Baglan, K. L., Stromberg, J. S., et al. (2002) 'Acute and subacute toxicity associated with concurrent adjuvant radiation therapy and paclitaxel in primary breast cancer therapy', *Breast J*, 8: 149–53.
52. Olsen, N. K., Pfeiffer, P., Johannsen, L., et al. (1993), 'Radiation-induced

brachial plexopathy. Neurological follow-up in 161 recurrence-free breast cancer patients', *Int J Rad Oncol Biol Phys*, 26: 43–9.

Section C

1. The Korean Breast Cancer Society (2006), 'Nationwide Korean Breast Cancer Data of 2004 Using Breast Cancer Registration Program', *J Breast Cancer*, 9 (2): 151–61.
2. The Korean Breast Cancer Society (2008), *Breast Cancer Facts & Figures*, Korean Breast Cancer Society, Seoul, Korea: 4–7.
3. Ji, Y. H., Kim, M. S., Yoo, S. Y., et al. (2007), 'National Statistics of Radiation Oncology in Korea', *J Korean Soc Ther Radiol Oncol*, 26 (2): 131–3.
4. Shanghai Municipal Center for Disease Control and Prevention (2008), *Shanghai Cancer Report*, Shanghai Municipal Center for Disease Control and Prevention, Shanghai.
5. Fan, L., Zheng, Y., Yu, K. D. et al. (2009), 'Breast cancer in a transitional society over 18 years: Trends and present status in Shanghai, China', *Breast Cancer Res Treat*, January 2009 (E-pub ahead of print).
6. Yu, K. D., Di, G. H., Wu, J., et al. (2007), 'Development and trends of surgical modalities for breast cancer in China: A review of 16 year data', *Ann Surg Oncol*, 14: 2502–9.
7. Kato, H., Sobue, T., Katanoda, K., et al. (2008), *Cancer Statistics in Japan*, in: <http://ganjoho.ncc.go.jp/public/index.html>.
8. Japan Ministry of Health, Labour and Welfare (undated?), *Vital statistics of Japan*.
9. Sonoo, H. and Noguchi, S. on behalf of the Academic Committee of the Japanese Breast Cancer Society (2008), 'Results of questionnaire survey on breast cancer surgery in Japan 2004–2006', *Breast Cancer*, 15: 3–4.
10. Japanese Breast Cancer Society (2006?): <http://www.jbcs.gr.jp/member_o/member/2006kakutei.pdf>.
11. Gebski, V., Lagleva, M., Keech, A., et al. (2006), 'Survival effects of postmastectomy adjuvant radiation therapy using biologically equivalent doses: A clinical perspective', *J Natl Cancer Inst*, 98 (1): 26–38.
12. Hui, Z. G., Li, Y. X., Yu, Z. H., et al. (2006), 'Survey on use of postmastectomy radiotherapy for breast cancer in China', *Int. J. Radiat Oncol Biol. Phys*, 66: 1135–42.
13. National Comprehensive Cancer Network (NCCN) (2009), *Clinical Practice Guidelines in Oncology*, NCCN, Chinese version (see: NCCN-CHINA. ORG).
14. Shikama, N., Mitsumori, M., Yamauchi, C., et al. (2006), 'Patterns of care

study for postmastectomy radiotherapy in Japan: Its role in monitoring the patterns of changes in practice', *Jpn J Clin Oncol*, 36 (8): 499–503.

15. National Institutes of Health Consensus Development Panel (2001), 'Development conference statement: Adjuvant therapy for breast cancer', *J Natl Cancer Inst*, 93 (13): 979–89.

16. Simonsen, L., Viboud, C. and Taylor, R. (2005), 'Effects of radiotherapy and of differences in the extent of surgery for early breast cancer on local recurrence and 15-year survival: An overview of the randomised trials', *Lancet*, 366 (9503): 2087–106.

17. Chen, J. Y., Jiang, G. L., Yu, X. L., et al. (2008), 'Outcomes of patients with early stage breast cancer treated with breast conservative surgery and whole breast irradiation', *Chinese Journal of Radiation Oncology*, 17: 444–9.

18. Chen, J. Y., Yu, X. L., Guo, X. M., et al. (2008), 'Does the surgery-radiation interval have an impact on treatment outcomes in pre-menopausal breast cancer patients treated with breast conservative surgery and adjuvant chemotherapy?: The Shanghai experience', *Int J Radiat Oncol Biol Phys*, 72 (1): Suppl. PS 194, abstract 2058.

19. Huang, X. B., Chen, J. Y., Jiang, G. L., et al. (2006), 'Factors influence the clinical volume delineation of intact breast in intensity-modulated radiotherapy of breast cancer', *Ai Zheng*, 25: 62–5.

20. Jin, Y. N., Wang, Y. J., Zhang, X. Q., et al. (2005), 'Clinical outcome and cosmetic results of conservative surgery plus radiation therapy in early stage breast cancer patients', *Chinese Journal of Radiation Oncology*, 14: 177–80.

21. Yamauchi, C., Mitsumori, M., Sai, H., et al. (2007), 'Patterns of care study of breast-conserving therapy in Japan: Comparison of the treatment process between 1995–1997 and 1999–2001 surveys', *Jpn J Clin Oncol*, 37 (10): 737–43.

22. Wendy, S., Michael, B., Charles, H., et al. (2000), 'A shorter fractionation schedule for postlumpectomy breast cancer patients', *Int J Radiat Oncol Biol Phys*, 47 (5): 1219–28

23. Whelan, T., MacKenzie, R., Julian, J., et al. (2002), 'Randomized trial of breast irradiation schedules after lumpectomy for women with lymph node-negative breast cancer', *J Natl Cancer Inst*, 94 (15): 1143–50.

24. Yarnold, J., Ashton, A., Bliss, J., et al. (2005), 'Fractionation sensitivity and dose response of late adverse effects in the breast after radiotherapy for early breast cancer: Long-term results of a randomised trial', *Radiother Oncol*, 75 (1): 9–17.

25. Owen, R., Ashton, A., Bliss, J. M, et al. (2006), 'Effect of radiotherapy

fraction size on tumour control in patients with early-stage breast cancer after local tumour excision: Long-term results of a randomised trial', *Lancet Oncol*, 7 (6): 467–71.

26. The START Trialists' Group (2008), 'The UK Standardisation of Breast Radiotherapy (START) Trial A of radiotherapy hypofractionation for treatment of early breast cancer: A randomised trial', *Lancet Oncol*, 9 (4): 331–341

27. Agrawal, R. K., Aird, E. G. A., Barrett, J. M., et al. (2008), 'The UK Standardisation of Breast Radiotherapy (START) Trial B of radiotherapy hypofractionation for treatment of early breast cancer: A randomised trial', *Lancet*, 371 (9618): 1098–107.

28. Lu, B. (2004), 'Hypofractionation in postoperative radiotherapy of breast cancer', *Chinese Journal of Radiation Oncology*', 13: 93–5.

29. Wu, J. X, Hui, Z. G., Yu, Z. H., et al. (2003), 'Post-mastectomy radiotherapy with different fractionated dose schemes in early breast cancer', *Zhonghua Zhong Liu Za Zhi*, 25: 285–8.

30. Vaidya, J. S., Baum, M., Tobias, J. S., et al. (2001), 'Targeted intra-operative radiotherapy (Targit): An innovative method of treatment for early breast cancer', *Ann Oncol*, 12 (8): 1075–80.

31. Holmes, D. R., Baum, M. and Joseph, D. (2007), 'The TARGIT trial: Targeted intraoperative radiation therapy versus conventional postoperative whole-breast radiotherapy after breast-conserving surgery for the management of early-stage invasive breast cancer (a trial update)', *Am J Surg*, 194 (4): 507–10.

32. Vaidya, J. S., Baum, M., Tobias, J. S., et al. (2006), 'Targeted intraoperative radiotherapy (TARGIT) yields very low recurrence rates when given as a boost', *Int J Radiat Oncol Biol Phys*, 66 (5): 1335–8.

33. Veronesi, U., Orecchia, R., Luini, A., et al. (2005), 'Full-dose intraoperative radiotherapy with electrons during breast-conserving surgery: Experience with 590 cases', *Ann Surg*, 242: 101.

34. Mussari, S., Della Sala, W. S., Busana, L., et al. (2006),. 'Full-dose intraoperative radiotherapy with electrons in breast cancer', *Strahlenther Oncol*, 182 (10): 589–95.

35. Magee, B., Swindell, R., Harris, M. and Banerjee, S. S. (1996), 'Prognostic factors for breast recurrence after conservative breast surgery and radiotherapy: Results from a randomised trial', *Radiother Oncol*, 39 (3): 223–7.

36. Formenti, S. C., Truong, M. T., Goldberg, J. D., et al. (2004), 'Prone accelerated partial breast irradiation after breast-conserving surgery: Preliminary clinical results and dose-volume histogram analysis', *Int J*

Radiat Oncol Biol Phys, 60 (2): 493–504.

37. Vicini, F. A., Chen, P., Wallace, M., et al. (2007), 'Interim cosmetic results and toxicity using 3D conformal external beam radiotherapy to deliver accelerated partial breast irradiation in patients with early-stage breast cancer treated with breast-conserving therapy', *Int J Radiat Oncol Biol Phys*, 69 (4): 1124–30.

38. Morganti, A. G., Cilla, S., Valentini, V., et al. (2009), 'Phase I–II studies on accelerated IMRT in breast carcinoma: Technical comparison and acute toxicity in 332 patients', *Radiother Oncol*, 90 (1): 86–92.

39. Kozak, K. R., Smith, B. L., Adams, J., et al. (2006), 'Accelerated partial-breast irradiation using proton beams: Initial clinical experience', *Int J Radiat Oncol Biol Phys*, 66 (3): 691–8.

40. Krishnan, L.; Jewell, W. R., Tawfik, O. W. and Krishnan, E. C. (2001), 'Breast conservation therapy with tumor bed irradiation alone in a selected group of patients with stage I breast cancer', *Breast J*, 7 (2): 91–6.

41. Lawenda, B. D, Taghian, A. G., Kachnic, L. A., et al. (2003), 'Dose–volume analysis of radiotherapy for T1N0 invasive breast cancer treated by local excision and partial breast irradiation by low-dose-rate interstitial implant', *Int J Radiat Oncol Biol Phys*, 56 (3): 671–80.

42. Vicini, F. A., Kestin, L., Chen, P., et al. (2003), 'Limited-field radiation therapy in the management of early-stage breast cancer', *J. Natl. Cancer Inst*, 95 (16): 1205–10.

43. Benitez, P. R., Chen, P. Y., Vicini, F. A., et al. (2004), 'Surgical considerations in the treatment of early stage breast cancer with accelerated partial breast irradiation (APBI) in breast conserving therapy via intersitial brachytherapy', *Am J Surg*, 188 (4): 355–64.

44. Fentiman, A. S., Poole, C., Tong, D., et al. (1996), 'Inadequacy of Iridium implant as sole radiation treatment operable breast cancer', *Eur J Cancer*, 32 (4): 608–11.

45. Fentiman, I. S., Deshmane, V., Tong, D., et al. (2004), 'Caesium 137 implant as sole radiation therapy for operable breast cancer: A phase II trial', *Radiother Oncol*, 71 (3): 281–285.

46. Kuske, R. R., Winter, K., Arthur, D. W., et al. (2006), 'Phase II trial of brachytherapy alone after lumpectomy for select breast cancer: Toxicity analysis of RTOG 95–17', *Int J Radiat Oncol Biol Phys*, 65 (1): 45–51.

47. Arthur, D. W., Winter, K., Kuske, R. R., et al. (2008), 'A phase II trial of brachytherapy alone after lumpectomy for select breast cancer: Tumor control and survival outcomes of RTOG 95–17, *Int J Radiat Oncol Biol Phys*, 72 (2): 467–73.

48. Perera, F., Yu, E., Engel, J., et al. (2003), 'Patterns of breast recurrence in

a pilot study of brachytherapy confined to the lumpectomy site for early breast cancer with six years' minimum follow-up', *Int J Radiat Oncol Biol Phys*, 57 (5): 1239–46.

49. Polgár, C., Major, T., Fodor, J., et al. (2004), 'High-dose-rate brachytherapy alone versus whole breast radiotherapy with or without tumor bed boost after breast-conserving surgery: Seven-year results of a comparative study', *Int J Radiat Oncol Biol Phys*, 60 (4): 1173–81.

50. Wazer, D. E., Berle, L., Graham, R., et al. (2002), 'Preliminary results of a phase I/II study of HDR brachytherapy alone for T1/T2 breast cancer', *Int J Radiat Oncol Biol Phys*, 53 (4): 889–97.

51. Wazer, D. E., Kaufman, S., Cuttino, L., et al. (2006), 'Accelerated partial breast irradiation: An analysis of variables associated with late toxicity and long-term cosmetic outcome after high-dose-rate interstitial brachytherapy', *Int J Radiat Oncol Biol Phys*, 64 (2): 489–95.

52. Kaufman, S. A., DiPetrillo, T. A., Price, L. L., et al. (2007), 'Long-term outcome and toxicity in a Phase I/II trial using high-dose-rate multicatheter interstitial brachytherapy for T1/T2 breast cancer', *Brachytherapy*, 6 (4): 286–92.

53. Polgár, C., Fodor, J., Major, T., et al. (2007), 'Breast-conserving treatment with partial or whole breast irradiation for low-risk invasive breast carcinoma – 5-year results of a randomized trial', *Int J Radiat Oncol Biol Phys*, 69 (3): 694–702.

54. Ott, O. J., Hildebrandt, G., Pötter, R., et al. (2007), 'Accelerated partial breast irradiation with multi-catheter brachytherapy: Local control, side effects and cosmetic outcome for 274 patients. Results of the German–Austrian multi-centre trial', *Radiother Oncol*, 82 (3): 281–6.

55. Kuske, R. R., Winter, K., Arthur, D. W., et al. (2006), 'Phase II trial of brachytherapy alone after lumpectomy for select breast cancer: Toxicity analysis of RTOG 95–17', *Int J Radiat Oncol Biol Phys*, 65 (1): 45–51.

46. Póti, Z., Nemeskéri, C., Fekésházy, A., et al. (2004), 'Partial breast irradiation with interstitial Co–60 brachytherapy results in frequent grade 3 or 4 toxicity. Evidence based on a 12-year follow-up of 70 patients', *Int J Radiat Oncol Biol Phys*, 58 (4): 1022–33.

57. Polgár C. and Major T. (2009), 'Current status and perspectives of brachytherapy for breast cancer', *Int J Clin Oncol*, 14 (1): 7–24.

58. Johansson, B., Karlsson, L., Liljegren, G., et al. (2009), 'Pulsed dose rate brachytherapy as the sole adjuvant radiotherapy after breast-conserving surgery of T1–T2 breast cancer: First long time results from a clinical study', *Radiother Oncol*, 90 (1): 30–35.

59. King, T. A., Bolton, J. S., Kuske, R. R., et al. (2000), 'Long-term results

of wide-field brachytherapy as the sole method of radiation therapy after segmental mastectomy for Tis, 1, 2 breast cancer', *Am J Surg*, 180 (4): 299–304.

60. Vicini, F. A., Beitsch, P. D., Quiet, C. A., et al. (2005), 'First analysis of patient demographics, technical reproducibility, cosmesis, and early toxicity: Results of the American Society of Breast Surgeons MammoSite Breast Brachytherapy Registry Trial', *Cancer*, 104 (6): 1138–48.

61. Niehoff, P., Ballardini, B., Polgár, C., et al. (2006), 'Early European experience with the MammoSite radiation therapy system for partial breast brachytherapy following breast conservation operation in low-risk breast cancer', *Breast*, 15 (3): 319–25.

62. Chao, K. K., Vicini, F. A., Wallace, M., et al. (2007), 'Analysis of treatment efficacy, cosmesis, and toxicity using the MammoSite breast brachytherapy catheter to deliver accelerated partial-breast irradiation: The William Beaumont Hospital experience', *Int J Radiat Oncol Biol Phys*, 69 (1): 32–40.

63. Tsai, P. I., Ryan, M., Meek, K., et al. (2006), 'Accelerated partial breast irradiation using the MammoSite device: Early technical experience and short-term clinical follow-up', *Am Surg*, 72 (10): 929–34.

64. Cuttino, L. W., Keisch, M., Jenrette, J. M., et al. (2008), 'Multi-institutional experience using the MammoSite radiation therapy system in the treatment of early-stage breast cancer: 2-year results', *Int J Radiat Oncol Biol Phys*, 71 (1): 107–44.

65. Vicini, F., Beitsch, P. D., Quiet, C. A., et al. (2008), 'Three-year analysis of treatment efficacy, cosmesis, and toxicity by the American Society of Breast Surgeons MammoSite Breast Brachytherapy Registry Trial in patients treated with accelerated partial breast irradiation (APBI)', *Cancer*, 112 (4): 758–66.

66. Li, J. B., Zhang, L., Lu, J., et al. (2008), 'Study on the target movement in external-beam partial breast irradiation with active breathing control after breast-conserving surgery', *Zhonghua Zhong Liu Za Zhi*, 30: 207–210.

67. Kosaka, Y., Mitsumori, M., Yamauchi, C., et al. (2008), 'Feasibility of accelerated partial breast irradiation using three-dimensional conformal radiation therapy for Japanese women: A theoretical plan using six patients' CT data', *Breast Cancer*, (15) 1: 108–14.

68. Benitez, P. R., Streeter, O., Vicini, F., et al. (2006), 'Preliminary results and evaluation of MammoSite balloon brachytherapy for partial breast irradiation for pure ductal carcinoma in situ: A phase II clinical study', *Am J Surg*, 192 (4): 427–33.

Section D

1. Singletary, S. E., McNeese, M. D. and Hortobagyi, G. N. (1992), 'Feasibility of breast-conservation surgery after induction chemotherapy for locally advanced breast carcinoma', *Cancer*, 69 (11): 2849–52.
2. Kuerer, H. M., Newman, L. A., Smith, T. L., et al. (1999), 'Clinical course of breast cancer patients with complete pathologic primary tumor and axillary lymph node response to doxorubicin-based neoadjuvant chemotherapy', *J Clin Oncol*, 17 (2): 460–9.
3. Chen, A. M., Meric-Bernstam, F., Hunt, K. K., et al. (2005), 'Breast conservation after neoadjuvant chemotherapy', *Cancer*, 103 (4): 689–95.

Chapter 7

Section A

1. von Minckwitz, G., et al. (2008), 'Integrated meta-analysis on 6634 patients with early breast cancer receiving neoadjuvant anthracycline–taxane $+/-$ trastuzumab containing chemotherapy', Oral presentation, San Antonio.
2. von Minckwitz, G. and Blohmer, J. U. (2005), 'In vivo chemosensitivity-adapted preoperative chemotherapy in patients with early-stage breast cancer: The GEPARTRIO pilot study', *Ann Oncol*, 16 (1): 56–63.
3. von Minckwitz, G. and Kümmel, S. (2008), 'Intensified neoadjuvant chemotherapy in early-responding breast cancer: Phase III randomized GeparTrio study', *J Natl Cancer Inst*, 100 (8): 552–62.
4. von Minckwitz, G. (2007), 'Evaluating the efficacy of capecitabine given concomitantly or in sequence to epirubicin/cyclophosphamide docetaxel as neoadjuvant treatment for primary breast cancer. First efficacy analysis of the GBG/AGO intergroup-study GeparQuattro', Poster # 79, SABCS.
5. Untch, M. (2008), 'Neoadjuvant treatment of HER2 overexpressing primary breast cancer with trastuzumab given concomitantly to epirubicin/ cyclophosphamide docetaxel±capecitabine. First analysis of efficacy and safety of the GBG/AGO multicenter intergroup-study GeparQuattro', Abstract, EBCC.
6. Buzdar, A. U., Ibrahim, N. K., et al. (2005), 'Significantly higher pathologic complete remission rate after neoadjuvant therapy with trastuzumab, paclitaxel, and epirubicin chemotherapy: Results of a randomized trial in human epidermal growth factor receptor 2-positive operable breast cancer', *J Clin Oncol*, 23 (16): 3676–85.
7. Shan, K. and Lincoff, A. M. (1996), 'Anthracycline-induced cardiotoxicity',

Ann Intern Med, 125 (1): 47–58.

8. Martín, M. and Esteva, F. J. (2009), 'Minimizing cardiotoxicity while optimizing treatment efficacy with trastuzumab: Review and expert recommendations', *Oncologist*, 14 (1): 1–11.

9. Keefe, D. L. (2002), 'Trastuzumab-associated cardiotoxicity', *Cancer*, 95 (7): 1592–600.

10. Gianni, L. et al. (2008), 'Neoadjuvant trastuzumab in patients with HER2-positive locally advanced breast cancer: Primary efficacy analysis of the NOAH trial', SABCS, Abstract no. 31.

11. Untch, M., Eidtmann, H., duBois, A., et al. (2004), 'Cardiac safety of trastuzumab in combination with epirubicin and cyclophosphamide in women with metastatic breast cancer: Results of a phase I trial', *Eur J Cancer*, 40: 988–97.

12. Buchholz, T. A., Lehman, C. D., et al. (2008), 'Statement of the science concerning locoregional treatments after preoperative chemotherapy for breast cancer: A National Cancer Institute conference', *J Clin Oncol*, 26 (5): 791–7.

13. Kaufmann, M. and Hortobagyi, G. N. (2006), 'Recommendations from an international expert panel on the use of neoadjuvant (primary) systemic treatment of operable breast cancer: An update, *J Clin Oncol*, 24 (12): 1940–9.

14. AGO Guidelines: <http://www.ago-online.de>.

15. Fisher, B. and Bryant, J., et al. (1998), 'Effect of preoperative chemotherapy on the outcome of women with operable breast cancer,' *J Clin Oncol*, 16 (8): 2672–85.

16. Kuerer, H. M., Newman, L. A., et al. (1999), 'Clinical course of breast cancer patients with complete pathologic primary tumor and axillary lymph node response to doxorubicin-based neoadjuvant chemotherapy', *J Clin Oncol*, 17: 460–9.

17. Liedtke, C. and Mazouni, C. (2008), 'Response to neoadjuvant therapy and long-term survival in patients with triple-negative breast cancer', *J Clin Oncol*, 26 (8): 1275–81.

18. Knauer, M. and Haid, A. (2007), 'Does combination of neoadjuvant and adjuvant chemotherapy improve outcome in operable breast cancer patients?' Poster #5065, San Antonio.

19. Yoneda, T., Michigami, T., Yi, B., et al. (1999), 'Use of bisphosphonates for the treatment of bone metastasis in experimental animal models', *Cancer Treatment Reviews*, 25: 293–9.

20. Bundred, N. J. and Campbell, I. D. (2008), 'Effective inhibition of aromatase inhibitor-associated bone loss by zoledronic acid in

postmenopausal women with early breast cancer receiving adjuvant letrozole: ZO-FAST Study results', Cancer, 112 (5): 1001–10.

21. Gasparini, G., Toi, M., Gion, M., et al. (1997), 'Prognostic significance of vascular endothelial growth factor protein in node-negative breast carcinoma', *J Natl Cancer Inst*, 89: 139–47.

22. Linderholm, B., Tavelin, B., Grankvist, K., et al. (1998), 'Vascular endothelial growth factor is of high prognostic value in node-negative breast carcinoma', *J Clin Oncol*, 16: 3121–8.

23. Toi, M., Kondo, S., Suzuki, H., et al. (1996), 'Quantitative analysis of vascular endothelial growth factor in primary breast cancer', *Cancer*, 77: 1101–6.

24. Eppenberger, U., Kueng, W., Schlaeppi, J. M., et al. (1998), 'Markers of tumor angiogenesis and proteolysis independently define high- and low-risk subsets of node-negative breast cancer patients', *J Clin Oncol*, 16: 3129–36.

25. Ademuyiwa, F. O. and Miller, K. D. (2008), 'Incorporation of antiangiogenic therapies in the treatment of metastatic breast cancer', *Clin Breast Cancer*, 8 (suppl. 4): S151–6.

Section B

1. Loibl, S., von Minckwitz, G., Raab, G., et al. (2006), 'Surgical procedures after neoadjuvant chemotherapy in operable breast cancer: Results of the GEPARDUO trial', *Ann Surg Oncol*, 13: 1434–42.

2. Huang, E. H., Tucker, S. L., Strom, E. A., et al. (2004), 'Postmastectomy radiation improves local-regional control and survival for selected patients with locally advanced breast cancer treated with neoadjuvant chemotherapy and mastectomy', *J Clin Oncol*, 22: 4639–47.

3. Oh, J. L., Dryden, M. J., Woodward, W. A., et al. (2006), 'Locoregional control of clinically diagnosed multifocal or multicentric breast cancer after neoadjuvant chemotherapy and locoregional therapy', *J Clin Oncol*, 24: 4971–5.

4. Rouzier, R., Extra, J. M., Carton, M., et al. (2001), 'Primary chemotherapy for operable breast cancer: Incidence and prognostic significance of ipsilateral breast tumor recurrence after breast-conserving surgery', *J Clin Oncol*, 19 (18): 3828–35.

5. Jatoi, I. and Proschan, M. A. (2005), 'Randomized trials of breast-conserving therapy versus mastectomy for primary breast cancer: A pooled analysis of updated results', *Am J Clin Oncol*, 28: 289–94.

6. Senofsky, G. M., Gierson, E. D., Craig, P. H., et al. (1998), 'Local excision, lumpectomy, and quadrantectomy: Surgical considerations', in S. L. Spear

(ed), *Surgery of the Breast: Principle and Art*, Philadelphia, Lippincott-Raven: 129–35.

7. Kaufmann, M., von Minckwitz, G., Smith, R., et al. (2003), 'International expert panel on the use of primary (preoperative) systemic treatment of operable breast cancer: Review and recommendations', *J Clin Oncol*, 21: 2600–8.

8. Krämer, S., Kümmel, S., Camara, O., et al. (2007), 'Partial mastectomy reconstruction with local and distant tissue flaps', *Breast Care*, 2: 299–306.

9. Sadetzky, S., Oberman, B., Zipple, D., et al. (2005), 'Breast conservation after neoadjuvant chemotherapy', *Ann Surg Oncol*, 12: 1–8.

10. Chen, A. M., Meric-Bernstam, F., Hunt, K. K., et al. (2005), 'Breast conservation after neoadjuvant chemotherapy', *Cancer*, 103: 689–95.

11. Tafra, L., Lannin, D. R., Swanson, M. S., et al. (2001), 'Multicenter trial of sentinel node biopsy for breast cancer using both technetium sulfur colloid and isosulfan blue dye', *Ann Surg*, 233: 51–9.

12. Jones, J. L., Zabicki, K., Christian, R. L., et al. (2005), 'A comparison of sentinel node biopsy before and after neoadjuvant chemotherapy: Timing is important', *Am J Surg*, 190: 517–20.

13. Miller, A. R., Thomason, V. E., Yeh, I. T., et al. (2002), 'Analysis of sentinel lymph node mapping with immeditate pathologic review in patients receiving preoperative chemotherapy for breast carcinoma', *Ann Surg Oncol*, 9: 243–7.

14. Kim, T., Guiliano, A. E. and Lyman, G. H. (2006), 'Lymphatic mapping and sentinel lymph node biopsy in early-stage breast carcinoma: A metaanalysis', *Cancer*, 106: 4–16.

15. Haid, A., Tausch, C., Lang, A., et al. (2001), 'Is sentinel lymph node biopsy reliable and indicated after preoperative chemotherapy in patients with breast carcinoma?', *Cancer*, 92: 1080–4.

16. Mamounas, E. P. (2006), 'Neoadjuvant chemotherapy in operable breast cancer', *Breast Care*, 1: 348–51.

17. Rastogi, P., Anderson, S. J., Bear, H. D., et al. (2008), 'Preoperative chemotherapy: Updates of National Surgical Adjuvant Breast and Bowel Project Protocols B–18 and B–27', *J Clin Oncol*, 26: 778–85.

18. Kuerer, H. M. and Hunt, K. K. (2002), 'The rationale for integration of lymphatic mapping and sentinel node biopsy in the management of breast cancer patients receiving neoadjuvant chemotherapy', *Semin Breast Dis*, 5: 80–7.

19. Xing, Y., Foy, M., Cox, D. D., et al. (2006), 'Meta-analysis of sentinel lymph node biopsy after preoperative chemotherapy in patients with breast cancer', *Br J Surg*, 93: 539–46.

20. Purushotham, A. D., Upponi, S., Klevesath, M. D., et al. (2005), 'Morbidity after sentinel lymph-node biopsy in primary breast cancer: Results from a randomized controlled trial', *J Clin Oncol*, 23: 4312–21.

21. Kuehn, T., Bembenek, A., Decker T, et al. (2005), 'A concept for the clinical implementation of sentinel lymph node biopsy in patients with breast carcinoma with special regard to quality assurance: Consensus Committee of the German Society of Senology', *Cancer*, 103: 451–61.

22. Lyman, G. H., Giuliano, A. E., Somerfield, M. R., et al. (2005), 'American Society of Clinical Oncology guideline recommendations for sentinel lymph node biopsy in early-stage breast cancer', *J Clin Oncol*, 23: 7703–20.

23. Julian, T. B., Krag, D., Brown, A., et al. (2004), 'Preliminary technical results of NSABP B–32, a randomized phase III clinical trial to compare sentinel node resection to conventional axillary dissection in clinically node-negative breast cancer patients', *Breast Cancer Res Treat*, 88 (suppl. 1): S11.

24. Krag, D., Weaver, D., Ashikaga, T., et al. (1998), 'The sentinel node in breast cancer: A multicenter validation study', *N Engl J Med*, 339: 941–6.

25. McMasters, K. M., Tuttle, T. M., Carlson, D. J., et al. (2000), 'Sentinel lymph node biopsy for breast cancer: A suitable alternative to routine axillary dissection in multi-institutional practice when optimal technique is used', *J Clin Oncol*, 18: 2560–6.

26. Mamounas, E. P., Brown, A., Anderson, S., et al. (2005), 'Sentinel lymph node biopsy after neoadjuvant chemotherapy in breast cancer: Results from National Surgical Adjuvant Breast and Bowel Project Protocol B–27', *J Clin Oncol*, 23: 2694–702.

27. Tafra, L., Verbanac, K. M. and Lannin, D. R. (2001), 'Preoperative chemotherapy and sentinel lymphadenectomy for breast cancer', *Am J Surg*, 182: 312–15.

28. Veronesi, U., Paganelli, G., Viale, G., et al. (2003), 'A randomized comparison of sentinel-node biopsy with routine axillary dissection in breast cancer', *N Engl J Med*, 349: 546–53.

29. Reitsamer, R., Peintinger, F., Rettenbacher, L., et al. (2003), 'Sentinel lymph node biopsy in breast cancer patients after neoadjuvant chemotherapy', *J Surg Oncol*, 84: 63–7.

Section C

1. Dowsett, M. and Dunbier, A. K. (2008), 'Emerging biomarkers and new understanding of traditional markers in personalized therapy for breast cancer', *Clin Cancer Res*, 14 (24): 8019–26 (review).

2. Toi, M., Nakamura, S., Kuroi, K., et al. of the Japan Breast Cancer Research Group (JBCRG) (2008), 'Phase II study of preoperative sequential FEC and docetaxel predicts of pathological response and disease free survival', *Breast Cancer Res Treat*, 110 (3): 531−9 (E-pub: Sept. 19, 2007).

3. Rouzier, R., Perou, C. M., Symmans, W. F., et al. (2005), 'Breast cancer molecular subtypes respond differently to preoperative chemotherapy', *Clin Cancer Res*, 11 (16): 5678−85.

4. Bear, H. D., Anderson, S., Smith, R. E., et al. (2006), 'Sequential preoperative or postoperative docetaxel added to preoperative doxorubicin plus cyclophosphamide for operable breast cancer: National Surgical Adjuvant Breast and Bowel Project Protocol B−27', *J Clin Oncol*, 24 (13): 2019−27.

5. Smith, I. C., Heys, S. D., Hutcheon, A. W., et al. (2002), 'Neoadjuvant chemotherapy in breast cancer: Significantly enhanced response with docetaxel', *J Clin Oncol*, 20 (6): 1456−66.

6. Fiorentino, C., Berruti, A., Bottini, A., et al. (2001), 'Accuracy of mammography and echography versus clinical palpation in the assessment of response to primary chemotherapy in breast cancer patients with operable disease', *Breast Cancer Res Treat*, 69 (2): 143−51.

7. Hlawatsch, A., Teifke, A., Schmidt, M., et. al. (2002), 'Preoperative assessment of breast cancer: Sonography versus MR imaging', *AJR Am J Roentgenol*, 179 (6): 1493−501.

8. Loo, C. E., Teertstra, H. J., Rodenhuis, S., et al. (2008), 'Dynamic contrast-enhanced MRI for prediction of breast cancer response to neoadjuvant chemotherapy: initial results', *AJR Am J Roentgenol*, 191 (5): 1331−8.

9. Johansen, R., Jensen, L. R., Rydland, J., et al. (2009), 'Predicting survival and early clinical response to primary chemotherapy for patients with locally advanced breast cancer using DCE-MRI', *J Magn Reson Imaging*, 29 (6): 1300−7.

10. Manton, D. J., Chaturvedi, A., Hubbard, A., et al. (2006), 'Neoadjuvant chemotherapy in breast cancer: Early response prediction with quantitative MR imaging and spectroscopy', *Br J Cancer*, 94 (3): 427−35.

11. Schwarz-Dose, J., Untch, M., Tiling, R., et al. (2008), 'Monitoring primary systemic therapy of large and locally advanced breast cancer by using sequential positron emission tomography imaging with [18F]Fluorodeoxyg lucose', *J Clin Oncol*, Dec. 15.

12. Duch, J., Fuster, D., Muñoz, M., et al. (2009), '(18)F-FDG PET/CT for early prediction of response to neoadjuvant chemotherapy in breast cancer', *Eur J Nucl Med Mol Imaging*, March 27.

13. von Minckwitz, G., Sinn, H. P., Raab, G., et al. (2008), 'Clinical response after two cycles compared to HER2, Ki–67, p53, and bcl–2 in independently predicting a pathological complete response after preoperative chemotherapy in patients with operable carcinoma of the breast', *Breast Cancer Res*, 10 (2): R30 (E-pub: April 1, 2008).

14. Ueno, T., Toi, M. and Linder, S. (2005), 'Detection of epithelial cell death in the body by cytokeratin 18 measurement', *Biomed Pharmacother*, 59 (suppl. 2): S359–62.

15. Mauri, D., Pavlidis, N. and Ioannidis, J. P. (2005), 'Neoadjuvant versus adjuvant systemic treatment in breast cancer: a meta-analysis', *J Natl Cancer Inst*, 97 (3): 188–94.

16. Partridge, S. C., Gibbs, J. E., Lu, Y., et al. (2002), 'Accuracy of MR imaging for revealing residual breast cancer in patients who have undergone neoadjuvant chemotherapy', *AJR Am J Roentgenol*, 179 (5): 1193–9.

17. Nakamura, S., Kenjo, H., Nishio, T., et al. (2002), 'Efficacy of 3D-MR mammography for breast conserving surgery after neoadjuvant chemotherapy', *Breast Cancer*, 9 (1): 15–9.

18. Andre, F., Mazouni, C., Liedtke, C., et al. (2008), 'HER2 expression and efficacy of preoperative paclitaxel/FAC chemotherapy in breast cancer', *Breast Cancer Res Treat*, 108 (2): 183–90.

19. Mazouni, C., Peintinger, F., Wan-Kau, S., et al. (2007), 'Residual ductal carcinoma in situ in patients with complete eradication of invasive breast cancer after neoadjuvant chemotherapy does not adversely affect patient outcome', *J Clin Oncol*, 25 (19): 2650–5.

20. Turnbull, L. (2008), 'Magnetic resonance imaging in breast cancer: Results of the COMICE trial', *Breast Cancer Research*, 10 (suppl. 3): P10 (from Symposium Mammographicum 2008, Lille, France, July 6–8, 2008).

21. Solin, L. J, Orel, S. G., Hwang, W. T., et al. (2008), 'Relationship of breast magnetic resonance imaging to outcome after breast-conservation treatment with radiation for women with early-stage invasive breast carcinoma or ductal carcinoma in situ', *J Clin Oncol*, 26 (3): 386–91.

21. Jeruss, J. S., Mittendorf, E. A., Tucker, S. L., et al. (2008), 'Combined use of clinical and pathologic staging variables to define outcomes for breast cancer patients treated with neoadjuvant therapy', *J Clin Oncol*, 26 (2): 246–52 (E-pub: Dec. 3, 2007, related articles, links).

22. Carey, L. A., Metzger, R., Dees, E. C., et al. (2005), 'American Joint Committee on Cancer tumor–node–metastasis stage after neoadjuvant chemotherapy and breast cancer outcome', *J Natl Cancer Inst*, 97 (15): 1137–42.

23. Li, X., Lewis, M. T., Huang, J., et al. (2008), 'Intrinsic resistance of tumorigenic breast cancer cells to chemotherapy', *J Natl Cancer Inst*, 100 (9): 672–9.

Section D

1. Hudis, C. (2007), 'Trastuzumab – Mechanism of action and use in clinical practice', *N Engl J Med*, 357: 39–51.
2. Osborne, C. K., Shou, J., Massarweh S., et al. (2005), 'Crosstalk between estrogen receptor and growth factor receptor pathways as a cause for endocrine therapy resistance in breast cancer', *Clin Cancer Res*, 11: 865s–70s.
3. Harris, L., You, F., Schnitt, S., et al. (2007), 'Predictors of resistance to preoperative trastuzumab and vinorelbine for HER2-positive early breast cancer', *Clin Cancer Res*, 13: 1198–207.
4. Perou, C., Sørlie, T., Eisen M., et al. (2000), 'Molecular portraits of human breast tumours', *Nature*, 406: 747–52.
5. Valabrega, G., Montemurro, F., Aglietta, M. (2007), 'Trastuzumab: Mechanism of action, resistance and future perspectives in HER2-overexpressing breast cancer', *Ann Oncol*, 18: 977–84.
6. Molina, M., Codony-Servat, J., Albanell, J., et al. 2001: 'Trastuzumab (herceptin), a humanized anti-Her2 receptor monoclonal antibody, inhibits basal and activated Her2 ectodomain cleavage in breast cancer cells', *Cancer Res*, 61: 4744–9.
7. Gennari, R., Menard, S., Fagnoni, F., et al. (2004), 'Pilot study of the mechanism of action of preoperative trastuzumab in patients with primary operable breast tumors overexpressing HER2', *Clin Cancer Res*, 10: 5650–5.
8. Nielsen, D., Andersson, M., Kamby C. (2009), 'HER2-targeted therapy in breast cancer. Monoclonal antibodies and tyrosine kinase inhibitors', *Cancer Treat Rev*, 35: 121–36.
9. Cho, H, Mason, K., Ramyar, K., et al. (2003), 'Structure of the extracellular region of HER2 alone and in complex with the Herceptin Fab', *Nature*, 421: 756–60.
10. Nahta, R., Hung, M., Esteva, F. (2004), 'The HER–2-targeting antibodies trastuzumab and pertuzumab synergistically inhibit the survival of breast cancer cells', *Cancer Res*, 64: 2343–6.
11. Bselga, J., et al. (2007), 'Objective response rate in a phase II multicenter trial of pertuzumab (P), a HER2 dimerization inhibiting monoclonal antibody, in combination with trastuzumab (T) in patients (pts) with HER2-positive metastatic breast cancer (MBC) which has progressed during

treatment with T', in 2007 ASCO Ann Meet Proceed, Part I, *J Clin Oncol*, 25 (18S) (June 20 suppl.): 1004.

12. Romond, E., Perez, E., Bryant, J., et al. (2005), 'Trastuzumab plus adjuvant chemotherapy for operable HER2-positive breast cancer', *N Engl J Med*, 353: 1673–84.

13. Piccart-Gebhart, M., Procter, M., Leyland-Jones, B., et al. (2005), 'Trastuzumab after adjuvant chemotherapy in HER2-positive breast cancer', *N Engl J Med*, 353: 1659–72.

14. Joensuu, H., Kellokumpu-Lehtinen, P., Bono, P., et al. (2006), 'Adjuvant docetaxel or vinorelbine with or without trastuzumab for breast cancer', *N Engl J Med*, 354: 809–20.

15. Procter, M. , et al. (2009), 'Assessment of trastuzumab-related cardiac dysfunction in the Herceptin Adjuvant (HERA) Trial with 3.6 years median follow-up', *J Clin Oncol*, 27: 15s (suppl. abstr. 540),

16. Goldhirsch, A., Ingle, J., Gelber, R., et al. (2009), 'Thresholds for therapies: Highlights of the St Gallen International Expert Consensus on the primary therapy of early breast cancer 2009', *Ann Oncol*, 20: 1319–29.

17. Perez, E., et al., (2007), 'Updated results of the combined analysis of NCCTG N9831 and NSABP B–31 adjuvant chemotherapy with/without trastuzumab in patients with HER2-positive breast cancer', in ASCO Ann Meet Proceed Part I, *J Clin Oncol*, 25 (18S) (June 20 suppl.): 512

18. Gianni, L., et al., (2009), 'Update of the HERA trial and the role of 1 year Trastuzumab as adjuvant therapy for breast cancer', *The Breast*, 18 (March suppl. 1): S11.

19. Slamon, D., et al. (2006), 'BCIRG 006: 2nd interim analysis phase III randomized trial comparing doxorubicin and cyclophosphamide followed by docetaxel (ACT) with doxorubicin and cyclophosphamide followed by docetaxel and trastuzumab (ACTH) with docetaxel, carboplatin and trastuzumab (TCH) in Her2neu positive early breast cancer patients', *SABCS*, 52

20. Joensuu, H., et al. (2009), 'Update of the FINHER trial based on 5 years of followup', *The Breast*, 18 (March suppl. 1): S10.

21. Wolmark, N., Wang, J., Mamounas, E., et al. (2001), 'Preoperative chemotherapy in patients with operable breast cancer: Nine-year results from National Surgical Adjuvant Breast and Bowel Project B–18', *J Natl Cancer Inst Monogr*, 96–102

22. van der Hage, J., van de Velde, C., Julien, J., et al. (2003), 'Preoperative chemotherapy in primary operable breast cancer: Results from the European Organization for Research and Treatment of Cancer trial 10902', *J Clin Oncol*, 19: 4224–37.

23. Buzdar, A., Valero, V., Ibrahim, N., et al. (2007), 'Neoadjuvant therapy with paclitaxel followed by 5-fluorouracil, epirubicin, and cyclophosphamide chemotherapy and concurrent trastuzumab in human epidermal growth factor receptor 2-positive operable breast cancer: An update of the initial randomized study population and data of additional patients treated with the same regimen', *Clin Cancer Res*, 13: 228–33,

24. Gianni, L., et al. (2007), 'Neoadjuvant trastuzumab (Herceptin) in locally advanced breast cancer (NOAH): Antitumor and safety analysis', in 2007 ASCO Ann Meet Proc Part I, *J Clin Oncol*, 25 (18S).

25. Bines. J. et al. (2003), 'Primary treatment with weekly docetaxel (Taxotere) and trastuzumab (Herceptin) for HER−2 overexpressing locally advanced breast cancer', *Eur J Cancer*, 1 (suppl. 5): S114.

26. Coudert, B., Arnould, L., Moreau, L., et al. (2006), 'Pre-operative systemic (neo-adjuvant) therapy with trastuzumab and docetaxel for HER2-overexpressing stage II or III breast cancer: Results of a multicenter phase II trial', *Ann Oncol*, 17: 409–14.

27. Van Pelt, A., Mohsin, S., Elledge, R., et al. (2003), 'Neoadjuvant trastuzumab and docetaxel in breast cancer: Preliminary results', *Clin Breast Cancer*, 4: 348–53.

28. Lybaert, W., et al. (2007), 'Docetaxel (T) + capecitabine (X) with or without trastuzumab (H) neoadjuvant therapy for locally advanced breast cancer (BC): Phase II study', in ASCO Annual Meeting Proceedings Part I. *J Clin Oncol*, 25 (18S, June 20 suppl.): 110–42.

29. Tripathy, D, et al. (2007), 'MCaGCe: Neoadjuvant capecitabine plus docetaxel ± trastuzumab therapy for recently diagnosed breast cancer: Phase II results', *Breast Cancer Res*, 106 (suppl. 1).

30. Limentani, S., Brufsky, A., Erban, J., et al. (2007), 'Phase II study of neoadjuvant docetaxel, vinorelbine, and trastuzumab followed by surgery and adjuvant doxorubicin plus cyclophosphamide in women with human epidermal growth factor receptor 2-overexpressing locally advanced breast cancer', *J Clin Oncol*, 25: 1232–8.

31. Coudert, B., Largillier, R., Arnould, L., et al. (2007), 'Multicenter phase II trial of neoadjuvant therapy with trastuzumab, docetaxel, and carboplatin for human epidermal growth factor receptor−2-overexpressing stage II or III breast cancer: Results of the GETN(A)−1 trial', *J Clin Oncol*, 25: 2678–84.

32. Han, H. S., et al. (2007), 'Dose-dense docetaxel, carboplatin and trastuzumab as neoadjuvant therapy for human epidermal growth factor receptor−2- positive stage II and III breast cancer', *Breast Cancer Res Treat*, 106 (suppl. 1).

33. Hurley, J., et al. (2007), 'Docetaxel, cisplatin, and trastuzumab as primary systemic therapy for human epidermal growth factor receptor 2-positive locally advanced breast cancer', *J Clin Oncol*, 24 (12): 1831–8.

34. Burstein, H., Harris, L., Gelman, R., et al. (2003), 'Preoperative therapy with trastuzumab and paclitaxel followed by sequential adjuvant doxorubicin/cyclophosphamide for HER2 overexpressing stage II or III breast cancer: A pilot study', *J Clin Oncol*, 21: 46–53.

35. Kelly, H., Kimmick, G., Dees, E., et al. (2006), 'Response and cardiac toxicity of trastuzumab given in conjunction with weekly paclitaxel after doxorubicin/cyclophosphamide', *Clin Breast Cancer*, 7: 237–43.

36. Anton, A., et al., (2007), 'Phase II study of a weekly liposome-encapsulated doxorubicin/docetaxel/pegfilgrastrim in combination with weekly trastuzumab as primary treatment in HER2 positive (HER2 +) early breast cancer patients (II − IIIa). Intermediate analysis of 26 patients. GEICAM 2003–03 study', *Breast Cancer Res Treat*, 106 (suppl. 1).

37. Cristofanilli, M., et al. (2006), 'A phase II combination study of lapatinib and paclitaxel as a neoadjuvant therapy in patients with newly diagnosed inflammatory breast cancer (IBC)', *Breast Cancer Res Treat*, 100: S5.

38. Shimizu, C, Masuda, N, Yoshimura, K, et al. (2009), 'Long-term outcome and pattern of relapse after neoadjuvant chemotherapy in patients with human epidermal growth factor receptor 2-positive primary breast cancer', *Jpn J Clin Oncol*, 39: 484–90.

39. Dawood, S., Gonzalez-Angulo, A., Peintinger, F., et al. (2007), 'Efficacy and safety of neoadjuvant trastuzumab combined with paclitaxel and epirubicin: A retrospective review of the M. D. Anderson experience', *Cancer*, 110: 1195–200.

40. Ellis, M. J., Tao, Y., Luo, J., et al. (2008), 'Outcome prediction for estrogen receptor-positive breast cancer based on postneoadjuvant endocrine therapy tumor characteristics', *J Natl Cancer Inst*, 100: 1380–8.

41. Korkaya, H., Paulson, A., Iovino, F., et al. (2008), 'HER2 regulates the mammary stem/progenitor cell population driving tumorigenesis and invasion', *Oncogene*, 27: 6120–30.

42. Li, X., Lewis, M., Huang, J., et al. (2008), 'Intrinsic resistance of tumorigenic breast cancer cells to chemotherapy', *J Natl Cancer Inst*, 100: 672–9.

Section E

1. Valenzuela, M. and Julian, T. B. (2008), 'Neo-adjuvant hormonal therapy', *Breast J*, 14 (3): 279–83.

2. Baum, M., Budzar, A. U., Cuzick, J., et al. (2002) 'Arimidex, Tamoxifen,

Alone or in Combination (ATAC) Trialists' Group. Anastrozole alone or in combination with tamoxifen versus tamoxifen alone for adjuvant treatment of postmenopausal women with early breast cancer: First results of the ATAC randomised trial', *Lancet*, 359: 2131−9.

3. Baum, M., Buzdar, A., Cuzick, J., et al. (2003), 'The ATAC (Arimidex, Tamoxifen Alone or in Combination) Trialists' Group. Anastrozole alone or in combination with tamoxifen versus tamoxifen alone for adjuvant treatment of postmenopausal women with early-stage breast cancer: Results of the ATAC (Arimidex, Tamoxifen Alone or in Combination) trial efficacy and safety update analyses', *Cancer*, 98: 1802−10.

4. Coombes, R. C., Hall, E., Gibson, L. J., et al. (2004), 'A randomized trial of exemestane after two to three years of tamoxifen therapy in postmenopausal women with primary breast cancer,' *N Engl J Med*, 350: 1081−92.

5. Goss, P. E., Ingle, J. N., Martino, S., et al. (2003), 'A randomized trial of letrozole in postmenopausal women after five years of tamoxifen therapy for early-stage breast cancer', *N Engl J Med*, 349: 1793−802.

6. Hodi, Z., Chakrabarti, J., Lee, A. H., et al. (2007), 'The reliability of assessment of oestrogen receptor expression on needle core biopsy specimens of invasive carcinomas of the breast', *J Clin Pathol*, 60: 299−302.

7. Early Breast Cancer Trialists' Collaborative Group (2005), 'Effects of chemotherapy and hormonal therapy for early breast cancer on recurrence and 15-year survival: An overview of the randomised trials', *Lancet*, 365: 1687−717.

8. Allen M. Gown (2008), 'Current issues in ER and HER2 testing by IHC in breast cancer', *Modern Pathology*, 21: S8−S15.

9. Oyama, T., Ishikawa, Y., Hayashi, M., Arihiro, K. and Horiguchi, J. (2007), 'The effects of fixation, processing and evaluation criteria on immunohistochemical detection of hormone receptors in breast cancer', *Breast Cancer*, 14: 182−8.

10. Goldstein, N. S., Ferkowicz, M., Odish, E., et al. (2003), 'Minimum formalin fixation time for consistent estrogen receptor immunohistochemical staining of invasive breast carcinoma', *Am J Clin Pathol*, 120: 86−92.

11. Lee, H., Douglas-Jones, A. G., Morgan, J. M. and Jasani, B. (2002), 'The effect of fixation and processing on the sensitivity of oestrogen receptor assay by immunohistochemistry in breast carcinoma', *J Clin Pathol*, 55: 236−8.

12. Arber, D. A. (2002), 'Effect of prolonged formalin fixation on the

immunohistochemical reactivity of breast markers', *Appl Immunohistochem Mol Morphol*, 10: 183–6.

13. von Wasielewski, R., Mengel, M., Nolte, M. and Werner, M. (1998), 'Influence of fixation, antibody clones, and signal amplification on steroid receptor analysis', *Breast J*, 4: 33–40.

14. Douglas-Jones, A. G., Collett, N., Morgan, J. M. and Jasani, B. (2001), 'Comparison of core oestrogen receptor (ER) assay with excised tumour: Intratumoral distribution of ER in breast carcinoma', *J Clin Pathol*, 54: 951–5.

15. Barnes, D. M., Harris, W. H., Smith, P., et al. (1996), 'Immunohistochemical determination of oestrogen receptor: Comparison of different methods of assessment of staining and correlation with clinical outcome of breast cancer patients', *Br J Cancer*, 74: 1445–51.

16. Harvey, J. M., Clark, G. M., Osborne, C. K., et al. (1999), 'Estrogen receptor status by immunohistochemistry is superior to the ligand-binding assay for predicting response to adjuvant endocrine therapy in breast cancer', *J Clin Oncol*, 17: 1474–81.

17. Cheang, M. C., Treaba, D. O., Speers, C. H., et al. (2006), 'Immunohistochemical detection using the new rabbit monoclonal antibody SP1 of estrogen receptor in breast cancer is superior to mouse monoclonal antibody 1D5 in predicting survival', *J Clin Oncol*, 24: 5637–44.

18. Arihiro, K., Umemura, S., Kurosumi, M., et al. (2007), 'Comparison of evaluations for hormone receptors in breast carcinoma using two manual and three automated immunohistochemical assays', *Am J Clin Pathol*, 127: 356–65.

19. Regitnig, P., Reiner, A., Dinges, H. P., et al. (2002), 'Quality assurance for detection of estrogen and progesterone receptors by immunohistochemistry in Austrian pathology laboratories', *Virchows Arch*, 441: 328–34.

20. McCarty, K. S. Jr., Miller, L. S., Cox, E. B. and Konrath, J. (1985), 'Estrogen receptor analyses: Correlation of biochemical and immunohistochemical methods using monoclonal antireceptor antibodies', *Arch. Pathol. Lab. Med*, 109: 716–21.

21. Horii, R., Akiyama, F., Ito, Y. and Iwase, T. (2007), 'Assessment of hormone receptor status in breast cancer', *Pathology International*, 57: 784–90.

22. Kurosumi, M. (2007), 'Immunohistochemical assessment of hormone receptor status using a new scoring system (J-score) in breast cancer', *Breast Cancer*, 14: 189–93.

23. Nadji, M., Gomez-Fernandez, C., Ganjei-Azar, P., et al. (2005), 'Immunohistochemistry of estrogen and progesterone receptors

reconsidered: Experience with 5,993 breast cancers', *Am J Clin Pathol*, 123: 21–7.

24. Collins, L. C., Botero, M. L. and Schnitt, S. J. (2005), 'Bimodal frequency distribution of estrogen receptor immunohistochemical staining results in breast cancer: An analysis of 825 cases', *Am J Clin Pathol*, 123: 16–20.

25. Allred, D. C. and Mohsin, S. K. (2005), 'ER expression is not bimodal in breast cancer', *Am J Clin Pathol*, 124: 474–5 [letter].

26. Kirkegaard, T., Edwards, J., Tovey, S., et al. (2006), 'Observer variation in immunohistochemical analysis of protein expression, time for a change?' *Histopathology*, 48: 787–94.

27. Mudduwa, L. and Liyanage, T. (2009), 'Immunohistochemical assessment of hormone receptor status of breast carcinoma: Interobserver variation of the quick score', *Indian J Med Sci*, 63: 21–7.

28. Sharangpani, G. M., Joshi, A. S, Porter, K., et al. (2007), 'Semi-automated imaging system to quantitate estrogen and progesterone receptor immunoreactivity in human breast cancer', *Journal of Microscopy*, 226: 244–55.

29. Rexhepaj, E., Brennan, D. J., Holloway, P., et al. (2008), 'Novel image analysis approach for quantifying expression of nuclear proteins assessed by immunohistochemistry: Application to measurement of oestrogen and progesterone receptor levels in breast cancer', *Breast Cancer Research*, 10: R89.

30. Ross, J. S., Symmans, W. F., Pusztai, L. and Hortobagyi, G. N. (2007), 'Standardizing slide-based assays in breast cancer: Hormone receptors, HER2, and sentinel lymph nodes', *Clin Cancer Res*, 13: 2831–5.

31. Hayashi, S. (2004), 'Prediction of hormone sensitivity by DNA microarray', *Biomed Pharmacother*, 58: 1–9.

32. Paik, S., Shak, S, Tang, G., et al. (2004), 'A multigene assay to predict recurrence of tamoxifen-treated, node-negative breast cancer', *N Engl J Med*, 351: 2817–26.

33. Usami, S., Moriya, T., Amari, M., et al. (2007), 'Reliability of prognostic factors in breast carcinoma determined by core needle biopsy', *Jpn J Clin Oncol*, 37: 250–5.

34. Hodi, Z., Chakrabarti, J., Lee, A. H., et al. (2007), 'The reliability of assessment of oestrogen receptor expression on needle core biopsy specimens of invasive carcinomas of the breast', *J Clin Pathol*, 60: 299–302.

Index